SECTARIAN REFORMERS IN AMERICAN MEDICINE, 1800–1910

AMS Studies in the Nineteenth Century
ISSN 0196-657X
Series ISBN-13: 978-0-404-61480-5

No. 41

John S. Haller, Jr.

Sectarian Reformers in American Medicine, 1800–1910

ISBN-13: 978-0-404-64471-0

Sectarian Reformers in American Medicine, 1800–1910

John S. Haller, Jr.

AMS Press, Inc.
New York

Library of Congress Cataloging-in-Publication Data

Haller, John S.

Sectarian reformers in American medicine, 1800-1910 / John S. Haller, Jr.
p. cm.— (AMS studies in the nineteenth century, ISSN 0196-657X ; 41)
Includes bibliographical references and index.
ISBN 978-0-404-64471-0 (cloth : alk. paper)

1. Medicine—United States—History—19th century. 2. Medicine—United States—History—20th century. 3. Health care reform—United States—History—19th century. 4. Health care reform—United States—History—20th century. 5. Alternative medicine—United States—History—19th century. 6. Alternative medicine—United States—History—20th century. I. Title.

RA395.A3H3435 2011

362.10973—dc23 2011048742

All AMS books are printed on acid-free paper that meets the guidelines for performance and durability of the Committee on Production Guidelines for Book Longevity of the Council on Library Resources.

AMS Press, Inc.

Brooklyn Navy Yard, 63 Flushing Ave. – Unit #221
Brooklyn, New York 11205-1073, U.S.A.
www.amspressinc.com

MANUFACTURED IN THE UNITED STATES OF AMERICA

CONTENTS

List of Illustrations vi
Introduction xi
Chapter 1. Orthodoxy and American Practice 1
Chapter 2. Old and New World Eclectics 15
Chapter 3. Jeremiads and Apostates 37
Chapter 4. Reform Literature 61
Chapter 5. Reform Colleges 87
Chapter 6. Reform Societies 101
Chapter 7. Between the Abrahams 117
Notes 137
Illustrations 155
Appendices
- A. Reform Medical Journals to 1909 189
- B. Reform Medical Colleges to 1915 245
- C. Reform Medical Societies to 1900 267

Index 311

LIST OF ILLUSTRATIONS

Fig. 1. Breathing a vein 155
Fig. 2. Des sang-sues 156
Fig. 3. Various types of bloodletting instruments (1) 157
Fig. 4. Various types of bloodletting instruments (2) 158
Fig. 5. Léon Rostan (1790–1866) 159
Fig. 6. Gabriel Andral (1797–1876) 160
Fig. 7. Armand Trousseau (1801–1867) 161
Fig. 8. Marshall Hall (1790–1857) 162
Fig. 9. Sir John Forbes (1787–1861) 163
Fig. 10. Benjamin Rush (1745–1813) 164
Fig. 11. Benjamin Waterhouse (1754–1846) 165
Fig. 12. Elisha Bartlett (1805–1855) 166
Fig. 13. Samuel Jackson (1787–1872) 167
Fig. 14. George McClellan (1796–1847) 168
Fig. 15. Samuel Thomson (1769–1843) 169
Fig. 16. Patent authorizing use of Samuel Thomson's system of medicine, 1843 170
Fig. 17. Advertisement for Dr. Cyrus Thomson's Infirmary in New York, 1843 171
Fig. 18. Wooster Beach (1794–1868) 172
Fig. 19. Wooster Beach's Reformed Medical College of the City of New York, 1830 173
Fig. 20. Alva Curtis (1797–1881) 174
Fig. 21. American Medical Institute and Botanico-Medical College of Ohio, 1843 175
Fig. 22. Thomas Vaughan Morrow (1804–1850) 176
Fig. 23. Joseph Rodes Buchanan (1814–1899) 177
Fig. 24. Metropolitan Medical College, New York City, 1852 178
Fig. 25. James McClintock (1809–1881) 179
Fig. 26. Eclectic Medical College of Philadelphia, 1860 180
Fig. 27. Samuel Hahnemann (1755–1843) 181
Fig. 28. Charles J. Hempel (1811–1879) 182
Fig. 29. Adolph Lippe (1812–1888) 183
Fig. 30. Homeopathic Medical College of Missouri 184
Fig. 31. "The Regulars in Consultation," 1841 185
Fig. 32. Homeopath and allopath arguing the virtues of their medical systems, 182? 186
Fig. 33. Similia similibus curantur, 1841 187
Fig. 34. Alexander Wilder (1823–1908) 188

For
Joe and Dot

Bleed the patient till he is white.

—François-Joseph-Victor Broussais

I am saying only what everybody knows to be true, when I say that the general confidence which has heretofore existed in the science and art of medicine, as this science has been studied, and as this art has been practiced, has within the last few years been violently shaken and disturbed, and is now greatly lessened and impaired.

—Elisha Bartlett

Introduction

In his book *Intellectuals* (1988), British historian Paul Johnson noted the decline of clerical power in the western world during the eighteenth century, replaced by secular intellectuals who had become a major force in the identification of society's ills and in the prescriptions for its cure. "Unlike their sacerdotal predecessors," he explained, the newer secular intellectuals "were not servants and interpreters of the gods but substitutes. Their hero was Prometheus, who stole the celestial fire and brought it to earth." European intellectuals who followed in the footsteps of these secular visionaries aspired to be the leaders of the new age, finding many of their shibboleths in the French Revolution and its sweeping out of the older order to make way for the new.[1]

Among the impassioned members of this new secular class in Europe and America were academically trained physicians who became archetypes in denouncing the past and constructing newer therapeutic systems of their own devising. These iconoclasts made frequent apologies for the instability of the practice of physic, stigmatizing as quackery or empiricism much that had gone before them. Believing that their predecessors had tinkered with false notions at the expense of over-purged and over-bled patients, they spurned the tyranny of existing schools for a more sensible treatment of disease. Almost without exception, however, "New Turks" became "Old Turks" and, while theories continued to change, therapeutic procedures remained surprisingly similar. Having disposed of animism, spagiric medicine, solidism, and humoralism as convenient objects of derision, the new iconoclasts were not without their own "fashions." Until the second half of the nineteenth century, medicine was a kaleidoscope of opinions, beliefs, laws, formulas, and procedures. Indeed, the age was rife with competing schools and overpowering egos. It resembled what Thomas Jefferson imagined when he observed that the many disciples of George Ernst Stahl

(1660–1734), Friedrich Hoffmann (1660–1742), Hermann Boerhaave (1668–1738), William Cullen (1710–1790), and John Brown (1735–1788) "succeed one another like the shifting figures of a magic lantern; and their fancies, like the dresses of the annual doll-babies from Paris, becoming from their novelty, the vogue of the day, and yielding to the next novelty, their ephemeral favors."[2]

What broke the mold of this seemingly endless cycle was the work of the positive school of medicine which flourished in France after the Revolution, fed by a persistent sense of doubt about the prevailing medical wisdom and by a desire to achieve a level of certainty in medical knowledge through the greater use of quantitative methods. Among the founders of this empirical methodology were Philippe Pinel (1745–1826) at La Salpêtrière, whose contributions to medical observation broke existing barriers; Xavier Bichat (1771–1802), whose classification of human tissues set new standards for postmortem examinations; Jean-Nicolas Corvisart (1755–1821), who reintroduced percussion and physical diagnosis; René T. H. Laennec (1781–1826), who invented the stethoscope and developed the discipline of pathological anatomy; and Gaspard Laurent Bayle (1774–1816), who applied these new methods to research on consumption. Others among this group of independent thinkers were Pierre C. A. Louis (1787–1872), author of works on consumption and typhoid fever, and who introduced the numerical and statistical method to the science of medicine; Jules Gavarret (1816–1890), who systemized Louis's methods; and Jean Cruveilhier (1791–1873), Pierre François O. Rayer (1793–1867), and Armand Trousseau (1801–1866), who were its exponents.

They and their successors introduced a new spirit into medicine and, with it, a broadening of diagnostic powers through more thorough clinical and pathological methods. Elsewhere the investigation of disease widened as Josef Skoda (1805–1881) in Vienna; Johann Lucas Schönlein (1793–1864) in Berlin; Robert James Graves (1796–1853) and Willliam Stokes (1804–1878) in Dublin; and Marshall Hall (1790–1857) in England built on the more exacting methods of clinical medicine introduced by the French. Among the results of this new spirit was the gradual arresting of the bloody lancet, staying the hand of the purger, and an end to indiscriminate dosing.

The dynamics of this scientific change quite naturally differed from country to country, tempered by geographical, historical, and institutional idiosyncrasies that ultimately affected the manner and form of the outcome. In America, for example, the demand for physicians to meet the nation's ever-expanding boundaries far exceeded the supply of doctors produced by its few university-based medical colleges, thereby opening the door to less rigorous educational forms and more innovative types of rank-and-file professionals. Similarly, the breakdown of distinctions between physician, surgeon, and pharmacist; the lack of any broadly accepted definition of the term "doctor;" and the predilection for local control in licensing meant that the scientific revolution in medicine (i.e., clinical and laboratory medicine) would take a less rigorous and more circuitous route than the state-centered systems of Europe.

In spite of these differences, it is a mistake to take a single-country approach to the age of scientific medicine. More so than any other discipline, medicine was transnational in scope, with theories, methods, and techniques that bridged geographic boundaries. This image, already evident among the system-builders of the eighteenth and early nineteenth centuries, multiplied with the development of clinical and laboratory science in the second half of the nineteenth century. The contributions from the different research fields in the biological and medical sciences—experimental physiology, cellular pathology, embryology, and zoology—were enough to connect diagnosis with causal theories and, in the process, reshape medical education.

Courses on the theory and uses of the microscope, chemical analyses of the body's secretions, as well as practical exercises on auscultation and percussion, were just the beginning salvos from these newer medical faculties. Scientific medicine became the centerpiece for medical reform, linking the interests of newer generations of researchers, establishing higher standards for academic appointments, constructing a more integrated approach to medical and clinical research, enhancing the place of the laboratory within the curriculum, and building associations of academically trained scientists to share information and articulate common interests. No longer was medicine held captive by the "system-builders," as no single system could encompass, let alone monopolize, the scientific agenda. In their place were images of newer diagnostic technology (i.e., stethoscope, microscope, thermometer) used in both the laboratory and the clinic in the service of scientific medicine. By the late nineteenth century, this early technology would multiply many-fold.

This book is intended to provide the reader with a perspective on this century of ferment in European and American medicine, a century when the energies of many illustrious—and some not so illustrious—doctors focused on the prospect of reform and when much of their literature promised to revolutionize the world with the outcome of their prodigious efforts. This was also a century whose literature, despite differences in perspective, credited the French Clinical School and German laboratory medicine for its most significant medical accomplishments.

Besides being a story about the culture of medical change, it is also about words—scientific, modern, regular, orthodox, reform, eclectic, sectarian, homeopathic, allopathic, and physio-medical—and how they affected individual and societal perceptions. The book is also about failure in that it recounts the history of medical eclecticism, a movement broadly identified in France, Great Britain, Germany, and America as building a new relationship between doctor and patient on the basis of accrued wisdom drawn from multiple sources and methodologies, using observation and experimentation. Having begun on an optimistic footing, and pursued with vigor by a many well intentioned and reform-minded physicians, medical eclecticism became a respectable movement although seldom identified by that name. In America, however, the term eclectic was seized upon by small group of botanics who, while giving lip service to its historical and philosophical roots, chose to build their own idiosyncratic definition of reform around their advocacy of herb-based medicines. Their pursuit of this more narrow agenda is a story worth telling, particularly since the principles the eclectics chose to forsake remain the foundation blocks of modern practice.

I have deliberately chosen to focus my efforts on the Thomsonians, eclectics, physio-medicals, and homeopaths, to the exclusion of other sectarian groups. This decision was by no means arbitrary since they alone were deemed large enough in size to be included in statistical information provided by the American Medical Association. While mention will surely be made of botanics, hydropaths, Grahamites, mesmerists, as well as other lesser known sectarians, the emphasis placed on the former is due to their larger membership, their establishment of more than a smattering of medical colleges, their founding of national associations and publications to represent their respective points of view, and the level and degree of their political influence.

The chapters unfold a story that recounts how the diversity of American culture, particularly during the first half of the nineteenth century, contributed to the openness with which its people embraced sectarianism in medicine.

Chapter 1 ("Orthodoxy and American Practice") explains the contextual nature of medical orthodoxy, the competition among its various system-builders, the aging materia medica, and the emerging crises of belief spawned in no small manner by medicine's feuds and failures. It also discusses the debate within American orthodoxy of less dependence upon Old World beliefs and the potential for a genuinely unique "American Practice."

Chapter 2 ("Old and New World Eclectics") traces the origins of eclecticism from its ancient roots to its blossoming in nineteenth-century France, Germany, and England. The philosophy migrated to America in the carpet bags of New England Transcendentalists who adopted it as part of their cerebral response to empiricism and materialism. It also arrived on native shores in the medical bags of students who had traveled abroad to observe and study the pathological investigations of the Paris Clinical School. The chapter also recounts the group of botanical reformers who transformed this movement into a narrow herb-based system of medicine.

Chapter 3 ("Jeremiads and Apostates") recounts the growing skepticism that crept into the teachings of America's leading medical educators, including their advocacy of a more positive medicine drawn not from speculation on "first causes" but from inductions drawn from physiology, anatomy, and pathology. It also recounts the emergence of medicine's more noted apostates who, having declared their independence from orthodoxy, adhered to economist Adam Smith's belief that the free marketplace was the most appropriate arena in which to sort out the differences between competing healing systems.

Chapter 4 ("Reform Literature") provides a broader literary context in which to understand the spread of sectarian ideas and how they flourished in an age that celebrated democracy, repudiated class and privilege, challenged authority, and gave vent to the nation's restlessness and hunger for learning.

Chapter 5 ("Reform Colleges") explains the efforts of sectarian reformers to build an authentic science around their ideas and theories and sustain it with an enduring educational structure. Although most of their colleges were short-lived, they reflected a search for professional identity as well as an expression of sectarian strength and regional pride.

Chapter 6 ("Reform Societies") begins with Alexis de Tocqueville's depiction of America's democratic society as seeking identity through voluntarism and the power and advocacy of professional organizations. It then recounts the aspirations of reform medicine to survive and prosper through the legitimization of local, state, and national assemblages.

Chapter 7 ("Between the Two Abrahams") recounts the fizzling out of America's reform movement and its slow descent into intellectual, fiscal, and political disarray. By the time of Abraham Flexner's landmark study of medical education in the United States and Canada and his visits to all 155 medical schools in 1909, sectarian medicine had all but forfeited its once prominent place in American culture.

One last comment is necessary to put this book in context. Over the course of more than two centuries, medical orthodoxy in American has managed to control the interpretation of its clash with sectarian medicine. As William G. Rothstein pointedly observed in his *American Physicians in the Nineteenth Century: From Sects to Science*, published in 1985, medical historians have been too generous in concluding that, alone among the botanics, eclectics, and homeopaths, "regular physicians . . . nurtured the seed of medical science when medical science was virtually nonexistent . . . cultivated its growth until it began to blossom, and therefore alone merits the fruit of praise and honor for its efforts." All other groups were seen as either retarding the growth of medical science or "watch[ing] it skeptically and disapprovingly.[3]

Even a cursory view of the language used by regulars to depict these competing schools makes evident the contextual nature of the relationship. "Cheat," "medical fanatic," "wild dreamer in science," "absurd theorizer," "scientific fool," "quack," "mongrel," "radical," "imposter," "ignoramus," "uneducated," and "irresponsible," are but a few of the terms used to injure the reputation and question the position these groups held on the etiology and nature of disease. Notwithstanding these pejorative terms, nineteenth-century Americans viewed medicine in much the same manner they viewed religion, accepting an essentially Protestant perspective which included a favorable disposition toward voluntarism and sectarianism. That being said, to ignore medicine's sectarians is a serious omission particularly since medical orthodoxy should be viewed during much of its early history as little more than a sect itself. Abraham Flexner said as much in his *Medical Education in the United States and Canada* (1910) when he wrote: "Prior to the placing of medicine on a scientific basis, sectarianism was, of course, inevitable. Every one started with some sort of preconceived notion; and from a logical point of view, one perception is as good as another. Allopathy was just as sectarian as homeopathy."[4]

While the founding of the American Medical Association in 1846 suggests a concern among established doctors for the general dereliction of medical education and practices, the nation's outspoken reformers insisted that the dangers threatening health care were due not to the lassitude of the many but the pretenses of the few. The belief that the nation had to be rescued from the iniquities of medical orthodoxy was manifested over and over again in the emotional outbursts of medicine's unconventional healers. Whether these unorthodox healers actually healed was not as important as their assertion that their common sense principles were essentially American in spirit and basically different from Old World beliefs. These assertions, although false in their particulars, helped to stimulate and validate their efforts. Recognized or not, Europe would continue to be the touchstone of their sometimes awkward and unbridled appetites.

No relationship, least of all one between majority and minority medical groups, should be viewed in terms of one side alone. Most of these movements held a number of relevant features in common; they could identify a vocal group of willing patients; draw upon multiple levels of political support; lay claim to certain common protections under the law; and reduce illness to several fundamental principles. Despite these multiple levels of commonality, medical orthodoxy used its formidable rhetoric and base of support to advance its agenda in a manner that explained its victory as a triumph of modernity over cultlike opponents caught in the snares of the past. Given the breadth and depth of the impact made by these apostates, their story justifies, if not demands, a more balanced accounting.

* * *

Those to whom I am indebted include Michael A. Flannery, Associate Director for Historical Collections at the Lister Hill Library of the Health Sciences, University of Alabama at Birmingham, whose observations and suggestions proved to be extremely helpful; Dennis B. Worthen, Scholar in Residence at the Lloyd Library and Museum in Cincinnati; Director Maggie Heran and staff members Carol Maxwell, Betsy Kruthoffer, Heather Snyder, Heather Newkirk, and Anna Heran of The Lloyd Library and Museum; librarians Kathy Fahey, Mary K. Taylor, Barbara Preece, Kimbra Stout, David Koch, and David Carlson of Morris Library, Southern Illinois University Carbondale; Connie Poole and the late Barbara Mason from the Southern Illinois University School of

Medicine, Springfield, Illinois; and the librarians and support staff of the Newberry Library; Johns Hopkins University Library; Ohio State University; Yale Medical Library; University of Chicago Library; the Widener Library of Harvard University; University of California, Davis; Flower Veterinary Library of Cornell University; Health Sciences Library of the University of Washington; National College of Naturopathic Medicine; John Hay Library of Brown University; University of Pennsylvania; Kent State University Library; University of Maryland Library; New York State Library, Albany; Historical Society of Pennsylvania; Meadville Theological Library; and the Theodore Lownik Library of Illinois Benedictine College.

As always, I am grateful to my wife, Robin, who offered inspiration, encouragement, criticism, and substantial assistance, including the reading of numerous drafts and indexing the finished manuscript.

Chapter 1. Orthodoxy and American Practice

By the end of the eighteenth century, western medical orthodoxy, including its practitioners and theoreticians working their trade in the New World, represented a compilation of wisdom that extended from ancient writers such as Hippocrates, Galen, and Celsus, into modernity. Constitutional pathology still held sway but had undergone progressive elaborations based on newer experimental observations. Dutch physician Hermann Boerhaave's (1668–1738) *Institutiones medicae* (1721), for example, did not so much challenge the humoral paradigm as support the ancient edifice with more modern knowledge. An advocate of the iatro-mechanical view, he conceived of the body as a complex system of solids and fluids whose structure varied according to sex, age, constitution, and disease. In his study of disease, he took particular interest in the fibers and sought to distinguish between those that were weak and those that were rigid or stiff. By effecting a synthesis between the works of William Harvey (1578–1657) and Antoni van Leeuwenhoek (1632–1723) on the circulation of the blood, and Marcello Malpighi's (1628–1694) demonstration of the capillary system, Boerhaave transformed the human body from a potpourri of Galenic concepts into a Newtonian-type machine whose fluids obeyed the laws of physics as they traveled through vessels of different diameters. The body was for him a system of pumps and chemical balances and Boerhaave's book became the standard-bearer for medical education and practice in the eighteenth century. He raised Leyden to its highest distinction and took on pupils from all parts of the world, including Peter the Great of Russia. So great was his influence, wrote historian Lester S. King, that he was able "to construct a polished doctrinal edifice, almost monolithic, that captured men's attention, satisfied their curiosity—and restricted their imagination."[1]

While newer empirical evidence brought variances to the doctrinal edifice of the humors, therapeutical methods showed little change as physicians returned over and over again to the age-old techniques of bleeding, purging, cupping, warm baths, blistering, mustard plasters, mercury, tartar emetic, opium and other agents to reduce the volume of fluids, release obstructing matter, divert blood from areas of inflammation, and relieve congestion. Except in cases of pain, malaria, smallpox, and syphilis for which physicians had identified specific treatments, doctors relied on an armamentarium of nonspecific medicines and measures designed to attack the patient's unitary disease state. Physicians were wedded to a rationalistic system for both their understanding of disease and their medical response, convinced that the body's natural resources were too weakened to fight disease unaided.

Western medicine afforded meager results notwithstanding the brilliance and industry of its devoted servants whose aim was to create systems of medicine that were both philosophical and complete. System-building was the chief product of the eighteenth and early nineteenth centuries. From Cullenism, Brounianism, Broussaianism, and Rushism among the proponents of orthodoxy, to Baunscheidtism, homeopathy, hydropathy, eclectism, mesmerism, phrenology, and physiomedicalism among reformers, European and American medicine displayed a chaotic self-image as the boundaries between orthodox and unorthodox therapies shifted ground.

In looking at medicine in the late eighteenth and early nineteenth centuries, it is fair to state that no one belief dominated therapeutic thinking. Instead a plethora of theories struggled to become the reigning interpretation or philosophy. None represented a clear majority in the schools, in the minds of physicians, or in the preferences of patients. Indeed, patients refused to draw hard and fast lines, preferring the political economist Adam Smith's argument for a law of free competition. It was he who suggested to physician William Cullen that men should be able to choose their doctor in the same manner that they chose their wife or tailor.[2] Thus, while one system eventually marginalized its competitors and wrote themselves into history in ways that made them appear always to have been the majority, so-called orthodoxy was neither original nor always the majority. Rather, it was one of several competing schools mistaking English philosopher Francis Bacon (1561–1626), who delineated the principles of inductive reasoning over the a priori methods of medieval scholasticism and other syllogistic ratiocinations, as its basis of thinking. Doctrinal disputes were far more broad-based, with battle lines more blurred, and the infighting more intense than commonly understood. However, with victory, the winners found it easier to make their views appear to have always been in the majority.[3]

Orthodoxy's System-Builders

Scottish physician William Cullen (1710–1790), a student at Edinburgh and a graduate of Glasgow in 1740, was an avowed "solidist" whose system rested on the theory of spasm and atony of the capillaries. The first medical professor in Great Britain to lecture in English, Cullen took exception to the doctrines of Boerhaave whose teachings dominated the schools. His theory, founded on the writings of both Friedrich Hoffmann and Albrecht von Haller, placed the foci of disease in the solid structures of the body which he divided into four classes: *pyrexiae*, or fevers; *neuroses,* or nervous disorders; *cachexiae*, or depraved conditions; and *locales*, or local complaints. More than any of his contemporaries, he stood at the crossroads between ancient and modern medicine.[4] Cullen theorized that health and disease were best defined by the body's irritability or nervous energy as controlled by the brain, independent of the mind and will. From his nosological study of fevers, he concluded that the pathogenesis of disease was "spasm" of the arteries which he treated with sedation and rest, bloodletting, purges, blisters, and the application of cold. Cullen held chairs of medicine and chemistry at both Glasgow and Edinburgh and became the favorite of American colonials seeking a proper Old World finish to their medical studies. His *Institutions of Medicine* (1772) dictated medical practice for nearly fifty years, including the theoretical basis for the popularity of bloodletting in Europe and America.[5]

Scottish physician John Brown (1735–1788), a tutor in Cullen's family, broke with his mentor and advocated a competing system in his *Elementa medicinae* (1780) published initially in Latin and subsequently in English. Although taught to treat patients with a combination of bleeding and strict diet, Brown reversed this fashionable but debilitating regimen on the assumption that life was the result of "incitability," a term he used to express the action of stimuli upon an organism. All living actions, Brown explained, proceeded from this inherent property which was called into action by various external excitants. It followed that both health and disease were the result of this forced state of life and defined by the degree or state of the organism's excitability.[6] When diseased, the organism's life force typically demonstrated a deficiency of external or internal stimuli; and when exhausted, life ceased. Diseases were either *sthenic*, resulting from excessive incitability, or *asthenic,* resulting from deficient incitability. Brown's system was simple and devoid of metaphysics. To be true to his calling, a physician had merely to determine whether a disease was general (constitutional) or local, and the degree to which it was sthenic or asthenic. Since most diseases were regarded as general, affecting the entire organism, rather than local in nature, anatomy was of little value and symptomatology of even less account. Everything fell back on the condition of the body, and because the majority of diseases were asthenic, stimulants such as opium, followed by wine (or other alcoholic liquors), musk, camphor, ether, and even electricity, became the treatments of choice to offset the body's debility. Brown also recommended rich and well-seasoned meats and soups in place of watery drinks and the reduction of food intake. Brown's ideas captivated the medical world, in part because they represented a distinct departure from the prevailing system of humoralism, and also because they offered an alternative to the abuses of bloodletting and polypharmacy. His milder treatment of disease was called Brunonian and was received more favorably on the Continent than in England or America. The feuds between the supporters of Cullen and Brown were fierce, eliciting riots and even duels—a foreshadowing of the tensions that would later arise between homeopathy and medical orthodoxy.[7]

The incitability theory of Brown was transformed into the irritation theory of French military physician François J. V. Broussais (1772–1838) whose *Examen de la doctrine médicale généralement adopte* (1816; 1834) and *De l'irritation et de la folie* (1828) marked yet another turbulent change in the *ancien régime* of medicine. Like Brown before him, Broussais was opinionated, self-righteous, and confident in his role as a reformer. Unlike Brown, he reversed asthenic and sthenic disease, judging the latter to be far more significant. He theorized that a state of irritation was key to inflammation and caused by either internal or external irritants. Irritation most frequently attacked the stomach and alimentary canal, and by sympathy, affected distant parts and organs. All pathology was inflammation, which was nothing more than gastro-enteritis. In this manner Broussais and his disciples explained everything from cancer to convulsions, melancholia, scarlet fever, and smallpox as having a gastric pathology. Like most of his contemporaries, Broussais gave little credence to the healing powers of nature, and instead, urged the physician to combat inflammation with the full measure of the medical arts. This meant relying heavily on the lancet and leech, barley water and other emollient drinks, and avoiding purgatives and emetics.[8]

Contemporaneous with Broussais was the work of Giovanni Rasori (1766–1837) of Milan who first practiced as a Brunonian but later reversed himself. For him and his disciple, Giacomo Tommasini (1768–1846), diseases were of two types: *stimulus* (sthenic) and *contra-stimulus* (asthenic). While Broussais relied on the sedative or contrastimulant effects of bloodletting, Rasori's weapons of choice were digitalis and tartar emetic. Large repeated doses of tartar emetic were prescribed for their sedative, rather than the usual emetic effect on the individual organs. Known as the founder of the counter-stimulant school, Rasori employed tartar emetic to treat epidemic fever victims in Genoa, prescribing it "with a view to an effect on the system and on the disease, entirely independent of any evacuation whatever." Accordingly, he gave his patients from twelve to thirty grains after one or more bleedings, and up to sixty grains or more in twenty-four hours, depending on the state of the disease. Rasori continued this regimen until convalescence. Like others of his generation, he denigrated the ability of nature to cure disease, relying instead on the artful intervention of the physician.[9]

Aging Materia Medica

Along with its host of schools, systems, and sects, Western medicine claimed ownership of a materia medica that seemed to defy definitional constraints. Physicians with practices large and small attacked cholera, croup, pneumonia, pleuritis, and other diseases with regimens that included general bleeding, followed by jalap, cream of tartar, calomel, ipecac, liberal use of blisters to rouse the patient, and then narcotics (referred to as anodynes). They then considered their duty done, having expended the full measure of their formal training. Little more could be asked of them.[10] If patient mortality was high, it was no more than what most doctors and patients expected. Medicine had come a long way from the polypharmacy of *Theriaca Andromachi* with its sixty-five ingredients, but this change was not all for the better.

Medical orthodoxy may have differed on the etiology and modus operandi of disease and especially its philosophical underpinnings, but as far as treatment was concerned, it was monotonously uniform across competing systems.

TREATMENT BY REGULARS

Remittent Fever—mercury, bleeding, blistering, and antimony

Inflammatory Fever—mercury, bleeding, blistering, antimony and salts [bleeding until fainting]

Yellow Fever—mercury, bleeding, blistering, and salts

Scarlet Fever—Mercury, bleeding, blistering, and antimony

Intermittent Fever—mercury, bleeding, blistering, jalap, antimony, copper, arsenic, quinine

Puerperal Fever—mercury, bleeding, blistering, and opium

Dysentery—mercury, bleeding, blistering, opium, sugar of lead, nitric acid, tobacco, leeches, balsam copaiva, aquafortis, and salts

Small Pox—mercury, bleeding, blistering, antimony, nitre, salts, pounded ice to the head, and lunar caustic

Measles—mercury, bleeding, blistering, opium, muriate of ammonia, squills, nitre, and ice water

Insanity—mercury, bleeding, blistering

Putrid Sore Throat—mercury, bleeding, blistering, antimony, and salts

Inflammation of the Larynx—mercury, bleeding, blistering, and antimony

Inflammation of the Heart—mercury, bleeding, blistering

Inflammation of the Intestines—mercury, bleeding, blistering, and opium

Consumption—mercury, bleeding, blistering, antimony, squills, laudanum, issues and seton

Mercury, in one form or another, remained the sheet-anchor for most diseases, often combined with opium to increase its absorption into the system. The amount used varied by region. In New England, doses of mercurous chloride ranged from a tenth of a grain to ten grains, while in the South and West, doctors prescribed sixty- and seventy-grain doses, often repeated, until patients had consumed upwards of five- or six-hundred grains. Midwestern physician Daniel Drake (1785–1852), an 1818 graduate of the University of Pennsylvania and critic of contemporary practice, fondly quoted a Louisiana physician who, in treating yellow fever, admitted: "I drew blood enough to float the steamboat General Jackson, and gave Calomel enough to freight her."[11]

Arsenic was another popular medicine, used principally for cutaneous disease, chronic affections of the nervous system, intermittent fever, chronic rheumatism, diseases of the bone, frontal neuralgia, and headache. While pure metallic arsenic had no therapeutic use, its arsenates and salts were employed as alteratives, antiseptics, antispasmodics, antiperiodics, caustics, cholagogues, depilatories, hematinics, sedatives, and tonics. Some sixty different preparations were tried therapeutically and probably twenty or more remained in use through the end of the nineteenth century, including Aiken's Tonic Pills, Andrew's Tonic, Arsenauro, Gross's Neuralgia Pills, Chloro-Phosphide of Arsenic, and Sulfur Compound Lozenges. The potash solution of arsenious acid was the most popular arsenic-based drug while preparations such as De Valagin's mineral solution (arsenious acid in dilute hydrochloric acid) and Donovan's solution (iodide of arsenic and mercury) were frequent substitutes. Copper arsenite, iron arsenate, quinine arsenate, sodium arsenate, strychnine arsenate, and the later cacodylates of sodium and mercury were also popular. Taken internally in either liquid or solid form, injected hypodermically, inhaled as a vapor, administered intravenously, applied externally, and on rare occasions even given in enemas, arsenic became one of the mainstays of the nineteenth-century materia medica.[12]

Yet another favorite was tartar emetic (antimony), prescribed in varying amounts both internally and externally to fight apoplexy, asthma, chorea, dyspepsia, epilepsy, gout, hepatic complaints, hysteria, inflammation of the brain, intermittent fevers, jaundice, ophthalmia, paralysis, pneumonia, rheumatic affections, scarlatina, and ulcers. In minute doses, physicians employed antimony to subdue the acute inflammatory action of pneumonia by inducing nausea to evacuate fluids in the chest. Doctors also used its emetic properties as a parturient in labor.[13] As noted earlier, however, in the 1820s and 1830s physicians turned to larger doses, adhering to Rasori's belief that the novel treatment produced neither vomiting nor sweating, "but merely a peculiar state of the system which appears to be incompatible with the existence of inflammatory action."[14] American physicians were quick to adopt Rasori's method for establishing a condition of "tolerance" in the body. St. Louis physician L. C. Boisliniere reported that his patients were able to sustain daily doses of forty to fifty grains of tartar emetic without vomiting or purging.[15]

Peruvian bark was used almost exclusively in the treatment of intermittent fevers, and for a host of other fevers as well. Derived from the bark of the cinchona tree, it was also known as "fever tree bark" or "Jesuit bark" and prescribed as both a preventive and a cure for malaria, certain agues, and indeterminant fevers. By the late eighteenth century,

Europeans were importing large quantities of the bark, often adulterated with Peruvian balsam. In 1820, two French chemists, Pierre Pelletier and Joseph Caventou, produced sulfate of quinine, or quinine extract, which greatly reduced the drug's uncertainty but which also, because of its purity, created many severe side effects.[16]

For the most part, drug therapy mirrored the gusto of the culture it served. Dr. Oliver Wendell Holmes caught the essence of this phenomenon when he wrote:

> How could a people which has a revolution once in four years, which has contributed the Bowie-knife and the revolver, which has chewed the juice out of all the superlatives in the language in Fourth of July orations, and so used up its epithets in the rhetoric of abuse that it takes two great quarto dictionaries to supply the demand; which insists in sending out yachts and horses and boys to out-sail, out-run, out-fight, and checkmate all the rest of creation; how could such a people be content with any but "heroic" practice? What wonder that the Stars and Stripes wave over doses of ninety grains of sulfate of quinine, and that the American eagle screams with delight to see three drachms of calomel given at a single mouthful?[17]

American Practice

For several generations following their New World beginnings, Americans struggled to define a place for themselves in the thought and culture of Western Civilization. The Puritans, as we know, gave a certain dignity to their role by portraying themselves as pursuing "errands into the wilderness."[18] Their protest having begun against the hegemony of the Roman Church and the compromises made by the Church of England, they were eager to find fulfillment in the virtues of their newly discovered lands than from Old World institutions and traditions. But this was no easy task, especially when the vogue of European savants was to view the New World as inferior in every respect—from the salubrity of the air and soil, to signs of physical degeneration in both animals and species of plants, to the unfavorable natural conditions that explained the weaknesses of the land's ignoble Natives.

The seeds for a distinctive American School of medical practice can be found in the works of theologians, naturalists, and popular writers who taught that God had provided each region of the world with its own medicines. Elizabethan herbalist Nicholas Culpeper (1616–1654), for example, in The *English Physician—Enlarged* (1653; 1st American edition, 1708) remarked that every geographic region of the world produced plants whose medicinal properties were capable of curing indigenous diseases. Culpeper's *Pharmacopoeia Londinensis* or, *London Dispensatory* (1649; 1st American edition, 1720) contained accounts of 369 plants with both their astrological and remedial character explained.[19] His accounts were shared broadly among Europe's immigrants and led to the introduction of many new therapeutical substances. Physicians and self-proclaimed healers in the colonial and early national period drew from an assortment of remedies in the vegetable kingdom, including yellow dock, sarsaparilla, wintergreen, birch bark, comfrey, sassafras, dandelion, snake-root, sweet fern, mandrake, marjoram, colt's foot, mistletoe, and Peruvian bark.[20]

Culpeper's intellectual heirs in New World plant investigation included John Josselyn's *New Englands Rarities Discovered: In Birds, Beasts, Fishes, Serpents and Plants of that Country. Together with the Physical and Chyrurgical Remedies wherewith the Natives Constantly use to Cure their Distempers, Wounds, and Sores* (1672); John Wesley's *Primitive Physic* (1747); Thomas Short's *Medicina Britannica* (1751) which included plants from America; William Buchan's *Domestic Medicine* (1st American edition, 1771); Benjamin Rush's *An Inquiry Into the Natural History of Medicine Among the Indians of North America: And a Comparative View of the Diseases and Remedies With Those of Civilized Nations* (1774); and Rev. Manasseh Cutler's *An Account of Some of the Vegetable Productions Naturally Growing in this Part of America* (1785). Others included Johann David Schoepf's *Materia Medica Americana* (1787); Samuel Stearns's *The American Herbal, or Materia Medica, Wherein, the Virtues of the Mineral, Vegetable, and Animal Productions of North and South America are Laid Open, so far as They are Known: and Their Uses in the Practice of Physic and Surgery Exhibited* (1801); Benjamin Smith Barton's *Collections for an Essay Towards a Materia Medica* (1798–1804); William P. C. Barton's *Vegetable Materia Medica of the United States* (1817); Jacob Bigelow's *American Medical Botany* (1817–20); and Wooster Beach's *American Practice of Medicine* (1833).

The earliest non-Native healers credited the tribes of the American forest for providing information on the medicinal effects of the native plants. In fact, it was not uncommon for early practitioners to spend time among Native American healers learning how the plants were to be used. This was certainly true for Jacob Tidd of Amwell in Hunterdon County, New Jersey, who, during his brief captivity by local tribesmen, learned their botanic methods of treatment. Many of the medicinal plants identified by Native American healers became mainstays of botanic and eclectic practice. These included Agrimonia, Aletris, Alnus, Apocynum, Asclepias tuberosa, Cactus, Chelone, Chenopodium, Chionanthus, black and blue Cohosh, Collinsonia, Podophyllum, Phytolacca, Iris, Leptandra, Helonias, Euphorbia, Xanthoxylum, Gentian, Equisetum, Lycopus, Hepatica, Hydrastis, Convolvulus, Arum, Arbutus, Geranium, Geum, Gaultheria, Sanguinaria, Lobelia, Dioscorea, Scutellaria, Spiraea, Summac, Golden rod, Viburnum, Galium, Erigeron, and Veratrum Viride.[21]

Not until the aftermath of the War of Independence were the connotations of American imperfection and deficiency overshadowed by a brash yet healthy assurance in the people's achievements and potentialities. Only then did Americans show sufficient confidence in themselves to look for symbols that would highlight their own indigenous experiences, hopes, and dreams. Within a generation of achieving their political independence, Americans had unleashed a literary genre that exuded a spirit of native genius, cultural and intellectual independence, and triumphant individualism. The cross currents of geography, republicanism, democracy, and national destiny combined to produce a gusty image of popular sovereignty that credited the nation's triumphs to both God and themselves.

Out of these experiences grew a sense of self-confidence that proceeded with stops and starts to discard the reign of scepter, belt, and crosier. Not just kings, but nobles and churchmen failed the test of relevancy in the decades that followed as the higher claim of individual conscience won out over privilege. The reign of the "People" and the "Common Good" became the sources of new power relationships. With them, the spirit of liberty found its way into religion, the law, and even into the art of healing. Where once the subtleties of scholasticism ruled supreme, new ideas and methods emerged to lay claim to hearts and minds.

For Europeans, this brashness counted for nothing. Sydney Smith, founder of the *Edinburgh Review,* published an essay in 1820 that displayed little more than contempt for America's accomplishments and potential. "In the four quarters of the globe, who reads an American book? Or goes to an American play? Or looks at an American picture or statue? What does the world yet owe to American physicians or surgeons? What new substances have their chemists discovered?" he asked. Such judgments, while by no means universal, were nevertheless symbolic of sentiments common among Europeans in the first half of the nineteenth century.[22]

It came as no surprise, then, that Europe's system-builders failed to transplant in their entirety to American shores. Already such Old World practices as primogeniture, entail, and established religion had undergone transformations in the freedom and vastness of the New World. The growth of Protestant sectarianism mirrored a new contract between corporate privileges and individual conscience. So too, with medicine which witnessed ministers, midwives, aurists, botanics, surgeon-dentists, occultists, farriers, bone-setters, and other domestic and part-time healers competing with apprenticed and academically educated physicians. Their active participation in healing was a distinguishing element in the early American landscape where local opinion and private judgment replaced formal qualifications and legal enactments in the use of the term "doctor."

Despite the siren appeals of Old World theorists, American physicians and itinerant healers seemed anxious to divest themselves of their reliance on the procession of teachers and theories emanating from Edinburgh, London, Milan, Paris, and other medical capitals and, instead, lay claim to new theories and remedies in the healing art. It was not difficult to imagine that Americans had their own great expectations for medicine. Having won political independence, was it not appropriate for the new world to achieve medical independence as well? In 1808, a writer in *Medical Repository* expressed the belief that Americans had for too long sought their science from Old World sources. It was now time "to turn their backs to the east, and direct their views to the inviting and productive regions of interior America."[23]

Thomas Jefferson, whose genius transcended numerous fields of study, held a view of the medical profession that was uncanny in its clarity of vision. In a letter to Dr. Caspar Wistar, Jr., of Philadelphia in 1807, he noted that most young men entering medicine were innocent of theory and "untainted with error." Nonetheless, few were able to maintain a "wise infidelity"; instead, they fell victim to the "bewitching delusions" of teachers who had long ago abandoned sober facts and now treated patients on the basis of some fashionable theory or illusionary hypothesis.

> Having been so often witness to the salutary efforts which nature makes to re-establish the disordered functions, he [the physician] should rather trust to their action, than hazard the interruption of that, and a greater derangement of the system, by conjectural experiments on a machine so complicated and so unknown as the human body, and a subject so sacred as human life.... One of the most successful physicians I have ever known, has assured me, that he used more bread pills, drops of colored water, and powders of hickory ashes, than of all other medicines put together. It was certainly a pious fraud. But the adventurous physician goes on, and substitutes presumption for knowledge. From the scanty field of what is known, he launches into the boundless region of what is unknown. He establishes for his guide some fanciful theory of corpuscular attraction, of chemical agency, of chemical powers, of stimuli, of irritability accumulated or exhausted, of depletion by the lancet and repletion by mercury, or some other ingenious dream, which lets him into all nature's secrets at short hand. On the principle which he thus assumes, he forms his table of nosology, analogy, to all the cases he has thus arbitrarily marshaled together.... The patient, treated on the fashionable theory, sometimes gets well in spite of the medicines.[24]

By the early decades of the nineteenth century, talk of an "American School" or "American Practice" of medicine seemed to take on more of an imperative among reform-minded physicians and forward-looking thinkers who, like Jefferson, believed that a "presumptuous herd of medical tyros let loose upon the world destroy[ed] more lives than all the Robin Hoods, Cartouches and Macheaths do in a century."[25] Most assuredly, this father of American democracy was ready to commit to a truly American practice of medicine, free from the impositions of European dogmas and unhealthy procedures: "I hope and believe that it is from this side of the Atlantic that Europe, which has taught us so many other things, will be led into sound principles in this branch of Science, the most important of all, being that to which we commit the care of health and life."[26] What Jefferson foreshadowed in his observations, others sought deliberately to realize.

Benjamin Rush

Before the 1793 outbreak of yellow fever in Philadelphia and other American cities, the Brunonian theory of irritability had reigned supreme among the nation's orthodox practitioners. This contributed to the general acceptance of a "typhus constitution" and thus, when yellow fever broke out, doctors first treated it as an asthenic affection and resorted to the use of opium. But constitutional differences, it was believed, abounded between and among the regions—and even among the races—causing easterners and westerners as well as northerners and southerners to insist on different therapeutic regimens.[27]

One individual who weighed heavily in the response to the Brunonian theory was Benjamin Rush (1745–1813) of Philadelphia who had once been a student of William Cullen at Edinburgh, but who chose a modified Brunonianism, recognizing not two, but only one state of tension seated in the walls of the blood vessels. Unlike Brown who employed a preponderance of stimulants to restore balance to the system, Rush's unitary disease state demanded a depleting and purging regimen to remove the system's excitability. All diseases were sthenic, resulting from the "morbid excitement" in the blood vessels: one disease, varying in terms of its excitability. Content with his ratiocination, Rush discarded nosology and relied on a limited number of evacuant procedures, chiefly bleeding and purging. Like his botanic contemporary Samuel Thomson (1769–1843), he reduced medicine to a few simple principles that "required no depth of thought, extended reading, or length of time, to master it."[28] The outcome of this therapeutic regimen was often reckless, with disciples in the West and South carrying his ideas to nihilistic proportions. Rush's influence continued long after his passing and contributed substantially to the marshalling of self-doubts that fed reformers and their many sympathizers. As late as 1841, a Dr. Sleigt of Philadelphia claimed that five-sixths of the blood was superfluous and capable of being drawn without damaging or threatening the life of the patient.[29]

A signer of the Declaration of Independence, Rush believed the document to extend to medicine as well as to religion and which must, without equivocation, emancipate society from the tyranny of existing philosophies.[30] Later, following the French Revolution, and in the discussions leading up to the preparation of the

Constitution, Rush was no less shy in his remarks. "The Constitution of this Republic should make special provision for Medical Freedom as well as Religious Freedom," he wrote. "To restrict the art of healing to one class of men and deny equal privileges to others will constitute the Bastille of medical science. All such laws are un-American and despotic. They are fragments of monarchy and have no place in a Republic."[31] As evident in his treatment of yellow fever, Rush did not hesitate to break with his British mentors to establish a more American view of disease. And, agreeing with the free-market ideas of Adam Smith, he declared himself in favor of a more benign approach to medical legislation. "Conferring exclusive privileges upon Bodies of Physicians, and forbidding men of equal talents and knowledge from practicing medicine within certain districts of cities and countries," Rush remarked, "are Inquisitions—however sanctioned by ancient charters and names—serving as the BASTILES of our profession."[32]

In some ways, Rush got what he asked as American medicine in the first half of the nineteenth century became less a profession than a conglomeration of identities, pretensions, competing systems, self-doubts, and complaints. Any link between professional identity and education, much less scientific knowledge, was a stretch since the term "doctor" or "physician" required neither a degree or a license to use. By the time of his death in 1813, and in the decades that followed, the medical marketplace had become overrun by all manner of healers making claim to special expertise in the treatment of disease. Medical research was nonexistent and medical school education was largely in the hands of private practitioners who supplemented their practices as teachers and mentors. A physician's acceptance in any community was based more on self-advertisement, reputation, and word of mouth than certification by a degree.

During the heady days of Jacksonian Democracy, American practitioners began asking why there was no "American School" or practice of medicine. Why should Americans remain in servile subjection to the European theories of Cullen, Hoffmann, Stahl, and Boerhaave? Why should Americans mimic Old World licensing privileges? Should not medical practice be in harmony with the principles of human freedom and the most liberal of thinking? Should not American practice draw its inspiration from the flora and fauna of the Western Hemisphere rather than depend upon the materia medica of the Old World?

* * *

In a particularly cogent chapter in his *The Therapeutic Perspective: Medical Practice, Knowledge, and Identity in America, 1820–1885*, historian John Harley Warner explained that the term "rational" carried a bifurcated meaning in medical circles during the first half of the nineteenth century. For some, it meant being "prudent or judicious," or the exercise of induction and "common sense" outside of any exclusive system of treatment. For most, however, the term had just the opposite connotation, meaning that physic was grounded in past rules (i.e., traditions) of practice and tied irrevocably with an exclusive system understood to be regular. By the same token, the term "empirical" denoted attributes that carried mostly negative connotations. Rather than understood as knowledge grounded in observation and experience, it was viewed as having no acknowledged explanation, no basis or principle upon which it acted, that is, making empiricism synonymous with quack or imposter. As explained by Warner, this "semantic muddle" rumbled through the underbelly of nineteenth-century medical writers, compromising communication and confounding the best of professional intentions. Only slowly did the terms acquire more cogent meaning as the word rational migrated to an increasingly negative connotation and empirical was transformed into a more positive clinical meaning.[33]

The timing of this change, while difficult to pinpoint with exactitude, derived in large measure from the ambitions and inhibitions of the Parisian Clinical School whose leading spokesmen defied the ontological explanations of diseases that had held sway for centuries. The French empiricist assault stripped medical rationalism of its authority and, with it, the systems of Cullen, Brown, Broussais, and Rush passed away, driven into obscurity by the very vocabulary that had once sustained them. By the 1840s, the assault on the system-builders was all but complete, with only homeopathy, the last of the systems, continuing to foster a therapeutic structure based on an ancient set of a priori abstractions deemed to be laws or principles. But even homeopathy, which resolutely professed to have embraced the ideal of empiricism while being rooted in rationalism, was ultimately forced to accommodate to the clinical findings of the Paris school.

The return in the late nineteenth century of the word rational in describing medicine did not represent a retreat into the world of the system-builders, but rather a restructuring of medical discourse based on an empirical body of knowledge founded in laboratory science. Advances in the fields of pathology, bacteriology, and immunology undermined whatever holdovers remained of the previous century's system-builders. The recognition of specific pathogens not only challenged the conception of disease as an aggregate of symptoms but shifted the focus of medicine to preventive measures. The use of the term rational no longer implied certainty in medical dogma but rather an ongoing discourse between tradition and change that respected what the past had proven to work for the patient's advantage while showing an openness to new knowledge founded on laboratory-based empirical evidence.

Chapter 2. Old and New World Eclectics

To partake in the nineteenth century's use of the word "eclectic" is to play with one of the subtleties that underscored the age. This was a term whose diaspora transformed it into a set of complementary as well as competing ideas. For some, the word became a metaphor for the collapse of old systems of thinking and the emergence of a thoroughly disciplined pragmatism; for others, it stood for the noticeable irreverence that accompanied western society's emerging democratic character; and for still others, it represented the sense of moral righteousness drawn from the Greek *eklektikos,* meaning to choose the best. Except in the most veiled and muted terms, it is difficult to connect these different threads into an organized pattern. The leaders of eclectic thinking were as different as their sympathizers, and while they were contemporaneous with each other, there was surprisingly little that could be described as collaborationist between or among them. To be sure, they were colorful in their irreverence and opposition to past authorities. Similarly, they were self-confident about what they were doing. Nevertheless, the century's eclectics were in large measure estranged from each other's causes, preferring to define their beliefs and practices with different if not competing sets of shibboleths.

Antecedents

In the world of medicine, the intellectual origins of eclecticism extend as far back as Athenaeus of Attaleia in the first century A.D. who believed in the existence of an immaterial spirit, or *pneuma*, which he considered to be the source of health and disease. Athenaeus built his philosophical system on a principle called *episythetic*, meaning accumulative or collective, drawing from all systems that which best served the needs of the patient. In later times, eclecticism was attributed to the alchemist and physician Paracelsus who opposed the reigning humoral theory of disease, teaching instead that diseases were specific entities curable by specific remedies. A school of medicine known as the Eclectic Conciliators, the most prominent of whom was Daniel Stennert of the University of Wittemberg in Germany, attempted to harmonize the conflicting teachings of Hippocrates and his successors with the views of Paracelsus and other more modern thinkers. These eclectics were so welcoming of new ideas that they accepted witchcraft, alchemy, psychic, and magnetic theories on equal terms with other more orthodox ideas.[1] Other medical men considered to be eclectic in their thinking included the Belgian anatomist Andreas Vesalius (1514–1564), author of *De humani corporis fabrica libri septem* (1543); English physician and anatomist William Harvey (1578–1657), who discovered the circulation of the blood; Dutch naturalist Antoni van Leeuwenhoek (1632–1723), who made simple microscopes through which he studied microorganisms; and Edward Jenner (1749–1823) who announced the discovery of vaccination in 1798.

One particularly important source of creative thinking came by way of the German publisher Christoph Wilhelm Hufeland (1762–1836) who, in 1793, was appointed professor of pathology and therapeutics in Jena, and three years later, physician-in-ordinary to the duke at Weimar. In 1801 he moved to Berlin to become physician to the king of Prussia, director of the Medico-Chirurgical Academy, and superintendent physician to the Charity. His eighty-two volume *Journal der praktischen Arzneykunde und Wundarzneykunst* (1795–1836) ranked among the best publications in Europe and compared favorably in popularity and respect with that of the *Edinburgh Medical and Surgical Journal* (1805–54). A seeker of truth, Hufeland was author of *Ideas on Pathology* (1795), *Minor Medical Writings* (1822–24), and *Enchiridion Medicium* (1836) which went through eight German editions, was translated into French by A. J. L. Jourdan, and published in English by William Radde of New York in 1842. According to Morris Fishbein, editor of *Journal of the American Medical Association* from 1924 to 1949, Hufeland was among a small coterie of German physicians and publicists who, in his challenge to past system-builders, helped lay the intellectual foundation for modern medicine. Given Fishbein's praise, it is worthy to note that Hufeland published many of the critical writings of Samuel Hahnemann, the founder of homeopathy and an arch enemy of medical orthodoxy.[2]

French Eclecticism

Eclecticism reigned as the academic philosophy of France for much of the nineteenth century before coming to an end during the Third Republic. Its spokesman, educational leader, and philosopher Victor Cousin (1792–1867), held a chair in philosophy at the Sorbonne from 1814 until 1821 and, from 1830 to 1851 was director of the École Normale Supérieure. In 1840, he was appointed Minister of Public Instruction in the French cabinet where he helped to establish the French system of instruction. Seeking to unify France following the Revolution, yet desirous of preserving the Revolution's greatest legacies, Cousin formulated a philosophy that sought to steer a course independent of the Catholic Church while, at the same time, bringing harmony out of competing systems of thought. Cousin held that no single philosophical system was entirely correct. Influenced by the common sense philosophy of Thomas Reid (1710–1796) and by the idealism of German philosophers G. W. F. Hegel (1770–1831) and Friedrich Wilhelm Joseph von Schelling (1775–1854), he sought to combine through historical intuition the best aspects of idealism, materialism, mysticism, and skepticism into a workable system of truth. Cousin's writings included *Cours de l'histoire de la philosophie* (8 vols., 1815–29); *Fragments philosophiques* (1826); *Du Vrai, du Beau et du Biue* (1836; tr. *Lectures on the True, the Beautiful, and the Good,* 1854); *Exposition of Eclecticism* (1839); a translation of Plato; and studies of educational systems.[3]

Cousin first used the term "eclecticism" in his Sorbonne lectures in 1818, referring to his belief that all philosophic systems contained elements of truth "which form[ed] the life and strength of each of them."[4] The task of the modern philosopher was to use the knowledge gained by the methods of observation and experimentation to bring the conflicting elements together into a coherent whole.[5] Eschewing both empiricism and skepticism, he praised the history of philosophy as the means by which one learned the best elements of past philosophical systems.[6] Cousin, who called his philosophy "eclectic spiritualism," explained that while every system contained error, this did not mean that it was impossible to distinguish truth from falsity. Indeed, it was possible to distinguish each system from the other and make use only of that which was true. Eclecticism was not the absence of system but the application of one that collected and combined the truths that were "scattered in different systems." Eclecticism was a system by which to judge other systems; it was a system as old as the mind of Plato and enriched by Leibnitz and the views of the newer German philosophers.[7]

For Cousin, the departure of all sound philosophy was the study of human nature, observation, and reasoning, which is why he had such widespread impact on France's educational system. This also explains why historian Erwin H. Ackerknecht identified Parisian medicine during the first half of the nineteenth century as not only "eclectic" in nature but "probably the richest and most brilliant period of them all." Medical eclecticism arrived on the scene during a period of feverish political and social upheaval brought about by the collapse of the *ancien régime*, the often mindless chaos of the Revolution, and the reconstruction of medicine during the Napoleonic aftermath. It was a time of general disgust in the abstractions of pre-Revolutionary rationalistic theories; a desire to provide practical care at the bedside of the sick; the beginnings of an emphasis on empiricism, albeit confused and inconsistent; the reorganizing of medical education around hospitals and clinics; and the simultaneous desire to identify and cultivate newer principles and practices, including the use of more moderate treatments of existing therapeutic measures. In short, it was an effort to fuse the best elements of skepticism, utilitarianism, and political liberalism. Among its more brilliant spokesmen were Auguste François Chomel, Pierre C. A. Louis, Gabriel Andral, Pierre François O. Rayer, Jean Baptiste Bouillaud, Pierre Adolphe Piorry, Léon Rostan, and Armand Trousseau.[8]

Auguste François Chomel (1788–1856), professor of clinical medicine at Charité, and later at Hôtel Dieu, was known for his careful examinations and diagnoses as well as his mild and expectant therapies. Having learned early in his career the dangers of dogmatism, he relied upon pathological anatomy and the rigors of the numerical method as the basis for his medical judgments. A student of Philippe Pinel whose *Nosographie Philosophique, ou la Methode de l'Analyse Appliquée a la Medecine* (1798) was the basic guide of practitioners for more than twenty years, and personal physician to Louis Philippe, he avoided fixed disease classifications and, instead, emphasized the importance of observation, diathesis, and questioning.[9]

Chomel's friend and colleague, Pierre-Charles-Alexandre Louis (1787–1872), defended Chomel in his conflict with Broussais and helped to develop the concept of disease specificity. His case histories and autopsy records at Charité laid the foundation for his groundbreaking studies on phthisis (1825), typhoid fever (1829), and bleeding (1835). A graduate at the Paris Ecole de Santé, who spent his career in Chomel's clinic, Louis's reliance on quantitative information (including his statistical study of bloodletting), and the thoroughness with which he addressed disease, gave his statements "a finality and certainty never attained before." The publication of his *Archives Générales* (1835) on the ineffectiveness of large bleedings signaled the beginning of the end of this ancient practice. Among his many disciples were thirty-seven American pupils, all of whom, as Oliver Wendell Holmes reported, returned with praise of his modesty, his "fearless[ness] in the face of authority," and his "unwearing[ness] in the pursuit of truth."[10]

French genius Gabriel Andral (1797–1876) identified himself as an "eclectic by necessity" when he questioned the benefits of bloodletting along with many other time-held beliefs. No doubt Andral advanced his career by marrying the daughter of P. P. Royer-Collard (1763–1845) who, along with Victor Cousin, helped found the French school system based on eclecticism. Not unlike Cousin, Andral was a compromiser, viewing eclecticism as a means of reconciling the competing camps of medical theorists without, at the same time, establishing a new orthodoxy. Trained at Charité under T. N. Lerminier, he was a colleague to Louis, A. C. Reynaud, Jules Gavarret, and Bouillaud, and rose quickly to the rank of professor of hygiene (1828) and medical pathology (1830). Primarily through his work on chest diseases, both the stethoscope and auscultation became widely accepted. He was also one of the early pioneers in clinical thermometry.[11]

Another of the French eclectics was Pierre François Olive Rader who held positions on comparative pathology at St. Antoine and Charité; and his two-volume treatise on kidney diseases (1839) broke new ground by adding chemistry and microscopy to his pathological studies. Yet another was Jean-Baptiste Bouillaud (1796–1881), professor of clinical medicine at Charité for nearly fifty years and whose work on heart disease brought him international attention. His *Traité clinique et expérimental des fièvres dites essentielles* (1826), *Traité du choléra-morbus* (1832), and *Clinique Médicale de l'hôpital de la Charité* (1837) added to his already illustrious reputation. Although drawn into numerous political entanglements and fixated on the beneficial effects of rapid bleedings (*saignées coup sur coup*) that seemed to draw him back into the older orthodoxies, his work on inflammations set new standards for the age.

Pierre Adolphe Piorry (1794–1879), who worked at Pitié, Salpêtière, Charité, and Hôtel Dieu and who adhered enthusiastically to the numerical method, was another of the French eclectics. A pathological anatomist, he focused, in his works, on the importance of clinical observation, experiments on cadavers, and thorough diagnostic techniques, including the use of thermometry and chemical and microscopic examinations of the blood and secretions.[12]

Léon Rostan (1790–1866), physician and professor of clinical medicine at the Salpêtrière, who held one of the more frequented clinics in Paris, also ranked high among the new breed of eclectic thinkers. An advocate of "organicism," which represented a materialistic view of life in contrast to the competing belief in vitalism, Rostan viewed disease as an abnormal state of an organ rather than an alteration of some vital property. Like Samuel Hahnemann, the founder of homeopathy, he was enamored with the effects of animal magnetism and believed exclusively in the use of specific medicines.

Armand Trousseau (1801–1867) studied medicine with Pierre Fidele Bretonneau (1778–1862) and coauthored with Hermann Pidoux a three-volume *Treatise on Therapeutics* (1835). On the strength of this treatise, he was appointed to the Faculté in 1839 and replaced Chomel as professor of clinical medicine at Hôtel Dieu in 1850. Besides his medical achievements, Trousseau was active in politics and, following the revolution of 1848, was elected representative in the Constituent Assembly. His interests were truly eclectic—from diphtheria to tracheotomy, pediatrics, neurology, the use of cod-liver oil for rickets, expectant treatment, and *vis medicatrix naturae*.[13] In their *Treatise on Therapeutics*, which included a 100-page introduction on the history of medicine, Trousseau and Pidoux became known for their medical skepticism. They provided a fresh look at the materia medica and, drawing upon the work of contemporaries, broke from the older system-builders to provide the newest thinking on the use of medicine's therapeutic anchors.[14]

Using historian John Harley Warner's definition of the Paris Clinical School as "a distinctive complex of institutional arrangements, clinical techniques and teaching practices, modes of organizing knowledge, and structures of medical perception that characterized Paris medicine between 1794 and the mid-nineteenth century," it is clear from the available evidence that western healing practices were strongly impacted by this eventful episode in French medicine.[15]

British Eclecticism

Because medicine and medical philosophy were such transnational topics of discussion, medical eclecticism was not limited to Continental Europe. British medical students before the 1850s still went to Paris and Italy for anatomical, pathological, and therapeutical experiences, but increasingly, they chose to combine their travel itineraries with experiences in Vienna, Heidelberg, Berlin, Bonn, and Giessen. German universities and clinics offered medical and surgical experiences that were popular among visiting students. The luminaries for the New Vienna School of positive medicine included Karl Rokitansky (1804–1878) in pathological anatomy and Johann Lucas Schönlein (1793–1864) in parasitic pathology. British students were repulsed by the German preference for expectant medicine (similar to that which they found in France) and returned home with a stronger professional awareness of contrasting medical systems, facilities, practices, and attitudes. While not overtly using the term eclectic in their public statements (they preferred the term *positive* medicine), Britain's medical reformers took a commanding view of the winds of change and proceeded to pick and choose the best practices from conflicting theories and schools.[16]

Many of the medical icons of early nineteenth-century Britain were quick to acknowledge the public's distrust of doctors and the problems inherent in medical education. Sir Thomas Watson (1792–1882), for example, believed it essential for young physicians to begin by "unlearning" what they had acquired from books and former teachers. While critics and reformers of medicine were not numerous, there were still those who were anxious to challenge the pillars of stability. Men like Sir John Forbes (1787–1861) translated the works of Laennec and Avenbrugger; William Stokes (1804–1878) of Dublin investigated the use of the stethoscope; and John Hope (1725–1786) and Peter M. Latham (1789–1875) looked into the discipline of morbid anatomy.[17]

Much of the skepticism evident among British physicians stemmed from the confessions of John Forbes, fellow of the Royal College of Physicians and physician to the Queen's Household. "In the present state of our knowledge," he once stated, "the Hygienic—Eclectic—Hippocratic—Rational system of curing disease is the only one that can be justified or safely followed."[18] In an extended article in the *British and Foreign Medical Review,* his book *On Homeopathy, Allopathy, and Young Physic* (1845), and *On Nature and Art in the Cure of Disease* (1858), Forbes endeavored to expose the prejudices of the profession, the incompetence and uncertainties of the medical art, and the importance of the powers of Nature. Beginning with an admission that every well-informed and experienced member of the medical profession was "painfully aware of the great imperfections of their Art," he proceeded to explain how ignorance of the natural course and progress of disease had interfered with the nature and art of medicine and had led to the "ridiculous promises" of charlatans and the "absurd and useless" doctrines uttered by Samuel Hahnemann and Anton Mesmer.[19] For too long, he acknowledged, the *post hoc ergo propter hoc* mode of reasoning had been used to justify the often conflicting modes of practice. Were such to be true, human sacrifices and the meddling of ancient deities and witch doctors would remain as efficacious as in prior centuries. In truth, however, the popularity of homeopathy over the previous thirty years, although attributed by its followers to Hahnemann's precepts and practices, was the result of the resources of Nature, aided by faith and a dietetic regimen.[20] Pleased with the progress made in general science, he longed for the expurgation of "imaginary specifics" from the materia medica; greater attention paid by physiologists and pathologists to the newer discoveries made by the microscope; the elimination of such "potent perturbative agencies" as bloodletting, emetics, and purgings; and, in general, avoiding the evils of "energetic and meddling practice."[21]

Accompanying Forbes's ideas were those of Marshall Hall (1790–1857) of Edinburgh who made his mark with investigations on puerperal cases and with his criticism of bloodletting. Hall, whose contributions to physiologic research marked him as a scientific leader of the age, warned of the evil effects of mercury. A lecturer on the theory and practice of medicine at the Webb Street School of Medicine and physician to the General and St. Mary's Hospitals, Hall was frequently mentioned in American reform journals as a representative of regular medicine's self-doubts as well as a sponsor of therapeutic changes similar to those advanced by sectarian critics. In 1839, the first American edition of his *Principles of the Theory and Practice of Medicine* was published by Charles C. Little and James Brown. Revised and enlarged by Dr. Jacob Bigelow and Dr. Oliver Wendell Holmes, the book included extensive new information on the advantages of studying disease with the aid of the numerical method of Louis; the benefits from using percussion and auscultation; the dangers of overusing certain remedial agents such as opium, mercury, antimony, and bloodletting; and the importance of recognizing the class of self-limited diseases.[22]

John Hughes Bennett (1812–1875), who took his degree at Edinburgh, then studied in Paris where he became interested in both the microscope and with clinical medicine, followed on the footsteps of both Forbes and Hall. Returning to Scotland, he became professor of the institutes of medicine at the University of Edinburgh in 1841 and, through several publications, including *Clinical Lectures on the Principles and Practice of Medicine* (1859) and *Text-book of Physiology* (1872), he questioned many prevailing practices. In 1866, at a meeting of the British Medical Association, he challenged the use of mercury and called for a special committee to investigate the propriety of its continued application.[23]

In his *Clinical Lectures on the Principles and Practice of Medicine*, Bennett explained how it was only with the recent improvement in optical instruments, making visible structures in both healthy and diseased conditions, that advances in the collateral branches of science had begun to create a truly scientific medicine. Although eighteen years had passed since the cell doctrine had been introduced into physiology and pathology, far too few medical men had come to recognize the importance of these findings in their everyday practices. Believing that science, which was "steady, certain, and progressive," and art, which was "vacillating, doubtful, and limited," should advance together "to their farthest limits," he hoped there would soon be fewer false facts and theories to detract from a doctor's practical skills.[24] Avoiding the evils of skepticism and its resulting discordance in the adoption of what was known as the expectant treatment popular in both France and Germany, Bennett sought improvement in both the art and science of medicine by way choosing an eclectic approach to change. For Bennett, both the laboratory and the hospital clinic were the bases of medicine's future accomplishments. The sooner students came to the realization that it was essential for them to learn percussion, auscultation, histology, and chemistry, the sooner would the science and art of medicine be secure.

> The only safe method of escape from this state of things, it appears to me, is by the earnest effort on the part of those who sincerely desire the improvement of our art, to establish the science of medicine upon something like a solid foundation. Let us, at all events, endeavor to realize our position, and to separate what is known from what is unknown. Among the known, let us determine what we have derived from scientific generalization, and what from blind experience; and in the vast field of the unknown, let us, if possible, agree as to the direction and manner in which we ought to work, in order to explore its extent, and contract its boundaries.[25]

Bennett's *Clinical Lectures on the Principles and Practice of Medicine* was especially popular among homeopaths because the author took special notice of recent changes in therapeutics occasioned by knowledge gained from diagnosis and pathology. To be specific, Bennett looked at the diminished use of bloodletting and other antiphlogistic remedies in the treatment of acute inflammation, and the influence of suggestion on certain diseases of enervation. This explanation was fundamentally opposite his colleague, William Pulteney Alison (1790–1859), who reasoned that bloodletting was no longer appropriate because the human constitution had altered fundamentally, forcing medical men to adjust their treatment—not their principles—from earlier years.[26] Notwithstanding Allison's ratiocination, Bennett said that inflammation was the same now as it had ever been; rather, the principles on which bloodletting and other antiphlogistic remedies had been practiced were in opposition to sound pathology. Homeopaths were grateful for Bennett's honesty and hoped that his truthfulness would lead him and other regulars ultimately to adopt homeopathic principles.[27]

Bennett's medical sentiments were admired by the so-called American School of eclectics. In fact, the Eclectic Medical School of Chicago, better known as Bennett Medical School, was incorporated by special charter in 1868 and named after John Hughes Bennett. The college's official organ, the *Chicago Medical Times*, was the second oldest eclectic journal in existence and boasted the largest circulation of any medical journal in Illinois. The college dropped "eclectic" from its title in 1909. In 1910, it absorbed the Illinois Medical College and the Reliance Medical College and became, by affiliation, the School of Medicine of Loyola University.[28]

American Eclectics

American philosopher Woodbridge Riley, author of *American Thought: From Puritanism to Pragmatism and Beyond* (1915), suggested that the advocates of eclecticism in the United States faced a less than friendly reception. In education, the term suggested "a polite form of literary piracy," while in politics, its partakers were accused of being mugwumps and disloyal to party identity.[29] Riley's comment, which certainly reflected the prevailing opinion in the second half of the nineteenth century, fails to capture the congeniality between European eclecticism and the American literary spirit in the first half of the century. For one thing, European eclecticism exuded a certain practicality that Americans found alluring. It was also democratic in tone, giving a degree of equality to all systems and expecting a spirit of give and take in the process of arriving at truth. And reflective of the eighteenth-century empiricists, it eschewed mystery for clarity, celebrated observation over tradition and belief, and the power of thought over instinct and inspiration.

European eclecticism had a particular allure among the early New England transcendentalists Ralph Waldo Emerson and Amos Bronson Alcott who encountered Cousin's ideas through Caleb Sprague Henry's *Elements of Psychology: Included in a Critical Examination of Locke's Essay on the Human Understanding* (1834). Henry, a professor of philosophy at the University of the City of New York, interpreted eclectic philosophy to audiences in the United States over a period of twenty years. Americans also discovered Cousin through George Ripley's *Philosophical Miscellanies* (1838), a compilation of writings from different European authors. George Ripley (1803–1880), a Unitarian minister and one of the founders of the Brook Farm commune, carried on correspondence with Cousin and it seemed, for a time, that Ripley found comfort in European eclecticism. According to biographer Charles Crowe, Ripley viewed eclecticism as "the crest of a reaction against empiricism and materialism—a response which began with [Victor de] Bonald, [Félicité de] Lamennais, and [Joseph] de Maistre; continued with [François-Pierre-

Gouthier] Maine de Biran and [Pierre-Paul] Royer-Collard; and culminated in the eclectics, Cousin, Theodore Jouffroy, and Benjamin Constant."[30] But as Crowe explained, Ripley "inherited some of Cousin's faults such as a tendency toward sentimentality, pretentiousness, superficial optimism, and the bland assumption that all truths had been set down leaving little more for the philosopher to do than clever editing.[31]

Of all people, transcendentalist Ralph Waldo Emerson criticized Cousin's eclecticism for being too eager in its claims. "I would say there is an optical illusion in it," Emerson wrote. "It avows great pretensions. It looks as if it had all truth, in taking all the systems, and had nothing to do but to sift and wash and strain, and the gold and diamonds would remain in the last colander. But Truth is such a fly-away, such a sly-boots, so untransportable, unbarrelable a commodity, that it is as hard to catch as light."[32] Emerson's comment is striking since his own philosophical elusiveness seems unmatched in American letters. If eclecticism was guilty of vagueness, the critical remarks emanating from the "Sage of Concord" were surely inconsistent with his own thoughts and preferences.

Despite Emerson's puzzling reticence regarding the claims of eclecticism, he unabashedly announced in 1837 the celebration of the "American Scholar" and the drawing to a close of the nation's "long apprenticeship to the learning of other lands." In an age when the human mind seemed unfortunately enshrined in the thoughts and deeds of a few individuals, Emerson found it comforting that his fellow Americans were beginning to listen to the spirit of the native freeman rather than to the "courtly muses" of the Old World.[33] Whosoever would be a man had to be a nonconformist who was, above all, true to himself.

> A foolish consistency is the hobgoblin of little minds, adored by little statesmen and philosophers and divines. With consistency a great soul has simply nothing to do. He may as well concern himself with his shadow on the wall. Speak what you think now in hard words, and tomorrow speak what to-morrow thinks in hard words again, though it contradict everything you said to-day.—'Ah, so you shall be sure to be misunderstood.'—Is it so bad, then, to be misunderstood? Pythagoras was misunderstood, and Socrates, and Jesus, and Luther, and Copernicus, and Galileo, and Newton, and every pure and wise spirit that ever took flesh. To be great is to be misunderstood.[34]

In a lecture before the Mechanics' Apprentices' Library Association of Boston in 1841, Emerson appealed to the new spirit of reform that was affecting all aspects of society. "What is man born for but to be a Reformer," he announced, "a Remaker of what man has made; a renouncer of lies; a restorer of truth and good, imitating that great Nature which embosoms us all, and which sleeps no moment on an old past, but every hour repairs herself, yielding us every morning a new day, and with every pulsation a new life."[35] In expressing this sense of restlessness and of eager expectancy in the future, Emerson was merely saying what most Americans were struggling to articulate. "We are all a little wild here with numberless projects of social reform," Emerson wrote to his friend Carlyle in 1840. "Not a reading man but has a draft of a new community in his waistcoat pocket."[36]

The preeminence of the wise and temperate Emerson gave balance to America's experiment in democracy. Like the European eclectics who drew from multiple sources for their truths, Emerson found his particular metaphysics outside the confines of any one system; his genius retained a freedom that defied too sharp a focus. "We do not go to hear what Emerson says," wrote James Russell Lowell, "so much as to hear Emerson."[37] As the high priest of American democracy he chose deliberately to found no identifiable party or disciplined group of believers. Instead, he chose to bring the people to themselves, believing in their own abilities. In the raw lumber of his thought were found an affirmation and personal conviction that telegraphed a message of confidence to all who listened to his words. His "The American Scholar," delivered before Harvard's Phi Beta Kappa society in 1837, became America's intellectual Declaration of Independence, while his essay on "Self-Reliance" paid tribute to the innate worth of each individual, urging the reader and listener to "Trust thyself."

Americans in Paris

Despite the mixed opinions expressed by Emerson toward European eclecticism, and his conviction that Americans must set their own course and destiny, others were not nearly so emphatic. The vagueness of Cousin's eclectic philosophy and the lack of original thought brought its eventual rejection but not before suggesting a process of intellectual distillation that appealed to a generation of American medical students who found post-revolutionary Paris an exciting, if not seductive, environment for their social and medical interests.[38] The Paris Clinical School had taken a commanding lead over London, Edinburgh, Glasgow, and Dublin as the place for American students to gather. Not only were there many more appealing distractions for students with even a modicum of curiosity and money in their pockets, but the opportunity to work with such giants as Louis, Andral, and Bouillaud provided experiences that they would remember for a lifetime. There in the Paris hospitals a combination of clinical anatomy and medical statistics triumphed over medicine's past attentiveness to speculative rationalism. In joining the results of bedside observation with that of the autopsy table and a healthy skepticism, French clinicians overturned centuries of past assumptions, including the use of such therapeutic heavyweights as bleeding, calomel, and antimony.

Just as in previous years when American students had flocked to the system theorists of London and Edinburgh, they now gathered in Paris at Charité, Hôtel Dieu, Hôtel Vénérienne, La Pitié, Enfans Malades, Salpetrière, and other hospitals to learn at the feet of medicine's newest and most influential clinicians. Among the Americans who received a portion of their medical education in these wards were Valentine Mott (1785–1865), Peter S. Townsend (1796–1849), and Alonzo Clark (1807–1887) of New York; Elisha Bartlett (1804–1855) of Rhode Island; John C. Warren (1756–1857), James Jackson, Jr. (1810–1834), Oliver Wendell Holmes (1809–1894), George C. Shattuck (1813–1894), and Henry Ingersoll Bowditch (1808–1892) of Boston; and Benjamin W. Dudley (1785–1870), William Wood Gerhard (1809–1872), Casper Wistar Pennock (1799–1867), Alfred Stillé (1813–1900), and John Godman (1794–1830) of Philadelphia; and Francis Peyre Porcher (1825–1895) and Peter C. Gaillard (1812–1889) of Charleston.[39] In these Paris hospitals they practiced at patients' bedsides with the stethoscope and auscultation, and tested their diagnoses on the cadavers that moved inexorably from charity wards to the anatomy labs. These fortunate American students were quick to discover that medical education was much more than didactic. It included the discipline of correlating knowledge of disease, empirical observation, accurate diagnosis, and effective treatment.[40]

Historian Richard Shryock explained this migration of American doctors on the basis of the perceived "scientific supremacy" of the Paris schools at the time of their visits. More recently, John Harley Warner has attributed the American preference for Paris over London medical education more on the "social structure" of the Parisian medical education system that, unlike London schools, was open, free, and accessible. Only when they returned home, he argued, did American doctors attribute their choice to the empiricist character of the French hospitals. By then, British medicine had become a "necessary foil" to the perceived leadership of Paris as a center of medical innovation and radical empiricism. This was despite the fact that American doctors almost uniformly considered London doctors to be better healers and were critical of the French ineptness in the physician-patient relationship, accusing them of being "less interested in healing the sick than in verifying their diagnosis at the autopsy table."[41]

The transmission of these ideas and methods that did much to build the foundation for America's modern clinical practices and investigations left a bifurcated legacy among historians. For example, Erwin H. Ackerknecht explained the emergence of modern medicine as a story of progress via the transmission by foreign medical students and practitioners of an anatomical/clinical paradigm constructed in the French hospitals. On the other hand, Michel Foucault in his *The Birth of the Clinic* (1963) identifies this same paradigm as having inadvertently created a darker side to this medical model by shifting medical attention from the patient as an individual, to the patient as a disease entity. But as Warner explains, each of the two authors has shown that, "by tracing the

French impulse in the United States, we can discover a formative stage in the emergence of modern American medicine, including enduring sources of both extraordinary clinical power and shortfalls in humane patient care." For Warner, the French Clinical School not only stood for "a celebration of empiricism and animus against rationalistic systems," but in its interpretation, declension, and incorporation into American medicine, revealed "at least as much about the values, assumptions, expectations, and apprehensions of the American culture itself."[42]

This would explain Warner's assertion that American physicians "were highly selective about which aspects of Parisian medicine they transmitted to America and which ones they eschewed." Seldom did American students bring back their experiences in whole; most often, they accepted French pathology, diagnosis, and surgery while rejecting French therapeutic practices as inappropriate for American medicine. No doubt the American penchant for active intervention vs. expectant medicine weighed heavy in their preferences. Besides, the pauperized patients found in the Paris hospitals were viewed as lacking analogy with American patients whose constitutions were deemed substantively different. As Warner suggests, American doctors viewed French therapeutic teachings as leading "to inferior practice that would engender public distrust of the regular profession and thereby foster sectarian power."[43]

It would seem, therefore, that while American students were drawn to the pathological investigations of the Paris Clinical School, they were visibly more reticent about its therapeutics. When all was said and done, Americans preferred a much more active, interventionist approach to cure than the more somnambulant methods of the French (and later, the German) clinical school. The former seemed fitting for the American environment while the latter was judged to be too severe and insensitive for a caring practitioner.[44]

In his research on the rhetoric of reform, Warner made it clear that reformers in both Great Britain and America used the "decline-of-science" argument and the ascendancy of French medical science as a catalyst for change. In Great Britain, it became a tool to challenge the entrenched medical elite, redistribute professional power, advocate competing programs, and champion general practitioners. By contrast, American rhetoric was used to denounce rationalism, open opportunities for competing sectarians, urge a reconstruction of practice along more empirical lines, and as a vehicle to further democratization.[45]

American reformers came to an early conclusion that the rationalistic systems of Cullen, Brown, Broussais, Rasori, and Rush were the cause of the profession's poor identity. As physicians began to express publicly their concerns with the progress of therapeutics and the materia medica, believing that their generation's medical practices had become chaotic, if not dangerous, they took a renewed interest in empiricism, a term that previously they had relegated to the hosts of irregulars who plied their trade in the towns and countryside. The negative implications of this term, once the pariah of medical discourse, became a more compelling description of medicine's therapeutic aspirations. Assaulted by a strong empiricist tradition coming from Paris, American reformers found themselves expressing a much healthier skepticism than when they first started practice. In fact, the very use of terminology denoting "system" brought furrows to the brows of the generation's newest physicians. So concerned were doctors over the state of contemporary medicine that their public remarks became less and less constrained as they took measure of their profession.

The "Other" Eclectics

As we now know, eclectic philosophy became the underpinning of the formidable educational system in France designed by Victor Cousin. It was this philosophy that eventually migrated into the Paris hospitals and clinics and brought so much brilliance to their experimentation. In Britain and Germany, eclecticism claimed an ancient heritage yet stood for a miscellany of information that invited an ever growing interest in the writings of social revisionists and innovationists. In America, especially along the Northeast seaboard, a group of literary eclectics represented an educated fraternity of sometimes brilliant conversationalists who drew repeated sustenance from their European cousins. The same was true of those American physicians who partook of Europe's hospital and clinic experiences and who returned home with novel ideas and practices. However, having tasted at the springs of French and British eclecticism, they preferred to speak of their experience without naming or adhering to its formal philosophy. This left so-called eclectic thinking to be captured by an unbridled group of rebellious botanics whose taste for eccentricity, perfectionism, and millennialism made them as distinctive in their amateurishness as they were in the paucity of their ideas. Earnest, but drawn into multiple diversions, digressions, and disappointments, they mouthed the words of Europe's eclectics, including the accomplishments of the Paris Clinical School, but failed to carry their pronouncements into practice. What energies they displayed were quickly dissipated in denominational rivalries and ignominious squabbles.

Unlike the early Greek and later European forms of eclectic thinking which historians generally characterized as historically significant, few have been willing to give much credence to this so-called American period of medical eclecticism. According to Morris Fishbein, there was little evidence that the American eclectics were even aware of their antecedents, paying greater attention instead to the development of a distinctive plant materia medica and a therapeutic process built around the idea of specific medication. In "vogue" for a time, America's eclectic ranks eventually "fell into the hands of exploiters and promoters."[46] More recently, historian James Whorton recounted in

Nature Cures: The History of Alternative Medicine in America (2002) eclecticism's origins in the 1820s and its bid to borrow freely from all schools and systems of practice, "taking anything that experiences showed to be effective and safe." While recognizing the school's pragmatic appeal, Whorton gives eclecticism even less credence than Fishbein, noting its internal dissensions and, in less than a page, relegating it to the medical dustbin.[47] Despite the finality of Fishbein's and Whorton's remarks, America's band of eclectic reformers persisted for more than a hundred years. And while they justifiably earned much of the derision that came their way, they nonetheless deserve a more balanced study, particularly since American eclecticism began as a continuum of European eclecticism before branching into something distinctly idiosyncratic.

Among the intellectual contributors to American Reform Practice, later known as eclecticism, was the restless eccentric, naturalist and philologist Constantine S. Rafinesque (1783–1841) who endeavored to establish medical practice on a foundation of vegetable products. Born the son of a French merchant in Constantinople, Rafinesque enjoyed the life of a traveler and collector. His parents moved to France following his birth and, during the turmoil of the French Revolution, moved first to Tuscany, and then to Philadelphia. During his teens, Rafinesque was apprenticed to the Clifford Brothers mercantile house in Philadelphia and later worked as secretary to the U.S. consul in Sicily where he carried on a lucrative trade in commodities. In 1802, Rafinesque met with minister and physician Manasseh Cutler (1742–1823) and was supported in his endeavors by Samuel Latham Mitchell (1764–1831), cofounder of the *United States Pharmacopeia* in 1820.[48] In his research, which included fifteen years of travel and observation in the trans-Appalachian West, Rafinesque showed a deep appreciation for the medicinal uses of plants by the Native Americans.[49]

With the assistance of his former employer, merchant John D. Clifford, a trustee of Transylvania University (1819–1826) in Lexington, Kentucky, Rafinesque was offered a professorship of botany and natural science in the college. Although he published extensively during these years, Rafinesque was openly scornful of regular doctors and managed to teach for only a few years before the unfortunate combination of an "acerbic personality" and "idiosyncratic opinions" conspired to alienate him from colleagues.[50] The experience was enough, however, for him to divide medical practitioners into three classes: *Rationals, Theorists*, and *Empirics*. Included among the Rationals were the *Improvers*, the *Eclectics*, and the *Experimentalists*. This, it appears, was perhaps the earliest use of the term eclectic in American reform medicine. According to Rafinesque, the Eclectics were "those who select[ed] and adopt[ed] in practice whatever is beneficial, and who change[d] their prescriptions according to emergencies, circumstances and acquired knowledge." The Theorists included the advocates of regular medicine, and the Empirics were typically designated as deceitful, dealing most frequently in patent medicines. The

Empirics also included herbalists, Indian and root doctors, steam doctors, and other assorted types.[51]

Rafinesque's two-volume *Medical Flora, or Manual of the Medical Botany of the United States of North America* (1828–30) found few friends among regulars but was highly esteemed by members of the botanico-medical movement, especially by Alva Curtis and his disciples in Columbus and Cincinnati, who saw it as a major contribution to the vegetable materia medica. In the words of historian Francis R. Packard, the book quickly became "the vade-mecum of the Botanic physicians."[52]

American eclecticism took yet another turn with the writings of Dr. Wooster Beach (1794–1868) of New York. Although Samuel Thomson and Beach claimed to be reformers of regular medicine, opposing orthodoxy's reliance of bloodletting, calomel, and other heroic poisons, their systems were distinctively different from each other. As noted earlier, Thomson reverted to a classic Hippocratic stereotype in framing his medical system; by contrast, Beach chose not to cultivate any fixed system but, instead, campaigned to free the practice of medicine from the dogmas and creeds of all past systems. Desiring to open the field of inquiry, he invited students to learn from clinical observation at the patient's bedside.

Beach, the founder of the so-called "Reformed System" of medicine, was a native of Trumbull, Connecticut, and learned the elements of botanic medicine from Jacob Tidd of Amwell, New Jersey. Beach moved to New York City where he attended a course of lectures and received a diploma at the University of the State of New York. Among his teachers were doctors Wright Post, David Hosack, and Valentine Mott. He took additional instruction from a Dr. Ferris and other botanic physicians in New York City and, in 1825, located his practice at 93 Eldridge Street where he taught private students and dispensed medicines. He also became interested in various social and religious controversies and, using Eldrigde Street as his base of operations, founded several journals (*Ishmaelite, Battle-axe, Medical Reformer*, and *Telescope*) which became vehicles for the dissemination of his views.[53]

In 1827, Beach opened the United States Infirmary on Eldridge Street where he treated patients. He served as attending physician at the infirmary and, in 1832, he was appointed health physician for the Tenth Ward where he treated more than a thousand cases of cholera. In 1829, Beach organized the Reformed Medical Academy which, in 1830, became known as the Reformed Medical College. Members of the faculty included Beach in theory and practice and surgery; Calvin Preston in anatomy and physiology; George W. Chevers in materia medica and therapeutics; J. F. Daniel Lobstein in obstetrics and diseases of women and children; and John C. Kelly in chemistry. Prominent among the school's students were Thomas Vaughan Morrow, Ichabod Gibson Jones, John King, John J. Steele, and James R. Wood, all of whom became noted eclectic reformers. The college was the rallying point for Beach's principles of reform medicine and, although a licensed regular, he set himself the task of reforming medical practice by insisting that it be based upon rational and inductive principles. "The science of medicine, like the doric column, should stand simple, pure and majestic, having fact for its basis, induction for its pillar, and truth alone for its capital," he wrote.[54] The same year Beach organized his school he also established a national society known as the Reformed Medical Society of the United States.

Beach's subsequent *Practice of Medicine* (1833), which went through numerous reprints and revisions, represented a compilation of his medical experiences and his preferred choice of selecting from all sources, irrespective of theory, those remedies that had proved the most useful.[55] He was also author of *An Improved System of Midwifery* (1847), *Medical and Botanical Dictionary* (1847), and *A Treatise on Anatomy, Physiology and Health* (1847).

Beach was identified as early as 1837 by a writer in the *Western Medical Reformer* as having all the attributes of an eclectic. The writer explained that since the science of medicine was founded upon observation, "the truth must be sifted from the mass." This became the task of an eclectic who could "combine, arrange and systematize facts when arrived at." For this purpose, argued the author, Wooster Beach was the ideal person to undertake such a task.[56] Although Beach preferred the terms "Reformed System" or "American School" to describe his particular approach to medicine, Dr. Isaac J. Sperry of Connecticut responded: "You are Eclectic!" Supposedly, Beach replied: "You have given me the word which I have wanted; I am an Eclectic!"[57]

While not highly educated, Beach was credited by friends and disciples as a compiler and collector of medical experiences. "His intuitive knowledge of the nature of disease, and of the action of remedies, and his skillful plan of treating all diseases," wrote H. E. Firth, "was appreciated by his friends, and even acknowledged by his opponents."

> When the history of eclecticism shall be written up by the medical historian, the name of Dr. Wooster Beach shall stand out in characters of living light. If future posterity shall do justice to his name, he shall yet live, in poetry, in song, and in eloquence. Unborn generations shall witness his renown. Sires, matrons and infant childhood in ages yet to come, shall contemplate the statute of Wooster Beach, crowned with laurels, and decked with the emblem of a nation's gratitude, with one hand holding his books on practice, and with the other pointing to a nation saved from the terrible ravages of mercury and the lancet.[58]

In 1845, Beach briefly joined the Eclectic Medical Institute of Cincinnati as professor of clinical surgery and medicine. He also lectured at Central Medical College of New York. In 1855 he was elected president of the National Eclectic Medical Association. In his later years, Beach traveled abroad, visiting hospitals, colleges, and infirmaries in England, France, and Germany. Like many of his eclectic colleagues, he viewed the medical profession as under the sway of Old School doctors who stood firm like the Catholic Church and the aristocracies of Europe against the boldly progressive movement of science, liberty, and humanity. Wherever Old School influence prevailed, the eclectics and homeopaths were there to collectively castigate it as "Old Hunkerism."[59]

In the New England states, the champion of reform medicine was the Baptist preacher and theologian Calvin Newton (1800–1853). A graduate of Union College in 1829, he studied for the ministry at Newton Theological Seminary, taught Hebrew and rhetoric at Waterville College, Maine, and served a pastorate at Bellingham. After more than a decade as a preacher, Newton turned to the study of medicine, attending lectures at Cambridge University and then at the Berkshire Medical College from which he graduated. While attending the latter institution be became an admirer of its president, Dr. Henry H. Childs (former lieutenant governor of Massachusetts in 1843–44) who often derided the regular medical profession for its ignorance and arrogance, professing that every physician should be eclectic in his openness to the armory of new weapons in the warfare against disease. Upon graduating in 1845, Newton styled himself an eclectic and, within a year, began publication of the *New England Medical Eclectic and Guide to Health*, aimed at uniting Botanic physicians under the banner of no single system of thought.

In a matter of months, Newton sought to establish a medical college in New England dedicated to the sentiments of Childs and others whom he most admired. He began by offering informal instruction to students at his office in Worcester. This was followed by encouragement from the Uxbridge Botanic Medical Society that directed Newton and another instructor to unite their efforts by establishing a school to teach the various branches of medicine. Accordingly, in March 1846, the Worcester Botanico-Medical College opened with the Uxbridge Society providing it with a fifteen-member board of trustees and with financial support. Although the name of the school gave it the appearance of being Thomsonian, Newton was determined to retain its eclectic character by ensuring that those who enrolled or supported the school were persons "who belong to no medical clique, and have no party end to answer."[60]

Because of his insistence on the term eclectic, Newton came under attack from Alva Curtis and the Independent Thomsonians whose schools typically included the words "botanico-medical college" in their title. Curtis was blunt in his criticism, accusing Newton of being part of "the poisoning, blistering, cupping, bleeding, mongrelizing Beachites or Eclectics," and threatened to open a rival school in Boston. Undeterred by the threat, Newton co-opted Curtis's efforts by appointing him as a member of his faculty. Curtis declined the offer but the appointment brought peace among the warring parties. In 1849, a bill to incorporate the Worcester Medical Institution passed the Massachusetts Legislature and was enacted into law by Governor George Nixon Briggs.[61]

Alexander Wilder, one of the earliest historians of reformed medicine, explained eclecticism in the context of the colonies' successful separation from the domination of Great Britain. "The reign of the scepter, the belt and the crosier" had ended, he opined, and with it, the "worn-out despotisms of the Old World." Eclecticism was America's declaration of independence from the tyranny of the existing schools of medicine. In their place, New World medicine, based upon freedom of choice, affirmed unequivocally the benefits of simple indigenous remedies and the reliance upon the faculties of observation. This was not a reformation but a revolution from the current state of medicine.[62]

The choice of the term eclectic by these early reformers was "not lightly or carelessly chosen," explained Wilder, but adopted with the clear purpose by those who originated the term. As noted earlier, Constantine Rafinesque was one of the earliest users of the term, applying it in his *Medical Flora of North America*. He considered the eclectics to be liberal, learned, and well informed, ready to adopt methods of treatment that had been found beneficial and willing to adapt their methods as circumstances and knowledge changed.[63] In writing to Wooster Beach in 1840, Rafinesque remarked: "I belong like yourself, to the Reformed School of Medicine and agree with you much better than with the Thomsonian, homeopathic and botanical empirics. Your system is a good one, if not perfect; it is better at any rate than most of the fashionable systems, Galenian, Brunonian or mineral."[64] A further clarification came from John Dill Robertson, M.D., of Chicago who, in 1902, remarked that "the word 'Eclectic' in a medical sense signifies everything that the term 'American' does in a political one." It was on the grounds of true eclecticism that real progress had been achieved in the past, and would continue to be in the future.[65]

Nevertheless, the term was not held in high esteem by all reformers. William H. Cook, dean of the Physio-Medical Institute (Thomsonian) in Cincinnati during the late 1860s, took issue with the principles of eclecticism, accusing its advocates of professing "a queer confusion of ideas." To Cook's way of thinking, the eclectics were simply another "clique" within the allopathic profession struggling for identity. Championing Samuel Thomson as his intellectual forbearer, Cook accused the eclectics of ingratitude and perfidy in claiming title to professional liberty when all that they did was borrow from Thomson—"whose memory they are in such haste to defame." Thus the claims of Beach and Newton were little more than admissions of ideas and concepts "pilfered from others."[66]

To Samuel Thomson alone, Cook argued, belonged the title of true eclectic. However, this was a name no longer held sacred because of the damage done to it by the eclectic fraternity. By professing to choose that which was good from any and all sources, the eclectics were merely claiming "what every man has done from the beginning of the world." Rather than laying down some first principles to guide them, they chose to have no "standard of faith" at all. By what, Cook asked, were they to be guided in making their choices? "If the judge has no law to govern him, how is he to render judgment?" By refusing to be held to any principle, how is it that an eclectic can claim adherence to anything in science? "This claim to superiority in 'choosing,'" he concluded, "appears a most attractive one to Eclecticism, but it is really its greatest weakness; for it announces them to be without a single principle of their own, leaves them without the simplest requisite for the formation of a system of science, and then makes them glory in their own shame—the shame of making a wholesale plagiarism of the discoveries and principles of others."[67]

Cook reminded American eclectics of a similar sect seventeen hundred years earlier which, like the current school, attempted to form a system by "choosing" whatever it considered to be good from other systems. But the old eclecticism flourished for no more than fifty years "and then died so deep a death that the fact of its existence is now known only through the writings of those whom it attempted to overthrow."[68] An outspoken medical reformer, Cook accused the eclectics of confusing what they considered their claim in medical matters and what was every citizen's civil liberty. In other words, the value of professional liberty which the eclectics claimed to be a distinctive part of their beliefs was no more than what every American enjoyed as a matter of constitutional right.[69]

Although it can be argued that the eclectics, perhaps alone among the reformers, viewed themselves as true medical protestants, this comment cannot be said of all of them. Dr. James McClintock (1809–1881), for example, was born in Lancaster County, Pennsylvania, and at the age of seventeen, commenced his medical studies under the preceptorship of Dr. John Eberle of Philadelphia. At the conclusion of his studies he became a pupil of Dr. George McClellan at Jefferson Medical College and assisted him in many of his surgical operations. During his pupilage at Jefferson, he enjoyed the advantages available at the Pennsylvania Hospital and Philadelphia Almshouse Infirmary. At the age of twenty, young McClintock served as assistant professor of anatomy at the college and, at the age of twenty-four, delivered his first course of lectures on midwifery. During the 1832 cholera epidemic, he was appointed physician to the City Cholera Hospital and served also at the City Prison. It was during this time that he introduced a patent remedy under the name of Dr. McClintock's Diarrhea Cordial and Cholera Preventive.

In 1838, McClintock opened a School of Anatomy in Philadelphia to provide supplemental education to students at neighboring medical schools. A year later, he was appointed an attending physician to the Almshouse Infirmary and, in the spring of 1841, joined the Vermont Academy of Medicine as chair of anatomy and physiology. Soon after he joined the academy, the school changed its name to Castleton Medical College and he was named both president and professor of anatomy and physiology.

In his introductory lecture on the "Art of Healing" delivered to the medical class at Castleton in March 1842, McClintock celebrated the transition of medicine from primitive beliefs to the Newtonian world of science and the enlargement of medicine's boundaries through the assemblage of facts by way of observation and induction. "The day for medical hypotheses is over," he announced. "Men may theorize elsewhere, but here [in medicine] they must not."

> The reproach of uncertainty has been deserved long enough; we must wipe it out by giving to our Art the only certainty of which it is susceptible, founded upon close and accurate investigation. Divest yourselves, then, of the beginning of all prepossession; swear in the words of no master; adopt the dogmas of no sect; attach yourselves to no exclusive system. Devote yourselves to the study, not of opinions, but of facts, not of schools, but of nature. It were bad enough to lose time my misdirecting your efforts; but worse, inconceivably, would it be, to lay the corner stone of your education in prejudice.[70]

In true form for the age, McClintock urged his students to honor the achievements of medicine's distinguished doctors but to beware "of being led by any name to the adoption of a mere theory." It was good to cherish the "great masters" as benefactors of mankind but it was equally important not to follow them. This applied not only to the ancient doctors of medicine but to men like Hoffman, Cullen, Brown, and Broussais. "In a word, gentlemen, we should be men of no sect, but men of science."[71]

In his lectures to students, McClintock paid homage to "the untiring industry and philosophic spirit of the French clinical physicians" for their work in special and pathological anatomy. For him, medicine would forever be indebted to the work of Bichat, Corvisart, Laennec, Andral, and others whose knowledge, skills, and experiences had enlightened the science of disease. These "strong minds" and "noble spirits" kindled a harvest of medical triumphs that were rich in information and satisfying to the soul.[72] In the hospitals of Paris so many aspiring doctors formed "habits of thorough study."[73]

At the completion of his 1842–43 course of lectures, McClintock returned to Philadelphia and reestablished his School of Anatomy. Claiming to have adhered to eclectic principles as early as 1842 while president of the college at Castleton, McClintock gave deference to homeopaths and other irregulars who had fought orthodox dogma. For these reform feelings, he anticipated being called a quack by those who considered themselves regular, allopathic, or orthodox.[74]

In 1846, Dr. Thomas D. Mitchell, professor of materia medica at Transylvania University in Lexington, Kentucky, suggested that McClintock establish a summer college in the city where lectures could be given between the course of lectures offered by other fully chartered medical colleges. Through the efforts of friends, a bill for incorporation for his Philadelphia College of Medicine passed both houses of the legislature and was signed by Governor Francis R. Shunk. Shortly afterwards, he returned to the legislature to ask for the right to lecture in the winter months as well, thus making the school equal in status with all other chartered colleges in the state.[75]

In his *Introductory Lecture* before the 1860–61 class at the newly chartered college, McClintock described for his students the various sects that had existed in medicine, including the older *Rationalists, Empirics, Methodics, Pneumatics, Expectants, Humoralists*, and *Solidists*, and the more recent *Allopathists, Homeopathists*, and *Eclectics*. Reared as a member of the oldest and most numerous group of allopathists, or regulars, he admitted to practicing its precepts "as faithfully as an honest, independent man can do."[76] When all was weighed in the balance, however, McClintock found himself much more attuned to the group known as eclectics. "Physicians of this class," he explained to the new medical class, "avail themselves freely of the labours of their predecessors, and contemporaries of all schools, and from the knowledge thus attained, added to the results of their own investigations, they have established a system of practice, approaching, I think, more nearly to scientific accuracy, than any other school."[77]

* * *

Perhaps the most telling observation regarding this group of botanic reformers came from Alexander Wilder, who announced at the World's Medical Congress of Eclectic Physicians and Surgeons in 1894 that eclecticism "was born on American soil, .. baptized by American blood [and] championed by Americans during its whole existence. It . . . is American in its conception, American in its practices, and I hope to heaven that it will always be American in its nature."[78] More of an admission than a comment, it gave painful confirmation to the parochial tendencies of the American eclectics and a disposition that, despite earlier statements in praise of the French Clinical School, made it abundantly clear that they gave little more than lip service to the broader intellectual origins of the movement. Throughout its history, American eclecticism remained an expression of a narrow botanic movement that was punctuated by acrimonious feuds, invested heavily in the theory of specific diagnosis and specific medication (two principles that were derived from homeopathy), and survived through the marketing success of the John Uri Lloyd's specific medicines which became the sectarian substitute for regular medicine's synthetic pharmaceuticals and academic medicine.

Because of the botanics' capture of the terminology, American regular doctors took deliberate steps to avoid using the word "eclectic" to describe their refusal to accept any hard and fast rules or adhere to any exclusive system or belief. Nevertheless, their lexicon is replete with language that clearly connoted this approach. Stuart Close, M.D., editor of the *Homeopathic Recorder* during the 1920s, regretted that mainstream doctors had been reluctant to call themselves eclectics since that was truly what they were. "It is the privilege of the avowed Eclectic in medicine to choose and use whatever means seem good to him, subject only to general professional and legal requirements and customs," he wrote. It was a shame, he concluded, that they had not taken the name which served them best.[79]

Chapter 3. Jeremiads and Apostates

American social critics have often referred to the period between 1820 and 1850 as one in which no single representative philosophy or public image could be identified. Instead, they have likened it to an age of adolescence, one that was "vigorous," "ungoverned," "stammering," and "risky."[1] However defined by its supporters and detractors, the first half of the nineteenth century was characterized by an enthusiasm that criticized all forms of orthodoxy, including religion, law, and medicine; advanced numerous new "isms" as replacements for older beliefs; eschewed reasoned discourse; and advocated a strong personal and social ethic. For America's medical jeremiads and apostates, the period was remarkable for both their numbers and the breadth of their lamentations and beliefs. Many remained in the ranks of regular medicine while others departed as disaffected patients, visionaries, ill-tempered antagonists, and shameless opportunists. As medical revisionists and innovationists, however, they played an important role in explaining how the meaning of science in medicine evolved over time and how the idea of reform was represented in medical language. So much so, that "to ignore the opponents of orthodoxy is not merely to commit enormous condescension towards them," wrote historian Logie Barrow, but "to suppress the very relationship of opposition, and thus to smother the light it can throw on what was being opposed."[2] Vocal—and sometimes even polemical—in their lamentations, they demanded equality before the law in the free expression of their beliefs and practices. As admirers of economist Adam Smith, they argued that the marketplace was sufficient to sort out the differences between and among the nation's healers. With this in mind, a sensitive rereading of the nineteenth century reform medicine is much needed since most historians have regarded this period of reform more a spectacle of cult or fringe therapies than a disquisition on the meaning of medicine. Such views, however, fail to acknowledge the subtleties that existed amid the clamor of these critics and their jarring sects.

Early Jeremiads

Exemplary of early American concern with past system-builders was the Rhode Island physician Elisha Bartlett (1804–1855) who graduated in medicine from Brown in 1828, pursued additional medical studies in Paris, and then took up his residence in Lowell, Massachusetts, where he became the city's first mayor and was later elected to a seat in the state legislature. He returned to medicine, holding teaching positions at the Berkshire Medical Institute, Dartmouth College, Vermont Medical College, Transylvania College, University of Maryland, the University of New York, and the College of Physicians and Surgeons in New York. Editor of the *Monthly Journal of Medical Literature* at Lowell, he authored several significant works including, *An Essay on the Philosophy of Medical Science* (1844); *Inquiry Into the Degree of Certainty in Medicine* (1848); and *The History, Diagnosis, and Treatment of the Fevers of the United States* (1850). Bartlett was a firm believer in "a radical reformation of educational principles and systems" and, pursuant of his objective, held Victor Cousin of France and the popularizer of phrenology Johann Gaspar Spurzheim (1776–1832) of Austria in high esteem. He also advocated both spiritualism and transcendentalism.[3]

First in *An Essay on the Philosophy of Medical Science*, and later in *An Inquiry Into the Degree of Certainty in Medicine,* Bartlett noted widespread skepticism among colleagues as to medicine's power to cure disease. Willing to admit that medicine's confidence level had been "violently shaken," if not "greatly lessened and impaired" by past system-builders, he refused to despair.[4] In fact, Bartlett was one of the strongest advocates of the Paris Clinical School and the concepts espoused by Louis and his contemporary, Jules Gavarret, of the numerical method. The use of this method gave a whole new meaning to the findings of medical science, the sorting out of the clues to the etiology of disease, and the legitimacy of specific therapies.[5] Having benefited from his student days in France, Bartlett made claim to a new degree of certainty that belonged to both the science and art of medicine. Referencing the work of Louis at La Pitié and James Jackson of Boston General Hospital on the effectiveness of bloodletting in pneumonia, and the work of both René T. H. Laennec and Rasori in the use of tartar emetic in the treatment of pneumonia, Bartlett was satisfied that the chances of recovery were "indefinitely increased."[6] Bartlett's enthusiasm for the numerical method led him to claim a level of medical sophistication that was unrealistic for the time, but he nonetheless paved the way for what historian James Cassedy described as a "new consensus of orthodox medical ideas, a set of beliefs widely known as 'rational medicine.'"[7]

Another of the American doubters was John Ware (1795–1864), Hersey Professor of the theory and practice of medicine at Harvard. He once remarked that the art of medicine was "so imperfect, and so much conjecture interferes with correct judgment in medicine, that the mind of the physician must necessarily be left in many cases . . . in a state of some uncertainty with respect to the character of the disease he is to treat, and the best course to be pursued in its management."[8] Ware was pleased, however, with the fact that a "strong impulse" existed in his day for the investigation of medicine as a science. Provided that the pursuit of science became not an end in itself but tied to the sufferings and lives of patients, the scientific investigation of medicine had a purpose. He often reminded his colleagues that: "It is well that one should look at diseases, and study them as objects of science; but the sick must not be treated so as to feel that they are regarded only in this light."[9] Physicians must never forget the "higher duties" which they owed to their patients.

Such was the condition of medical education, he felt, that many new and competing sects had been founded because of a "love of novelty or of notoriety, or from the desire of gain, or on account of the ease with which distinction is obtained among the proselytes of a sect." Homeopathy, the most respectable of these groups, had risen out of the medical profession itself and because it had "done so much to shake the confidence of mankind in the old school." Although its theories seemed no more at variance with medical knowledge than the earlier systems of Boerhaave, Cullen, and Brown, the fact remained that homeopathy left its patients with nothing more than the "resources of nature."[10] No matter what sects arose, concluded Ware, the profession was strong and enduring and would select and absorb all the truth, "rejecting the falsehood which has arisen within and around it." New sects would no doubt arise and "so far as they advocate any just opinion, or originate improvements in practice, or illustrate important errors, the lessons they teach will survive amid the accumulated treasures of medical knowledge."[11] Here, in so many words, was the essence of Victor Cousin's eclectic philosophy.

Among the more notable teachers in America whose challenging questions fell on a receptive generation of students struggling to make sense of the information before them, none was more forceful than Dr. Samuel Jackson (1787–1872) of the University of Pennsylvania, whose annual introductory lecture on the institutes of medicine was frequently published at the request of his students. In 1830, he spoke to the medical class on the competing sources of medical knowledge—from the sanctioned learning of the past, to the lessons of teachers, and that obtained through "matured experience" and "disciplined observation." He acknowledged that uncertainties and imperfections in medicine were legion and attributed them to the manner in which medical science had been cultivated. Like Thomas Jefferson, he likened medicine to a "region of romance, filled with chimeras, and peopled with the vain phantoms of imagination." Added to this was the search for "first causes" that had led earlier physicians on futile crusades to blend the psychological and spiritual with the physiological, corporeal, and organic natures of man. This had resulted in a confusion of opinions, doctrines and practices.[12] True, supernatural agencies were no longer invoked as frequently as in earlier times, but Jackson recognized that physicians still searched for first causes and sometimes appealed to abstract forces or powers to satisfy that craving. He pointed to the metaphysical speculations of Samuel Hahnemann, Rasori, and Broussais as representing what he hoped would be the last of these efforts and that, in their place, an era of "demonstrative or positive medicine had commenced." By this he meant replacing the "presumptuous speculations on the nature of first causes" with inductions drawn from physiology, anatomy, pathology, and modifications in the different organs caused by medicinal and remedial agents.[13]

In 1832, Jackson wrote *Principles of Medicine, Founded on the Structure and Functions of the Animal Organism*, establishing him as one of the leaders in American medical education. In it, he described the three contemporary systems of medicine: *physiological, symptomatic*, and *organic*. Physiological medicine, the most pretentious of the three, determined the nature of disease by divining the character of the organism's vital actions. With this information, which was little more than a collection of hypotheses, physicians had built "monuments" to their unbridled egos. These metaphysical systems were not only more dogmatic but significantly defective in their application. Elements of physiological medicine had prevailed through history, with modifications by Flemish physician and chemist Jan Baptista Van Helmont (1577–1644) and German physician Georg Ernst Stahl (1660–1734) in the form of an *archaeus* and *vis medicatrix*, and later perfected by German physician Friedrich Hoffmann (1660–1742), and English physiologist and poet Erasmus Darwin (1731–1802). Mingled in later years with positive science, physiological medicine continued in vogue with the doctrines of Broussais, whose physiology and philosophy of irritation contained many truths but enforced in "too dogmatical a spirit."[14]

Symptomatic medicine, the second of the competing systems, held that the sum of the symptoms constituted the disease and furnished the indications of practice. Predominant in Britain, Germany, Italy, France, and the United States, symptomatic medicine was "allied intimately with ontological views of disease," but was not without "serious defects." According to Jackson, symptoms did not in themselves constitute the basis for either a sound or safe method of medical practice. Symptoms were certainly signs "addressed to the senses," but were often deceptive, manifesting in organs other than the seat of the disorder. Being the "effects" of a cause, symptoms had to be traced to their source. "The uninformed vulgar can perceive the symptoms of disease as well as the physician," Jackson pointed out, "but it is the instructed physician alone who can appreciate their meaning, obtain from them correct ideas, and act on them with certainty for the attainment of beneficial ends." The symptom-complex considered so essential to the homeopathic disciples of Samuel Hahnemann was clearly the means by which knowledge of a disease was acquired; but symptoms were not the disease itself. The conclusions deduced from them required a fuller knowledge of the structure of the organs.[15]

For himself, Jackson preferred the newer system of organic medicine that had grown out of pathological anatomy, a special branch of medical science popular in the hospitals of Paris. He hoped that American physicians would embrace this department of science and contribute to its advancement. At the time, however, he regarded William E. Horner (1793–1853) of Philadelphia and author of *A Treatise on Pathological Anatomy* (1829), as the only American who had directed any attention to the subject. Jackson felt that the principal impediment to the organic system was the lack of facilities to investigate the tissues and organs through autopsy. Notwithstanding the importance of organic medicine, alterations of structure due to disease did not reveal the antecedent cause—the disease itself. Nor did pathological anatomy provide any certitude for correct treatment. "Our means of restoration to the natural state are feeble, limited, and not often successful," he admitted. In other words, organic medicine led to no clear indication of therapeutic regimen. This frustration led to Jackson's decision to proceed with caution and to approach his work with a "philosophical eclecticism" that freed him from adhering to any one system.[16] Jackson's use of the term eclectic should not go unnoticed. As mentioned earlier, this word was in common parlance among reform-minded physicians in England, France, and the United States, and suggested a breaking away from the metaphysical thinkers of the past and present.

Of all his writings, Jackson's *A Lecture on Medical Education, Introductory to the Course of the Institutes of Medicine, in the University of Pennsylvania, for the Session 1833–34* became the representative statement of American medicine's appeal for reform. In it, Jackson pointed out that medicine, though long studied by some of the greatest minds, began as the "grossest empiricism" before passing into "darkness and superstition." Consequently, he urged students not to "repose implicit faith in the opinions, the dogmas, or even the facts" they were learning, but to "regard everything with the skeptic's eye."[17] Indeed, the older the opinions, facts, and doctrines, the more likely they were to be untrue. He warned students that medicine was not simply a collection of maxims and precepts handed down from past generations, requiring only "a limited degree of intelligence to put into successful operation." The objectives of a truly sound medical education required the learner to form sound habits of investigation; to compare and arrange facts in appropriate classes; and to have an appreciation for the power of numbers. Medicine could be treated both historically and philosophically, but Jackson gave greater weight to philosophy that emphasized the investigation and verification of facts by observation and experiment. Only when the facts were confirmed, could "the creative spirit of philosophy" cause "form, existence, order, [and] harmony [to] rise successively into being." Then, would true science take shape.[18]

> The history of mankind presents a series of delusions, that have ruled his intellect, that have made him a slave to the passions, the

> prejudices, or the designs of a few; that have stifled knowledge and extinguished truth; that have arrested the progress of civilization, and almost created a doubt as to the universality of the attribute of rationality. . . . The important object of education should be to avert this unhappy state of intellectual nullity—to form the habit of investigation, to conduct the mind to the comparison of things, estimating their similitudes and differences, arranging them in their respective and appropriate classes, and expressing them in precise formulae. A just education is much less the communication of knowledge, than instruction in the methods of acquiring knowledge—by examination and reflection—experience and induction.[19]

Jackson urged his students to ignore all reverence for authority. The way to truth was through a healthy skepticism, refusing to allow authority to take root. "Whatever doctrine you find in books, or hear in lectures," he told the students, "subject it to the ordeal of observation, experiment and reason."[20] Reform was both a necessity and a requirement for remedying the current state of medicine. This meant not only teaching and studying medicine as an inductive science, but forcing a "new re-organization of medical instruction," including the elimination of old courses; the introduction of new subjects, including new branches and departments; and a lengthier period of instruction.[21] No longer could reform be postponed, even though it imposed "new sacrifices, new duties, new tasks, [and] new labors" on teachers and students. Public confidence had been shaken as regular practice degenerated into blind routine. "Can it be denied," Jackson asked, "but that the only difference between regular practice and empirical practice, is a routine treatment of merely different remedies, and not always to the disadvantage of the empirical method?" Only by raising the level of medical instruction would the public's confidence be reassured. "Let medicine be, what in reality it is," he urged, "a science of calculation, of combination, of induction, the elements of which are deduced from the phenomena of organized beings, and the relations of exterior agents with them." Doing so would raise medicine above the "illusory pretensions" of the empirical arts.[22] Until then, medicine would remain an endless list of facts reported "by doubtful authorities, too often loosely observed, and more imperfectly recorded."[23]

A staunch admirer of the Paris Clinical School, Jackson urged students to abandon authority as the "supreme arbiter" and admonished them to use their minds to judge the validity of belief by working with approximations and probabilities. Health and disease were worthy objects of calculation and, if properly assessed, could be examined and understood with a much greater degree of certainty than presently achieved. What made Jackson's remarks so prescient to the age of French eclecticism and to his students was his description of the medical faculty and curriculum of the Academy of Paris. The faculty consisted of twenty-four professors and an equal number of adjuncts (agrégés), a program of instruction that consisted of thirteen courses divided into the winter and summer seasons, and an additional forty to fifty private lectures delivered by adjuncts.[24]

The Thomsonians

Perhaps the most successful of America's earliest apostates was the traveling healer Samuel Thomson (1769–1843) of Alstead, New Hampshire. From 1805, the year he began practicing medicine, until his death in 1843, he designed and implemented a health management system that was spread by hundreds of agents into every state; adopted by the five tribes of the Cherokee Nation; carried by the Mormons into Utah; advocated through more than eighty magazines and journals between 1822 and 1860; and transported as well into Canada and England. Rather than follow the traditional physician's path of treating patients and then billing them, he sold "rights" to his patented course of treatment, thereby making every right-holder his or her own physician. To accomplish this, he employed the courts to protect his intellectual property and built a medical empire that was estimated at nearly four million followers.[25]

Like Dr. Benjamin Rush of Philadelphia whom he greatly admired, Thomson called attention to three classes of men—priests, lawyers, and physicians—who over the centuries had wrested power from the "common people." Priests had kept the Scriptures in the dead languages so the people could not read them; lawyers had made themselves the keepers of the government's secrets; and physicians had wrapped the mantle of Latin around their prescriptions to hide their discoveries from common knowledge. All three of these classes had outlived their usefulness and now, having broken the bonds of servitude to England, the people of the United States were positioned to move forward with these powers now vested in themselves.[26]

Like Rush, too, Thomson viewed disease as a single unit, consisting of a reduction in life's vital action. Although debility appeared under different guises, the nature of disease was the same in all, that is, the loss of body heat. "So long as the fire keeps up that state and degree of warmth essential to the living state of the animal body," Thomson reasoned, comparing the human body to the operation of a steam engine, "so long as the fire is kept good in the boiler, to keep the engine at work, so long the pump will go." Given that the human constitution was the same for all, differing only in temperament, it followed that the loss of natural heat was due to obstructed perspiration caused by the formation of cankers, a grayish substance that lined the stomach and intestines. The removal of this obstruction and the restoration of digestion would, in turn, restore natural perspiration and body heat.[27]

Thomson's contribution to medical reform was his patented course of vegetable medicines. It consisted of a six-step process beginning with his emetic herb (*Lobelia inflata*) which he administered in a variety of forms to cleanse the stomach, promote perspiration, and relax the muscular system; cayene pepper (*Capsicum annuum*) to generate and hold heat in the stomach until the system cleared of instructions; steaming or vapor bath followed by emetics and enemas to clear the stomach and bowels of canker; bitters to restore the debilitated organs to their proper functions; restorative tonics (poplar bark, bayberry, peach meats, or meats of cherry stones) to strengthen the stomach and bowels; and finally, Thomson's Compound Tincture of Myrrh and *Capsicum* (better known as "Rheumatic Drops") to remove pain and promote natural heat. Those who purchased a "right" to Thomson's course of treatment and pledged not to reveal or otherwise expose any part of the information contained in his *New Guide to Health* (1822) were considered members of the Friendly Botanic Society of the United States and entitled to free communication with other purchasers of "rights" as well as assistance in relation to botanic practice.[28]

During Thomson's lifetime, numerous physicians and professors gave testimony favoring his reform system of medicine. They included Professor Powell of Vermont University; pioneer on smallpox vaccination Benjamin Waterhouse (1754–1846) of Cambridge; Professor William Tully (1785–1859) of Yale College; and Dr. William Robinson, a friend of Rush, who wrote and lectured on the benefits of the system.[29] In addition, anatomist and surgeon, Dr. George McClellan (1796–1847), founder of Jefferson Medical College of Philadelphia and father of the Union general, was often quoted by sectarians as having said: "I have used steam, cayenne and Lobelia and found them useful to remove disease."[30]

Benjamin Waterhouse of Cambridge praised Thomson for his native intelligence, his independence from popular superstition and prejudice, and his determination to be guided only by the laws of truth and justice. For too long, Thomson's steam and puke practice had faced foolish censure and wanton condemnation irrespective of the honest inquiry he had made to understand disease. In one of his earliest applications of the term eclectic, Waterhouse addressed Thomson as: "My sagacious, industrious and much-respected Empiric or Eclectic, if you like the latter term better."[31] He used the word "eclectic" with the clear intent of denoting the ancient philosophy that selected from various systems such opinions and principles that were judged sound and rational. Clearly, observed Waterhouse, Thomson fit the description.

After reading Thomson's *New Guide to Health*, Waterhouse concluded that Thomson was no quack. Rather, he was a man of "good capacity" and "persevering temper" who, over the course of more than twenty years, had arranged his experimental knowledge into a system similar to both Galen's and Hippocrates's. Although Thomson probably never read either of their writings, the belief system of Hippocrates appeared in all his theories. Placing observation and his own experiences over the pride of the "privileged order of practitioners," Thomson had developed a system of medicine that was free of harsh minerals and liberal use of the lancet.[32] Believing Thomson to have been "cruelly persecuted," Waterhouse urged doubters to read his works, test the article lobelia which Thomson had introduced to the materia medica, and give recognition to a man who accumulated knowledge by his own experiences. Unlike quacks who kept the components of their medicines secret and advertised them as remedies for almost every disease or disorder, Thomson revealed his discovery of the plant lobelia, recounted how it was prepared, and explained its medicinal virtues. Thomson was an experimenter who had built his medical system on lines directly opposite the Dogmatists and deserved to be read.[33]

Among Thomson's many disciples was Samuel Robinson who delivered a series of fifteen lectures before members of Cincinnati's Friendly Botanical Society. An impassioned speaker, he spoke of the need for the Common Man to take control of his God-given talents and, spurning the schools and colleges, to rely on himself for a more superior form of training—experience. A strong believer in the "tribunal of public opinion," Robinson held that God had lodged common sense in the "mass of the assembled multitude." In other words, *Vox populi, vox Dei*—the voice of the people is the voice of God. Thomson, a man of the people, was a mere ploughman farmer—unlearned in the schools and colleges—but trained by thirty years of observation, reason, and experimentation. To him was given the task of removing the veil that for so long had hidden the mysteries of healing. Ignorant of books, but not of experience, Thomson stood before the "tribunal of the whole world" to profess his discoveries and relief to the wretched.[34] Within weeks of Robinson's lectures, Horton Howard, a printer and Thomsonian agent from Columbus, Ohio, published Robinson's *Course of Fifteen Lectures* (1829), making it the earliest apologia for Thomsonism. Six authorized editions eventually went to press, with individual printings as high as eight thousand.[35]

What makes Robinson's lectures so significant in the literature of reform medicine is that he attempted to position Thomsonism *within* the broad fabric of medicine, and particularly within the context of the Paris Clinical School. While most observers of medical history would consider Robinson's objective somewhat of a "stretch" in reasoning, he nevertheless took pains to explain the competing systems of Cullen, Brown, Rush, and others, focusing finally on Thomson's thirty years of observation and practice. He noted that Thomson's ideas were surprisingly similar to those of Rush and consistent with the beliefs of both ancient and modern physicians. "The more we examine Thomson's system," he wrote, "we find its principal features agree with the most popular and received opinions of ancient or modern times."[36] Robinson was particularly fond of making the connection between Thomson's use of botanicals and the refusal of the French clinicians to drench patients with harsh medicines. Republicanism and French clinical medicine had remarkable staying power among America's early botanic reformers. "Between the physician who theorizes in his study, and the one who establishes his theory on facts and experience, the difference is as wide as between a novelist and a writer of true history," wrote Robinson. The genius of both Thomson and the French eclectics was that their practices derived from the Baconian emphasis upon trials, observations, and experiences, and not upon the "intolerable lumber" of earlier authorities.[37]

Thomson endeavored to keep close rein on his reform movement but, in 1838, a schism occurred between the liberal and conservative wings of his Friendly Botanic Society, causing both groups to establish separate organizations. The strict or hard-line Thomsonians required members to sign an oath adhering to pure Thomsonian practice and condemning all who practiced "mixed" medicine. The oath also forced agents and patent holders to purchase only genuine medicines and use only franchised medicine stores and infirmaries. The Independents, on the other hand, concentrated their efforts on erecting infirmaries and medical colleges and on expanding the number of general practitioners without worrying that their medicines came from unauthorized agents. The quality of the medicines, not their authorization, determined their value. Less concerned with maintaining strict orthodoxy, the Independents were more liberal in defining the credentials of their members, and more open to "improvements" in botanic medicine, including greater knowledge of anatomy and physiology.

By the 1850s, what remnants remained of the strict Thomsonians had migrated into the fold of the physio-medicals, a conservative, vitalist-based, medical system that died soon after the closing of its last medical college in 1911. As for the Independents, they continued for several more decades before eventually merging with the more liberal eclectics.

The Botanics

Among those physicians who preferred using only herbal-based medicines was Dr. Elisha Smith (d. 1830) who practiced in New York City and was the recognized founder of the branch of medicine know simply as botanic. Except to participate in political lobbying activities against potentially punitive legislation, Smith and his followers remained distant from other sectarians. His *Botanic Physician: Being a Compendium of the Practice of Physic Upon Botanical Principle, Containing All the Principal Branches Necessary to the Study of Medicine*, published in 1830, drew heavily on William Buchan, James Thacher, Constantine Rafinesque, and Samuel Henry, and provided one of the earliest statements of botanic philosophy distinct from Thomsonism. Smith's favorite treatments included strengthening bitters, syrups, and cathartics and, although a firm believer in vegetable medicines, he did not rule out the use of moderate bleeding or mineral drugs (with the exception of mercury). Unlike Thomson, he stressed the need for botanic physicians to be educated in all branches of medicine.[38] Smith was a supporter of reform medicine and served as president of the New York Association of Botanic Physicians. Following his death, his son, Dr. Isaac S. Smith, founded a medical college in 1836 that operated for ten years before closing.[39]

Smith was not alone in believing that botanics should follow no one individual or system. John B. Howell (d. 1839), a native of England, had studied medicine with a Dr. Thornton of London before coming to American in 1793 and pursuing his profession. As president of the Pennsylvania Associate Medical Society of Botanic Physicians, he was one of the early botanic practitioners who not only recognized the need to draw from both ancient and modern savants but to remain independent from the system-builders in thought and deed. His society, along with the short-lived semimonthly magazine, *The Botanic Medical Reformer and Home Physician* (1840–42), edited by his student Dr. Thomas Cooke (d. 1855), sought to steer a course independent of the Thomsonians and their rivals, the eclectics. Their efforts, however, failed in that both Thomsonians and eclectics attempted to lay claim to Cooke's journal.[40] In time, Cooke allied himself with the eclectics and, in 1850, he along with Joseph Sites and P. F. Sweet obtained a charter from the Commonwealth of Pennsylvania to open the Eclectic Medical College of Pennsylvania. The professors of the school included Cooke, Sites, Stephen H. Potter, Henry Hollembaek, Thomas J. Chase, and St. John H. Mintzer. The college merged in 1864 with Penn Medical College founded on the combined principles of eclecticism, homeopathy, and the chrono-thermal system of Samuel Dickson of London.

The Homeopaths

Homeopathy represented an effort to find a way out of the perceived nihilism of the day by looking not to the new school of Paris Clinical Medicine but rather by returning to the ancient theories (i.e., no two similar diseases can exist in the body at the same time) and finding a stronger rationale for them. The term *homeopathy*, meaning *like*, or producing of an effect like the disease, differed from *antipathic*, or *opposite*, producing an effect opposite the disease; and *allopathic*, or *another*, producing an effect different from, but not opposite to the disease. The doctrine of homeopathy was therefore couched in the term, *similia similibus curantur,* or likes cure likes.

Alone among America's earliest sectarian medical groups, homeopathy experienced the most bifurcated relationship with regular medicine. With a solid majority of its physicians having graduated from regular medical schools before changing allegiance, they knew well the culture of allopathic medicine and therefore took doubly hard the public posture of the American Medical Association which treated them as traitors to medical orthodoxy. Unlike Samuel Hahnemann (1744–1843) who saw himself as a true Protestant seeking an irrevocable break from medical orthodoxy, America's homeopaths were much more benign in their intentions, inclined to view themselves as specialists within the broad body of medicine. Only when their efforts failed did they choose to seek a more established existence with their own colleges, hospitals, and dispensaries. Even then, however, many remained hopeful that they would eventually merge in a more enlightened and respectful relationship with regular medicine.

Homeopathy, whose elements had ancient origins, but which was introduced formally as a system of universal application in the teachings of Hahnemann, made significant inroads into nineteenth-century medical practice in both Europe and America. "The medical art stands in need of a thorough reform from head to foot," proclaimed Hahnemann in 1808. "The evil has become so crying that the well-meaning mildness of a John Huss no longer avails, but the fiery zeal of a rock-firm Martin Luther is needed to sweep away the monstrous leaven." For too long medicine had operated on opinions, each of which "was ingenious and learned in proportion as it was valueless." Every physician acted according to the manner he was taught by his particular school or "as his fancy dictates," and each found an infinite number of opinions and authorities on whom to base his decisions.[41]

In his *Organon of Homeopathic Medicine* (1810), Hahnemann challenged the imperfect manner in which so-called Old School, orthodox, or regular doctors had approached disease. Although supposedly founded upon scientific principles and known among the faculty of medicine as the "rational art of healing" because it supposedly removed the morbid causes of disease by following nature, medical orthodoxy had succeeded instead in forming but an "obscure and imaginary picture" of disease. Encouraged by conjectures as to the relative sensibility, irritability, or nutrition of the body's organs, it had jumped to hypothetical reasonings that pointed out the best remedy in a particular case of disease. Thus had arisen the debilitating and repetitious practices of evacuations by means of emetics, purging, bloodletting, sweating, and all forms of applications to the body's surface. Believing for example that the human body held a plethora or superabundance of blood, orthodoxy prescribed a regimen of bleeding, cupping, and leeches that deprived the patient of blood essential for existence. Instead of a small dose of aconite for an inflammatory symptom, allopathic doctors went about their business of bleeding patients until they were near death in order to remove the presumed plethora. Similarly, to draw off morbid or peccant matter from the chest and lungs, Old School physicians produced artificial ulcers (issues and setons) or blisters (cantharides) to purify the system. Despite competing theories of disease causation, doctors were uniformly content to promote urine, perspiration, expectoration, or purgation until the patient's condition changed. "But the essence of diseases, and their cure," wrote Hahnemann, "will not bend to our fancies and convenience." The true causes of disease, he argued, were not material but rather "dynamic aberrations" or "immaterial changes" in the body's vital power.[42]

When dealing with the particulars of a disease, Hahnemann was no different from regular physicians in taking into account the patient's constitution, disposition, occupation, mode of life, habits, age, etc. But unlike Old School physicians, Hahnemann argued that the totality of symptoms represented the disease itself, constituting "the true and only form of it which the mind is capable of conceiving." Since it was impossible for the physician to see or understand the "spiritual essence" or "vital power" which produced the disease, it was enough to know its effects (the entire group of symptoms) and to treat them accordingly. The power of the physician's art was to be directed solely to the totality of symptoms in disease.[43]

As a scientific basis of practice, homeopathy was best expressed in the fixed law or principle known as *similia similiabus curantur,* meaning that medicines would cure diseases arising from morbific causes whose symptoms resembled the effects of the medicines themselves upon healthy persons of similar temperaments and habits. Hahnemann discovered this principle upon learning that the drug *Cinchona* cured certain forms of intermittent fever which, from experimenting on himself, he determined to be characterized by a particular group of symptoms produced by the same remedy when he was in good health. By the 1850s, the pathogeneses of more than four hundred remedies had been studied and had shown no deviation from the principle.[44]

In 1838, Hahnemann added to his law of similars with the principle of *dynamization*, explaining that while a true dilution consisted of adding water to a medicinal substance such as salt until it finally lost its taste, a dynamization took the latent state of a crude substance and excited its inmost powers to act spiritually over the body's vital forces. "I have been the first to discover and to promulgate this awakening of the latent dynamic properties of medicinal drugs," Hahnemann wrote, "which is effected either by the process of trituration or succussion." For that reason, he considered it improper to use the term dilution even though every new potency of drug had to be mixed with alcohol or sugar of milk to set free "the very inmost power of the drug." By employing vigorous shakes and proper care in the preparation of their medicines, physicians were able to add "exceedingly powerful" potencies to their drug armamentaria. While Hahnemann feared that more than two shakes of a dilution would make it more highly potentized than needed, others among his followers prepared their medicines with upwards of 60,000 shakes.[45] Hahnemann reasoned that those homeopaths who had failed to obtain the desired effects from their higher potencies had erred in the process of potentializing of their drugs.[46]

Until 1829, Hahnemann seemed not to approve the dynamizing of medicines higher than the 36th and 60th power. "There must be some end to the thing, it cannot go on to infinity," he wrote. He preferred the rule that all homeopathic remedies be attenuated and dynamized up to the 30th power.[47]

3rd................................millionth
6th................................billionth
9th................................trillionth

12th................................quadrillionth
15th................................quintillionth
30th................................decillionth

For Hahnemann, medicinal substances were not dead masses but "dynamically spiritual" forces that could be increased in potency to an almost infinite degree. For example, two shakes of a drop of the juice of *Drosera rotundifolia* could act as a specific remedy for whooping cough; but fifteen shakes actually endangered the life of the child being treated.[48] To be sure, differences existed among Hahnemann's followers as to the selection of high or low dilutions of medicines, but they generally agreed that cures were effected by all levels of dilutions, including the most infinitesimal dosages. Homeopath I. G. Rosenstein, for example, dismissed critics of infinitesimal dosages as ignorant of modern physics. "Is the activity of medicinal substances, or the doses which homeopathy prescribes, more repugnant to reason than the velocity with which light traverses space?" he asked. Certainly not. Homeopathic remedies were merely "stripped of their bodies" so that their spirit could be employed, thus becoming more palatable to the organism. He challenged those who refused to admit to their efficacy to explain how cholera, smallpox, scarlet fever, or the plague had become such fearful scourges without any visible or perceptible cause. Why should medical skepticism be reserved for the doctrine of infinitesimals when other forces with invisible causes were admitted, he asked. Clearly nature's greatest powers were "concentrated in atoms."[49]

From the perspective of homeopathy, numerous benefits had arisen from the advent of the new school, including the disuse of bleeding, cups, setons, and issues; the use of smaller doses of medicines in general practice; reducing the foreboding anxiety prevalent in the physician-patient relationship; placing greater emphasis on vitality; and giving greater emphasis on a nutritious diet, free of most spices. Why, reasoned homeopaths, should there not be a single law of cure like there was a law of gravitation? Why were homeopathic physicians considered illiberal if they used medicines that cured using *similia similiabus curantur*? Why should homeopaths be considered dishonest because they believed in different principles? Why was it ridiculous to maintain that medicinal atoms could exert an influence in health?[50]

For Charles Hempel of Philadelphia, it was wrong to place Hahnemann with the "common multitude of medical Reformers;" instead, he insisted that Hahnemann be viewed as a discoverer. Before him, there was medical empiricism, but no science and no art. "Hahnemann did not reform existing abuses; he discovered the Law of Cure as it is written upon Nature's Eternal Pages," Hempel wrote. "He proclaimed the law; he showed its applicability in all cases [and he] constructed a new Materia Medica."

> Friends, we desire to impress upon your minds the sublime grandeur of our position. We are no tame reformers. We are laborers of a new

> vineyard, ploughing a new field, sowing a new seed and reaping a new harvest. May you ever lose sight of this radical distinction which separates the philosophical thinkers of our School from the orthodox followers of our ancient God. May the spirit of the new medical Gospel descend upon you in all its unfading beauty and regenerating power. May you be blessed with a full perception of the great Truth that a new Intelligence has shone upon the dark page of Medicine, and that Homeopathy is not simply a formula for a different use of drugs, but a new Philosophy of Medicine, based upon a new order of Perceptions and Relations and involving the very Principles which not only govern the phenomena of Material Order, but determine the physiological harmonies of all living organisms.[51]

Homeopathy was also viewed as a form of spiritual ministration. "When the old system [allopathy] shall have quite vanished from the earth, and the new one [homeopathy] shall be established," explained the Reverend Thomas R. Everest, then "will the Gospel of the kingdom of grace be preached as Jesus ordered it to be preached, and received as God intended it to be received."[52] Accordingly, a number of homeopathic drugs were prescribed to produce (and thereby cure) certain moral and religious defects or states. For example, Gottlieb Jahr's *Manual of Homeopathic Medicine* made note of sulfur creating a feeling of "despair of eternal salvation;" pulsatilla producing "despair of eternal happiness;" lachesis producing "absence of religious feeling;" and aconite producing "an irresistible desire to blaspheme and swear." Thus, by treating patients who suffered from these mental states with medicines that produced similar states in otherwise healthy persons, homeopaths were able to direct their healing abilities to psychological, spiritual, and other non-materialistic etiologies.[53]

The principal medicinal plants proven by Hahnemann and his immediate disciples were indigenous to Europe. With the abundance of medical plants of the United States left out, it was important for American homeopaths to identify and prove the remedies from their own vegetable kingdom. For that reason, homeopathy relied on botanics as well as the works of Samuel Thomson, Horton Howard, and Wooster Beach for some of their earliest remedies. They also borrowed from eclectics Thomas Vaughn Morrow, Lorenzo E. Jones, William Sherwood, John King, and Charles S. Cleveland who had introduced many native remedies into practice. Homeopath Charles F. Millspaugh would eventually bring these various sources together in his two-volume *American Medicinal Plants: An Illustrated and Descriptive Guide to the American Plants Used as Homoeopathic Remedies: Their History, Preparation, Chemistry and Physiological Effects* (1887). By the 1892 edition, the term "homeopath" was dropped from the subtitle.[54]

The first homeopath in the United States was Dr. Hans Birch Gram (1786–1840) who settled in New York City in 1825. His successful practice, along with the enthusiasm he instilled in his students, came at a time when regulars and their patients were beginning to question the very foundations of medical orthodoxy. Unlike regions in the Middle West and frontier where the heroics of both medicines and men seemed to be the order of the day, homeopathy appealed to the more settled communities. From New York, homeopathy spread through Gram's disciples into surrounding states. Dr. Federal Vanderburg (1788–1868), a student of Gram in New York, moved to Connecticut where he quickly obtained a following. One such physician was a Dr. Gregg of Massachusetts, who, on learning from Vanderburg, introduced the system into Boston around 1837–38. Before long, homeopathy had spread along the eastern seaboard states, and moving south and west, found friends and hospitable neighbors in those areas that had begun to settle into a more relaxed and educated lifestyle.

Independent of Gram's and Vanderburg's influence, homeopathy moved into Pennsylvania and Ohio through the influence of German and Swiss immigrants. The next account of it being practiced in the United States is in 1836 by a Dr. Martin, a native of France, who settled in New Orleans. Other introductions of the practice followed. Although ridiculed by regular faculty and apothecaries, patient lists grew as, year by year, homeopathic cures became known. Between 1835 and 1837, a *Corresponding Journal for Homeopathic Physicians*, edited by Constantine Hering and published by the North American Academy of Homeopathy at Allentown, Pennsylvania, became the primary source of communication between American and German homeopaths. In 1837, a little more than a decade after Thomsonism was introduced into Baltimore, a Dr. McManus brought homeopathy to Maryland. Homeopathy found roots in Vermont in 1838; in Rhode Island, Delaware, Ohio and Kentucky in 1839; in New Jersey, Maine, New Hampshire, and Indiana in 1840; in Michigan in 1841; in Georgia and Wisconsin in 1842; in Alabama in 1843; Illinois, Missouri, and Tennessee in 1844; In Texas in 1848; and in Minnesota in 1852.[55]

The earliest homeopathic organizations were formed in Philadelphia (1833) and New York City (1834) and consisted of both physicians and laymen. Many of homeopathy's "domestic" or "lay" doctors served the rural and country districts long before being replaced by those educated in more traditional ways. No doubt the latter's involvement was due to the popularity of the Friendly Botanic Societies of the Thomsonians that had contained a combination of general botanic practitioners and individual patent owners. Their reputation was also enhanced by the series of cholera epidemics that ravaged the country in the 1830s and 1840s.[56] The first homeopathic pharmacy opened in Philadelphia in 1835; the first dispensary in New York ten years later, called the New York Homeopathic Dispensary; and the first hospital in 1850 and located in Philadelphia.[57]

Although homeopathy's leading principles varied over the years, the ten precepts laid out by E. E. Marcy in 1852 seem to best represent the consensus at the time.

1. The conservative forces of the organism are always brought to bear against all deleterious influences acting upon the tissues. If the disturbing cause be slight, nature alone suffices to bring about a curative reaction; but when the morbific impression is so intense as to resist the restorative efforts of nature, the homeopath deems it necessary to call in the aid of medicines.

2. In his remedial measures the homeopath recognizes but one law of cure, viz., similia similiabus curantur.

3. The only real cure ever made by drugs, are accomplished in accordance with the homeopathic law, whether made by physicians of the old or the new school—by crude drugs or by dilutions.

4. No two diseases, whether morbific or medicinal, can affect the same structure at the same time.

5. The vital force reacts with much less power against impressions made by morbific agents, than against those caused by specific medicinal influences. Disorders, therefore, caused by the former, tend to run on to the disorganization of the affected parts, while those produced by the latter, speedily result in spontaneous recoveries.

6. Homeopathic medicines expend their entire force upon those parts alone which are actually diseased; and it is for this reason that very minute doses are adequate to produce those impressions which result in spontaneous curative reactions.

7. A medicinal action, sufficient to cure disease, may be produced either by the tincture or by a dilution of the appropriate remedy,—our only object being, to substitute a healthy drug action in the place of a morbid one. Experience, however, has amply demonstrated, that in a majority of instances diluted drugs act more mildly, more speedily and more safely in provoking curative reactions,

than crude medicines, the first impressions of which are more active than is absolutely necessary for curing, although not usually so active as to give rise to serious results.

8. Drugs never lose their identity, individuality, or specific modes of action, whatever may be the form they are made to assume . . . . It is for this reason that homeopathists, from the time of Hahnemann to the present day, have employed, in their provings of drugs, every variety of form and dose, and numerous experimenters of different ages, sexes, temperaments, countries, and occupations, in order that the most complete pathogeneses might be obtained.

9. The susceptibilities of the tissues of the organism to medicinal impressions, are proportionate to the amount of inflammation, irritation, or nervous erethism present in each case; and as no two maladies or groups of symptoms every correspond in all respects, it follows that a great variety of strengths may be employed with advantage in our remedial applications.

10. In regard to doses, the homeopath has but one object in view, viz., the selection of that strength or attenuation which will most safely, mildly and speedily cure the disease. As this is purely a matter of experience and of facts, and not at all connected with the homeopathic theory of cure, its entire reasonableness must commend itself to the judgments of candid men.[58]

Homeopaths saw themselves as "honest laborers after the truth," who sought to "clear away the rubbish of former theories" that included the humoral doctrines of Boerhaave, the nervous doctrine of Cullen, the gastro-enteric doctrine of Broussais, and the dothin-enteric doctrines of Brettoneau, Bouillaud, Andral and Louis. For their part, homeopaths did not show much deference to the efforts of the French in pathological anatomy. True, the Paris Clinical School had enabled physicians to compare abnormal tissues with healthy ones and give a scientific estimate of those changes, but pathological anatomy "can accomplish nothing beyond this since autopsies yielded "very imperfect information." Homeopaths did not condemn out of hand the classification of diseases but insisted that any classification worth its salt had to be based on the totality of symptoms and not simply a particular grouping of symptoms. Anything less suggested the blind allegiance to certain remedies. Only the sum of those symptoms affecting the organic economy, the moral tendencies, and the intellectual faculties could bring about a more relevant nosology suitable to homeopathy.[59]

By 1851, there were about 600 homeopathic physicians in the United States out of an estimated 40,564 doctors of all stripes. This suggests that one out of every sixty-eight physicians was homeopathic—a small number when compared to fifty years later when homeopathic doctors numbered approximately one out of every thirteen physicians. In 1851, homeopaths had one national medical society, the American Institute of Homeopathy, with a membership of 250; eight local societies; and ten state societies. Homeopathy also had two medical colleges, one in Philadelphia, and the other in Cleveland; one homeopathic hospital located in Philadelphia; and six medical journals.[60]

When Massachusetts honored the centennial birthday of Samuel Hahnemann in 1855, the event was celebrated at the Tremont Temple, one of the largest public halls in Boston. Delegates were present from Maine, Massachusetts, New Hampshire, Vermont, and Rhode Island. Participants included Dr. Samuel Gregg of Boston, the mayor of Boston, Professor Jeffries Wyman of Harvard Medical School, and Winslow Lewis, president of the Boylston Medical School. The banquet at Faneuil Hall included the Lieutenant Governor, numerous members of the Senate and House of Representatives, State officers, clergymen, editors, and several liberal minded allopathic physicians.[61]

Homeopathy suffered from numerous corruptions among its own practitioners. Some, for example, professed to practice homeopathy but resorted as well to the use of the lancet, cups, leeches, emetics, and cathartics. These had chosen a "mixed" practice in order to retain "old patrons," demonstrate their open mindedness to all allopathic practice, and "to indulge their indolence." Others regarded hydropathy as a handmaid of homeopathy and made free use of cold showers, wet sheets, and other techniques employed by the disciples of the Austrian Vincent Priessnitz (1799–1851). There were even those homeopaths who decided to take the best from every medical system. These "eclectico-homeopathists" as they were called, chose among competing systems for whatever seemed to work. "The libel, so industriously circulated by the 'mixing' set," predicted J. P. Dake, M.D., would eventually turn on itself. For the faithful followers of Hahnemann, no alliance should ever contradict the principle of *similia similibus curantur.*[62]

Mesmer and Swedenborg

There also existed an etheric side to reform medicine that drew its inspiration from the experiments of the Viennese physician Franz Anton Mesmer (1734–1815) and his science of animal magnetism. Mesmer's ideas, which tended to be secular in nature, found fertile ground among a host of disciples who gave public demonstrations before American and European audiences. Mesmer's magnetic healings relied on a strong rapport between the healer and patient, shifting the subject's attention away from consciousness to an inward sensibility of the body and the flow of energy or vital force passing through and activating the body. Here was a marriage of matter and spirit, joining physiology with the power of the mind.

Joseph Rodes Buchanan, dean of the Eclectic Medical Institute from 1850 to 1856, saw in animal magnetism the building block for his "sarcognomy," a neurological system using percussion, friction, and "dispersive passes" from the healer to produce physiological effects on the body. During the years he was on the faculty of the Eclectic Medical Institute of Cincinnati, students were routinely introduced to this innovative new science through the pages of Buchanan's *Journal of Man* in 1849, his *Outlines of Lectures on the Neurological System of Anthropology* (1854), and articles in the *Eclectic Medical Journal.*

Homeopathy was also very much influenced by Mesmer and his movement, the efficacy of which, observed Hahnemann, "not but madmen can entertain a doubt." Influencing the body of the patient by means of touch ("gliding the hands slowly over the body from the crown of the head to the soles of the feet"), the mesmerizer distributed vital power to the part affected and uniformly through the body. The most effective mesmerizers, wrote Hahnemann, were men in "the full vigour of life" but who were able to "suppress all their desires," including sexual intercourse. Such men contained "an abundance of the subtle vital energy" and rather than employing it in the production and secretion of semen, used it to communicate with patients through the "medium" of touch and "a strong intention of the mind."[63]

But there was a more mystical and Gnostic dimension to reform medicine, found in the writings of the Swedish scientist and mystic Emanuel Swedenborg (1688–1771) who, as explained by Alexander Wilder, was born in the age of Harvey, Descartes, Vesalius, and Boerhaave "when the notions of scholars were bursting from their cocoons of the previous centuries."[64] With feelings that seemed to have no boundaries, he opened communication with the spirit world and taught others to do the same. In time, his treatises on medicine and physiology, including *The Animal Kingdom* (1843), *Prodromus, or the Forerunner of a Reasoning Philosophy* (1795), *The Future Life* (1844), and *Arcana Coelestia* (1849) were matched with a flurry of books on the spirit world, including conversations with spirits and angels. No matter that his doctrines and sermons touched on so many errant heresies, more than any other thinker, he epitomized the enlarged view of nineteenth century intellectuals who saw themselves as having discovered a truly synoptic understanding of life and sensation.

Swedenborgianism proved attractive to all manner of dissenters—from New England Transcendentalists and faith healers, to eclectics, homeopaths, and communitarians like the Fourierists. Unlike mesmerism, it drew its sustenance from a combination of physics, astronomy, anatomy, and the more mystical aspects of Christian scripture. Here, the body found health (harmony) through contact ("correspondence") with other minds and successive levels of consciousness or spirituality. Gone were the Calvinistic doctrines of sin, reprobation, and hell. In their place were themes of perfectionism, illuminism, and universalism. Just as disease represented a discordance between an individual's bodily realm and metaphysical orders of reality, so health represented the outcome of a concordance between the physical body and its spiritual nature.[65]

A number of America's eclectics and homeopaths were avowed Swedenborgians and, having ignored the confines of orthodox religion, located the body's physical and spiritual harmony in "vitalism," a metaphor for the inner connection between body and soul, matter and spirit. It came as no surprise that both Hahnemann and Swedenborg were students of the physician, alchemist, and occultist Paracelsus (1493–1541), holding that disease was a specific entity—a dynamic aberration of the spirit—cured by specific remedies. With medicines administered in the proper amount (attenuation) to unlock a drug's dynamic powers, a homeopath could affect a unhealthy organ's essential or vital energy, restoring harmony to the body's system. It was thus easy for homeopathic patients to see metaphors in Swedenborg's mystical worldview that linked the body's physical and spiritual harmony with the inner recesses of the mind and with a higher spiritual reality. Here was a medical system that stressed the primacy of spirit over matter, projected a vision of an orderly and predictable universe, and avoided the showy ostentations of the clairvoyants, séances, and table rappings.[66]

Although the boundaries between regular and reform medicine seem easy to establish, particularly among those who were ideologically inclined, the actual differences are much less obvious. Certainly mesmerism and Swedenborgianism were distinctive in character, but the therapeutic practices that separated regulars from eclectics, homeopaths, Thomsonians, and physio-medicals were far less evident. To be sure, reform medicine's description of regular medicine, although false in its particulars, was clear and unambiguous. For reformers generally, regular medicine was heroic, unpleasant, dictatorial, costly, and depletive of the body's vital energy. Irrespective of this rhetoric, however, reformers and regulars were not so easily distinguished since, in the absence of good science, therapeutics rested on a very idiosyncratic foundation, namely the physician's choice of identification. Arguably, greater differences existed among regional medicinal preferences, price of service, and anomalies within the physician-patient relationship than among those resulting from differences in therapeutic theory.[67]

In each of these groups, education and social standing—of both physician and patient—played a role. As noted earlier, homeopathic physicians were generally well educated, with most having received their medical education at a regular college. Their patients were typically religious (many adhered to Swedenborgian beliefs), urban, highly literate, and socially prominent within the middle and upper classes. By contrast, the

Thomsonians were more likely found among the lower socio-economic levels, while the eclectics and physio-medicals were common among the lower middle class and in the smaller towns and rural hamlets. These categories, however, were by no means firm as numerous examples exist showing significant deviancies.

* * *

America's apostates made much of the critiques of Bartlett, Ware, and Jackson. They noted that medicine taught at the University of Pennsylvania differed significantly from that of Jefferson Medical College, its cross-city competitor. Their rival teachings bore "no more resemblance to each other than a dissecting case does to a galvanic battery," claimed William A. Gardiner, editor of the *Philadelphia Journal of Homeopathy*.[68] The same criticism applied to that which was taught and practiced in nearly every other regular medical college. "Instead of being founded upon any well-defined scientific principles," he observed, medicine rested upon the "opinions of each individual professor." So-called orthodoxy was just another form of sectarianism; it neither deserved nor earned any special place in American culture.[69]

While Gardiner's allegations seem a bit overdrawn, and were certainly denounced by the Philadelphia's regular physicians, his criticism was reminiscent of an observation made nearly sixty years later by Abraham Flexner in his *Medical Education in the United States and Canada* (1910) that until the establishment of scientific medicine, regular medicine had been just as dogmatic as the so-called sectarian or alternative systems of medicine.[70] Professors were intent on professing, and in the absence of good science and convincing data, relied heavily on personal testimony and reputation. In such circumstances, medical knowledge and discourse had became the product of a very idiosyncratic form of education. This, plus the trenchant self-criticism and self-doubts enunciated by teachers in their lectures and private utterances, did much to create an atmosphere of rebelliousness among America's medical leadership and, in turn, among the newest generation of medical graduates.

Bleeding, blistering, vomiting, purging, and sweating were the offspring of constitutional pathology, identified by medical orthodoxy as the only efficacious methods for restoring the diseased body to health. While most physicians maintained their allegiance to orthodoxy, the repetitious nature of their lamentations suggests a sense of increasing frustration with the slow pace of reform. This was evident not only among those who had augmented their education with work in Great Britain and on the Continent, but also among those who remained at home. These physicians, many of whom held important positions in their societies and medical colleges, were not without influence. Like the remarks of Bartlett, Ware, and Jackson, their questions, concerns, and outright doubts became food for thought for generations of students and, not surprisingly, a number of them would eventually abandon regular practice. While only a modicum of regulars chose to follow the siren appeals of the Thomsonians, hydropaths, botanics, and eclectics, a significant number would leave medical orthodoxy for the benign therapies of homeopathy. In fact, no less that three-fourth's of the homeopathic physicians in 1852 were themselves graduates of regular colleges, a statistic that loomed ominously over the medley of opinions and testimonies leveled against them by regulars.[71]

Increasingly, American physicians became more contemptuous of the brittle boundaries between orthodox and unorthodox therapies. A feeling of dissatisfaction, if not confusion, resonated among their candid and sometimes indiscreet remarks on the art and science of medicine. As one critic caustically observed, when two physicians met together at the bedside of a patient, they "could not look each other in the face without laughing at the absurdity of their profession and its pretensions."[72]

Chapter 4. Reform Literature

In the decades prior to the Civil War, the publishing houses in New York, Philadelphia, Boston, Baltimore, Cincinnati, and Charleston flourished as changes in technical production, advertising rates, methods of news-gathering, and even the selling of subscriptions revolutionized the printing industry and ushered in the age of mass print media. In 1830, book sales totaled $3.5 million. School books accounted for roughly one-third; another third was divided among classical, legal, theological, and medical topics. By 1840, sales had reached $12 million. Of this, $5 million went toward school books and $1.6 million for medical, theological, legal, and miscellaneous topics. How Americans formulated their culture amid the competing forces of materialism, optimism, restlessness, aggressiveness, and religiosity came to life in the written works of the age.[1]

From *The Knickerbocker Magazine*, founded in New York in 1833, to Francis Parkman's *Oregon Trail* (1849), to the contributions of Washington Irving, James Fenimore Cooper, William Cullen Bryant, Walt Whitman, Nathaniel Hawthorne, Henry Wadsworth Longfellow, and John Greenleaf Whittier, American writers and poets were acquainting their contemporaries with the wealth and variety of their literature. Cooper, the tyro of early American narrative, helped define American nationalism, growing self-consciousness, and the bumbling democracy of the early nineteenth century. Exuding both aristocratic prejudices and a fondness for democratic principles, his *The Pioneers* (1823) and *Notions of the Americans* (1828), his defense of America against foreign critics in *A Letter to His Countrymen* (1834), the five novels of his Leatherstocking series, and his political primer *The American Democrat* (1838), gave vent to a spirit of self-expression that represented a strong statement of American literary independence. His words, like those of his contemporary writers, caught the ear of a busy yet restless nation, sending waves of social sentiment pouring into a myriad of reforms.

This was a period in the nation's history when Americans exercised a healthy distrust of Europe along with an inflated view of their own achievements and potentialities. America exuded a portrait of self-sufficiency that celebrated democracy, repudiated class and privilege, and entrusted the future in plain and simple men of intelligence. It was a time when authority was challenged by the growth of voluntary societies; the spread of sectarianism and unorthodox tendencies; challenges to rationalism and Calvinism; a new emphasis on intuition, antinomianism, and self-reliance; and a fashionable but strident humanitarianism that hailed all types of reform as cures for the nation's growing pains.

The widespread hunger for education produced other venues for public learning including the Lowell Institute of Boston, the Peabody Institute of Baltimore, the Cooper Union of New York, and innumerable books for the adult education market. Orville Roorbach's *Bibliotheca Americana* (1852) provides a revealing look at the books in print in the United States during the period 1820 through 1852. A large number of how-to handbooks and manuals were published. From Jacob Abbott's *Rollo* books (28 vols.) and George Ackerley *On the Management of Children in Sickness and in Health* (1836), to Timothy Shay Arthur's *Advice to Young Men* (1842), Henry Ward Beecher's *Lectures to Young Men* (1846), and William A. Alcott's *Young Man's Guide* (1844), Americans were a curious people whose interest in practical things abounded.[2]

As early as the 1840 census, the nation claimed nearly 50,000 primary and common schools, 3,200 academies and grammar schools, 171 colleges and universities, and nearly 3,000 libraries. For skeptics like Oliver Wendell Holmes, who viewed the general public as "hopelessly ignorant," his New England world, like the ancient Greeks, was divided into Brahmins and barbarians. Thus, his remarks were generally predictable; Holmes was simply reflecting his own particular class bias.[3]

Another source of education came by way of the Lyceum movement which originated among the mechanics' institutes in England and migrated quickly into America's antebellum culture. Its mover and shaker was Yale graduate, Josiah Holbrook (1788–1854) of Derby, Connecticut, who organized the first lyceum society in 1826 in the town of Millbury, Massachusetts. Before long, lyceum clubs were appearing across the landscape, providing professional and semi-professional lecturers the opportunity to share their wisdom on such diverse subjects as glaciers, genius, mesmerism, chemistry, religion, archeology, history, and all manner of reforms. Issues of incarceration, revivalism, spiritualism, magnetism, somnambulism, spirit-rapping, abolitionism, temperance, women's rights, education, perfectionism, and medical reform rose and fell amid the clash of democratic symbols, relying upon the lecture circuit to capture a share of the public mind. By the mid-1830s, some three thousand lyceums were functioning in the United States. Among the stable of lecturers were Ralph Waldo Emerson, E. P. Whipple, G. W. Curtis, Orville Dewey, Horace Greeley, Joel Headley, Bayard Taylor, and Henry David Thoreau. Emerson's *Representative Men* (1850), *English Traits* (1856), *The Conduct of Life* (1860), and his two books of essays published in 1841 and 1844 originated out of this national movement of popular lectures. The lyceum's heyday was the thirty years leading up to the Civil War; nevertheless, it continued into the post-Civil War years where it afforded easy income for such popular satirists as Mark Twain.[4]

Journals are a neglected aspect of our literary history despite their being the medium through which much of nation's early discourse reached public consumption. Magazines of all types were introduced to feed popular tastes. Some were financially successful and long-lived, while others fought indifference, mismanagement, or more successful rivals. Publications like the *Atlantic, Graham's Magazine, Harper's Monthly Magazine, Godey's Lady's Book, Southern Review, Knickerbocker, United States Magazine and Democratic Review, New England Magazine, American Magazine, North American Review,* and *Southern Literary Messenger* were indicative of the more successful publications, whose formula for fiction, poetry, ornate engravings, and other eye-catching pieces gained for them reputation, financial success, and a loyal readership. The lack of international copyright laws gave publishers and editors broad latitude in supplying readers with the works of European authors with little out-of-pocket expense. As the titles suggest, the success of many magazines was helped along by the fostering of a distinct regional consciousness. This characteristic was not only evident among publishers and writers from the South and North with their muted sectional differences, but between the Middle West and East where pride and rivalry abounded.

Reform Medical Journals

American medical reform journals (see *Appendix A*) were many and diffuse, with no single region, individual, or publication, laying claim to being an exclusive representative. By any form of measurement, this literature was considerable, spanning the full spectrum of medicine—from regular or allopathic, to botanic, eclectic, physio-medical, homeopathic, hydropathic, and other, lesser-known sects. Among the characteristics of the medical reform journals were to be found a generally scornful attitude toward allopathy; a catering to female readership; an openness to letters and commentaries by readers; angry protests against legal discrimination; a willingness to publish original poetry, particularly in the form of an acrostic or mnemonic; and a desire to provide a continuing update on newly published reform literature.

While New York City was the literary capital of the nation for the publication of reform medical journals, Philadelphia, Chicago, Cincinnati, St. Louis, and Boston were not far behind. The reform journals of the eastern seaboard had a look and feel of homogeneity, while those in the Middle West and South carried more of a regional flavor. In general, the journals were born of a consciousness among a definable group of reformers who had a mission, and with it, a utilitarian need for a common body of scholarship that could serve as an authoritative guide and set of intellectual standards. Although their editors sometimes published foreign authors, the emphasis was clearly upon native writers and especially those living near to their place of publication.

Exemplary of these journals was the *Reformed Medical Journal* of New York published in 1832 by doctors Wooster Beach and H. D. Sheppard under the patronage of the Reformed Medical Society of the United States. Its issues bristled with heated attacks against Old School orthodoxy and its reliance on calomel and bloodletting. Its pages were filled with comments on the treatment and death of George Washington; the opinions of Thomas Jefferson on the prevailing medical theories; reprintings of the writings of Rafinesque, John Wesley, Samuel Thomson, Horton Howard, and the German doctor, publisher, and reformer Christoph Hufeland; commentaries on steam medicine; mortality accounts on the spread of cholera and yellow fever; and reporting on the most recent medical legislation.

The publishers and editors of these journals helped build an image of reform doctors as a progressive class operating on the fringes of a tradition-bound profession. Instead of defending older structures and systems, these publishers and editors provided a framework within which they hoped readers could understand and appreciate newer concepts in healing. Added to this was their desire to make laymen a vital part of their reading audience. As the correspondence between readers and editors suggest, every reader was made to feel as though he or she was an active participant in and a contributor to the topics under discussion.

The reform medical journals were typically modeled on the more established journals. Each issue contained several essays that focused on a wide range of topics: a review of the literature; letters and comments to and by the editor; proceedings and medical society news; extracts from other journals; poetry; vital statistics; miscellaneous anecdotes; and necrology. Some editors assumed the role of consulting physicians and, for a fee, included letters from patients and healers describing difficult case histories and soliciting advice on proper treatment. Occasionally there were serial articles but these were the exception rather than the rule. All were consequential in giving context and character to the publication.

One also finds an unusual degree of consistency in ownership and editorship of these reform journals. Names like W. A. Chatterton, Halsey and King, S. H. Potter, J. G. Wesselhoeft, William Radde, Boericke and Tafel, R. S. Newton, and W. Paine appear frequently among the reform journals, lending a certain contextual uniformity to their social and political views. For example, John Milton Scudder was editor of numerous eclectic publications, while Alva Curtis published and edited a host of botanical journals. The homeopathic and Swedenborgian publications of Boericke and Tafel, along with their sale of homeopathic medicines, made them the undisputed leader of sectarian medical literature with offices in Philadelphia and New York, and later in Chicago, Baltimore, Pittsburgh, Cincinnati, San Francisco, and Washington, DC.

Editors whose lifelong interests were in medical reform used their journals to publish essays, reviews, translations, reports, poetry, and editorial commentary on subjects of their particular interest. Some magazines were more scholarly than others, but generally, they appealed to both the academically oriented healer as well as the domestic healer. At times, editors ventured beyond their immediate issues, shifting their attention and their emphasis to various fringe issues (i.e., phrenology, mesmerism, or vegetarianism) as tastes changed. In this regard, their journals became a historical record of the American reform movement and its chameleon-like attributes.

Journals that tended to be overzealous in their focus were usually the instruments of particular publishers such as Samuel Thomson of Boston, publisher/editor Alva Curtis of Cincinnati, or Fowler and Wells of New York who produced a long line of books on phrenology, physiology, temperance, hydropathy, hygiene, and other reform topics. Thomson gave his own name to his journal and set out through various editors whom he hired and fired to present and defend his medical views in a manner that was both instructive and combative. As Thomson was forever fighting his wayward agents as well as politicians, lawyers, regulars, other competitors, his journal became a vigorous critic of all monopolies and an equally vigorous advocate of republican government. While Thomson insisted on a focused approach to reform medicine, publisher and editor Alva Curtis, an energetic writer and speaker, advanced the cause of reform medicine by incorporating a variety of ancillary reform movements, including Grahamism, hydropathy, phrenology, mesmerism, nervauric treatment, and sarcognomy.

Fashionable lecturers of the 1840s proclaimed their dogmas to multitudes of listeners, prescribing no end of rules for eating, drinking, reading, exercise, and sex. Among them were the Grahamites, whose eating and living preferences carried with them a certain political correctness. "I have met with a good many of these priests of starvation," recalled homeopath I. G. Rosenstein, M.D. of Louisville. "Beans, roots, potatoes, and bran bred, is all they want." Rosenstein preferred not to dictate diet. "In a country like ours, where every one is not only his own judge in politics and religion," it was better to preach Nature's natural appetites and it was just as preferable to convince people to use their reasoning to restrain from unnatural desires and the detrimental consequences of untempered appetites.[5]

More than any of the sectarian journals, those based on the principles of homeopathy were willing outlets for theological and philosophical ideas, including Swedenborgianism; long translations from the metaphysical writings of German authors; and rantings against Cartesian and materialistic interpretations of medicine. With the split emerging between the high and low dilutionists, these characteristic elements served to reduce rather than expand readership. Fearing a loss of readers, a number of the reform journals in homeopathy refused to take sides in the argument, insisting that individual judgment took precedence over narrow ideological views.

One of the lasting contributions made by reform journals is that they helped to whet the public's appetite on matters of health and hygiene. Along with newspapers, they tracked the spread of cholera and yellow fever from city to city; shared the latest information on potential cures or preventatives against these epidemic diseases; enlightened readers on the evils of heroic regimens and the benefits of kindlier medicines; fought the muscular power of organized medicine; and attacked the evils of alcoholism, stimulating drinks such as coffee, and fried foods.

Reform Poetry

Along with the sentimental novel, poetry was read by all classes of people and strongly appealed to the gentler and more melancholy side of American culture. Women authored a disproportionate amount of the poetry published in the popular magazines with topics ranging from a crushed flower and a bride's farewell, to the death of a child or a household pet, or pious reflection focused on some high moral purpose. In an age when poetry was considered both an art form and a popular means of entertainment, family members would often put whole stanzas to memory, delighting friends and relatives with their prodigious efforts.

In medicine as in politics and religion, poetry became a useful tool of wags, cynics, critics, crowd pleasers, and pedants whose verses were told and retold across the American landscape. The following poems on the "Pathies" were printed repeatedly in journals and newspapers, and recited before enthusiastic audiences at lyceums and town halls.[6]

HOMEOPATHY
Take a little rum,
The less you take the better;
Mix it with the lakes
Of Werner and of Wetter.

Dip a spoonful out—
Mind you don't get groggy—
Pour it into the lake
Winnipisiogee.

Stir the mixture well,
Lest it prove inferior;
Then put half a drop

Into Lake Superior.

Every other day,
Take a drop, in water;
You'll be better soon,
Or, at least, you ought to.

ALLOPATHY
Take some calomel,
The more you take the better;
Mix it with a drop
Or two of cistern water.

Feed some to your dog;
It will make him vomit,
And, may be, see stars,
And perhaps a comet.

Once in each half hour
Take a rousing potion;
Stay a tumbler full,
If that suits your notion.

Should you chance to die,
As you're almost sure to,
You may safely say,
That it did not cure you.

HYDROPATHY
Take a dripping sheet
And closely wrap it round you,
Then jump into the bed
In which the doctor found you.

Cover up your head,
And your wife, don't fret her,
But pile the blankets on,
If you would be better.

When you've lain awhile,
And grown a little hotter.
Out of bed again

And ply the "scrub and water."

Try it every day,
Morning, noon and "later,"
And you'll live or die,
Just as true as "nature."

SENSCOPATHY
Take the open air,
The more you take the better,
Follow nature's laws
To the very letter.

Let the doctors go
To the Bay of Biscay.
Let along the Gin,
The Brandy, and the Whiskey.

Freely exercise,
Keep your spirits cheerful,
Let no dread of sickness
Make you over fearful.

Eat the simplest food,
Drink the pure cold water.
Then you will be well,
Or, at least, you ought to.

The following selections address Thomsonism and its founder, Samuel Thomson, who, over a period of several decades, melded his followers into a militant corps of dedicated believers, using them to lobby successfully state legislatures to pass medical acts favorable to their cause. He authorized agents, infirmaries, and medicine depots in every state and territory; organized the first national convention of botanic healers fifteen years before the American Medical Association could muster its own corps of regular doctors; and popularized a distinctive six-step "course" of medicine that became the regimen of choice for families in every part of the country. By 1840, Thomsonism had become a household word for several millions of people, including a sizable number of adherents in Canada and Great Britain. Unlike the more standard poetry of the day, the poems addressing Thomsonian medicine were written predominantly by men (principally Thomson and his agents) and intended for medical purposes rather than for any moral, ethical, or pious objective. Overall, Thomson's poetry was a well of good-tempered ridicule aimed at orthodoxy, using the collective wit of its authors to attack orthodox medical practices and effectively gain friends and disciples. Thomson and his reformers were a force to be reckoned with in the first half of the nineteenth century, capturing the minds and hearts of untold numbers of American families.

Thomson's own poetry served as a vehicle of medical instruction, teaching families in mnemonic fashion how to monitor sickness and proceed with a course of medicine. After selling an individual a "right" to his patented six-step therapeutic regimen, Thomson would leave with each purchaser a poem to be put to memory and which, when recalled, would provide a set of directions. In this manner, individuals or family members had only to recite the poem in order to understand and follow the rightful order of Thomson's six-step regimen.

BOTANIC DIRECTIONS
Disorder comes by losing inward heat:
That motion stop which render health complete;
The system clogs, the juices putrify;
For want of motion only, people die.
Th' Emetic proves itself designed,
A gen'ral medicine for mankind,
Of ev'ry country, clime, or place,
Wide as the circle of our race;
In ev'ry cause, and state, and stage,
Whatever malady may rage;
For male, or female, young or old,
Nor can its value half be told.
To use this med' cine do not cease,
Till you are helped of your disease;
For nature's friend this sure will be,
When taken sick on land or sea.
Let comp'sition be used bold,
To clear the stomach of a cold;
Next take the compound strong and free,
And keep as warm as you can be;
A hot stone at the feet now keep,
As well as inward warmth repeat,
The fountain 'bove the stream keep clear,
And perspiration will appear:
When sweat enough as you suppose,
In spirits wash and change your clothes,

And then set up if you should choose,
Or else in bed in calm repose,
Should the disorder reinforce,
Then follow up the former course,
The second time I think will do,
The third to fail I seldom knew.
Now take your bitters by the way,
Two, three, or four times in a day,
And if your appetite be good,
Then you may eat most kinds of food,
Physic I'd have you seldom used;
Injections in its stead would choose,
For if you physic much in course,
It will disorder reinforce.
If any one should be much bruis'd,
Where bleeding frequently is us'd,
A lively sweat upon that day,
Will start the blood a better way.
Let names of all disorders be,
Like to the limbs joined on a tree,
Work on the root and that subdue,
Then all the limbs will bow to you,
So as the body is the tree,
The limbs are cholic, pleurisy,
Worms and gravel go, and stone,
Relieve the fountain and they're gone.
My system's founded on the truth,
Man's Air and Water, Fire and Earth,
And death is cold, and life is heat,
These tempered well, your health's complete.
(Dr. Samuel Thomson)[7]

In 1838, the editor of *The Southern Botanic Journal* published a poem by Dr. A. A. Clark, a botanic physician, in hopes that it would provide readers with both an appreciation of Thomsonism's literary importance as well as a means for remembering the steps for his cure.

DR. THOMSON'S MATERIA MEDICA
The coffee first steep, the pure number three,
With warm number two, then use them both free;

To clear off the cold and raise up the heat,
Now place a *freestone* quite warm at the feet;
The inward warmth raising, now often repeat,
And change the first stone when losing its heat.
The fountain above *all obstructions keep clear,*
And free perspiration will surely appear.

Then take the emetic, the pure number one,
Until its full duty is faithfully done;
The stomach quite cleansed, and head just as free
From filth, pain and torment you'll equally be;
Then lying awhile in the sweetest repose,
You'll now wash all over and change all your clothes;
Again to your bed, both pure, clean and white,
And sleep in good comfort the rest of the night.

Now take the wine bitters, remember, I say,
Two, three, or four times in the course of the day;
Your appetite then, will surely prove good,
And you must appease it by *sweet, wholesome* food;
But vile sickening physic, I never would choose
To have you at first or at last to make use;
For, if you do take it, you may reckon in course,
The same vile disorder it will reinforce.

But should the disorder still not loose its force,
Pursue as directed, the former full course;
In nine of ten cases, I think it will do,
The third as to fail, I seldom have knew;
The *Thomsonia Emetica* was surely designed,
A general specific for all human kind;
For every kingdom, country and place.
As, wide as the circle that man does embrace.

In every case, and station and stage,
Whatever malady may be known to rage;
For male or for female, for young and for old,
Nor can its great value half ever be told;
To use this sure medicine, then never do cease,
'Til you are completely relieved of disease;
For nature's true friend it ever will be,

Its virtue and excellence you surely may see.

If any one's mangled, or very much bruised,
When taking of blood is so frequently used,
A good lively sweat on the very same day,
Will start circulation a much better way;
Let names of disorders, as they certainly be
Like limbs that are joined to the trunk of the tree,
Work on the root, the first cause to subdue,
Then sure all the branches will bow unto you.

Just so is your body, like the tree you may see,
The limbs are the chronics, and vile pleurisy.
Consumptions and dropsies, the gout and the stone,
Remove the first cause and they're perfectly gone.
The Thomsonian system is founded in truth;
Man's air, and he's water, he's fire, and he's earth;
And death is from cold, and life is from heat,
Then temper them well and your health is complete.

If fire from the elements abstracted should be,
Stillness and silence would reign you may see;
All life would then cease, you surely do know
Not a vestige of breathing would man ever show;
The earth, the sea, and all that remained,
As solid as marble would ever be chained;
The air that is fluid, to rock would be turned,
And all that now breathes in death would be turn'd.

Creation, a blank would ever remain,
Vitality gone from the earth and the main;
The whole would remain an immovable mass,
And death universal all kingdoms would blast,
Now think of these things, ye men of the schools,
Before you pronounce *us* illiterate fools;
The wisdom of ages are supporting this cause,
This system must stand, and here I will pause.[8]

Thomson's poetry avoided the easy sentimentality of the day, substituting a more didactic idiom that stressed the evils of privileged rank, the pretensions of book learning, defiance against unfair laws, and the importance of republicanism in all facets. The following poem expresses his contempt toward priests, lawyers, and doctors. Similar to what he explained in his *New Guide to Health*, the poem reflects his strong opposition to the credentialed professional classes.

THREE CRAFTS
Attend good people and draw near,
Till you this fact are brought to hear;
How nat'ral rights of human kind,
By crafts, for money kept you blind.

How selfish are the crafts combined,
Engaged 't oppress the human mind;
Physic, Divinity, and Law,
They chief of all our labors draw.

The nests of college birds are three,
Law, Physic and *Divinity;*
And while these three remain combined,
They keep the world oppressed and blind.

On lab'rers' money Lawyers feast,
Also the Doctor and the Priest;
Although their offices are three,
They will oppress where'er they be.

Men do consent like Balaam's ass,
To bear their burdens when they pass;
They ride men hard, and sometimes beat,
And drink their wine and eat their meat.

We greatly do ourselves misuse,
Our rights and liberty abuse;
While they do eat our meat and bread,
And give us poison in their stead.

They strive to keep the people blind,
With whims like these fill up their mind;
That they have power and full control,
Over the body, will, and soul.

The *Priest* pretends to save the soul—
Doctors to make the body whole;
For money *Lawyers* make their plea;

We'll save it, and dismiss the three.

This is the way the craft has gained;
When sick, we for the doctor send;
He says, "there is no chance to live,
Unless I deadly poison give."

When this is done, the sick grow worse,
Which takes the money from their purse;
He says, "I've great regard for you,"
But money is the most in view.

When'er the sick are like to die,
Call in the Priest, the doctors cry;
The Priest will come, and with them pray,
And clear the doctor every way.

He then doth say "don't trust in man,
There is a great and wiser plan;"
The one who freely by his will,
Doth doctors authorize to kill.

He says that man should not complain,
What way God sends death in his name,
If by the doctors, two or one,
They always say, "his will be done."

They also say, he has done well,
No man of skill could him excel;
His time is come, the Lord hath sent,
No doctor could his death prevent.

But nature's doctors have no chance,
No diploma can they advance;
The doctors cry out, quack and kill!
They don't allow such do God's will.

No quack can have a right to kill,
Unless he's passed the college-mill;
Should he the butcher then excel;
The people say 'tis very well.

Craft tell the doctor, make your bill,

And let the lawyer write the will;
And then to execute the same,
The lawyer takes it in his name.

Soon as the man is dead and gone,
The will is read—the work goes on,
The doctor brings a shocking charge;
The lawyer says it's none too large.

Because we three have all agreed
To charge the people as we need;
We claim the power and full control,
Over the body, will, and soul.

All three of us as one agree,
To take away true liberty,
And keep it from such people's hands,
As dare dispute our high demands.

Should any nat'ralist arise,
To clear the veil from off your eyes;
With all their power they'll run them down,
By crying *quackery* and *clown*.

If you would find where quackery lies,
You'll find the quack is he that cries;
And he must be a knavish clown,
Who would cry useful knowledge down.

We shall no longer disagree;
We know where quackery must be;
They must be quacks who do profess,
To cure with ratsbane, in distress.

Come freemen all unveil your eyes,
If you this slavish yoke despise;
Now is the time to be set free,
From Priests' and Doctors' slavery.

The craft is three in every stage,
On tory limbs and monarch's rage;
Their power is lost, we've spoil'd the tree,
Of *Hartford* tory monarchy.

Did twenty lawyers there agree,
To form a great conspiracy?
The clergy met at their own place,
To bind us freemen in disgrace.

The doctors with the same intent,
Petitioned to the government,
To make a law to stop the plan,
Of equal rights in every man.

What could the doctors' object be,
Except a general massacre;
When chiefly poison they applied,
And most of all their patients died.

What must have been the people's fate,
If the three crafts had gained of late;
Had lost our right to make the law,
We should like beasts their burdens draw.

In every town the college-mill,
The people by the law must fill;
They must attend each month at least,
The public chest must pay the Priest.

The doctors with the priests combined,
For to oppress the human kind;
And make their charge as they will,
The lawyer he collects their bill.[9]

With so many learned doctors practicing their own species of rationalism, it is not surprising that the medical profession failed to elicit an abiding confidence in early nineteenth-century American culture. As Thomas Jefferson and others attested, a large number of physicians were pitifully ignorant, drastic in their healing regimens, alarming in their pretense of understanding the keys to health and disease, and rapacious in their pecuniary interests. Based on erroneous philosophy, medicine tended to relieve patients more effectively of their pocketbooks than of their ailments. When physicians insisted upon treating patients with regimens that all but guaranteed failure, these ineffective treatments robbed physicians of their status in society, and more importantly, invited a host of reformers anxious to test their theories and skills among a desperate and willing population.

Troubled by the harsh treatments given to presidents George Washington and William H. Harrison by Old School doctors, Thomsonian disciple Richard J. Duke of Virginia penned this poem in the hope that readers would prevent their friends and loved ones from the use of bloodletting, calomel (mercurous chloride), and opium derivatives.

THE DEEDS OF ALLOPATHY
The Bible says, "Blood is the life,"
Oh, use not then the dreadful knife
To draw life's crimson flood away,
But cause the murderous hand to stay.

Give not your children calomel,
Or soon you'll toll their funeral knell;
Of laud'num, too, be well aware,
To children it's a deadly snare.

(Richard J. Duke)[10]

Regular medicine faced strong opposition throughout the early decades of the nineteenth century. Challenged by in-house critics as well as by numerous apostates, medical orthodoxy struggled to find its bearings amid the changes and tensions of the age. Substantive opposition to the Galenic tradition had come by way of the political revolution of late eighteenth century France, the creation of hospitals and medical schools, and the dominance of a new generation of empirically oriented teachers who chose to ignore the siren appeals of the older system-builders. Preferring less theory and more facts, and a healing art that rested on individual case histories built on observation at the bedside, medicine looked for guidance from a new breed of doctor who stressed the importance of disease identification on the basis of more precise clinical examinations.

As noted earlier, the so-called Paris Clinical Period in American medicine witnessed efforts within and outside established medical circles to bring about reform. Those who worked inside the medical establishment were genteel in their criticisms, preferring to work at the margins and contenting themselves with limited victories rather than frontal assaults. This effort brought with it a healthy skepticism of traditional remedies and therapeutics, a more focused interest on specific diseases, less concern for the body's overall state, and a desire to support nature's own healing processes. Here was a genuine effort to overthrow metaphysical concepts of disease that had reigned unchallenged for centuries. Those outside apostolic medicine—botanics, Indian doctors, eclectics, Thomsonians, physio-medicals, homeopaths, and hydropaths—were more pointed in their criticisms and depicted regulars in the narrowest and most contemptuous manner. There was a true medical Protestantism in their demeanor, believing it necessary to break completely from the ruling medical establishment. The poetry of Thomson and his followers is again representative of that Protestantism and obvious in its vehemence.

The following poem depicts the struggle between medical regulars and the reformers, with the latter group steadily growing in strength and numbers.

TO PHYSICIANS
Come, honest Physicians, lay by your suspicions;
There is no great secret in plain, simple truth.
Without boasted vainness, we tell you in plainness,
True medical science is but in her youth.
We've long been deceived—past ages are grieved,
To find all there medical skill was so weak,
And many inventions, from honest intentions,
Have grown into errors too gross for to speak.

Behold ancient sages, through all the dark ages,
Confus'd and perplexed by mysteries of cure,
No system erected, that could be protected
By reason and truth, which will always endure.
Since good Hippocrates, lived good Cincinnatus,
And Galen, and Celsus, and Plato, and Stahl—
Sydenham and others—all high learned brothers—
But Cullen and Brown at last rivaled them all.

When Doctors we mention, we have no intention
Of casting reproach upon those in the rear:
For Cullen's Nosology, needs no apology—
The Medical Science he split like a hair.
Though many are named, all cannot be famed,
With Harvey and Brown, for the good they have done,
By rending tradition and dark superstition,
To clear out the way for the true light to come.

The true light of nature has now become greater
Than all the high learning the schools do possess;
And plain, common talking, either standing or walking,
Reveals the whole mystery of cure we confess.
The Greeks, while they reigned, the science maintained,
By plain, simple teaching, quite common to all:
Their good sense and reason, would have thought it treason,

To leave their own language the dead to recall.

Rush, in his discourses, the system divorces,
As very uncertain and fickle withal.
A temple uncovered, his genius discovered,
With cracks at the bottom and all through the wall.
He lectured and battered—all systems he scattered;
Like atoms, they flew from his voice through the air.
A final new building, without gloss or gilding,
He knew would be hard, yet confessed would be fair.

Now Thomson's foundation, in this mighty nation,
Is laid on a basis both firm and secure.
No useless appendage, can be of advantage,
To those who would learn the true science of cure.
No clinical lectures, or wholesale conjectures,
Are used by Thomson disease to dispel:
His eye never glances at blisters or lances,
Nor teaspoonful doses of raw Calomel.
He takes his position, with good Composition:
Some good Number Two will increase vital heat.
Numbers One, Two and Three, he then mixes with tea,
Which will scour the stomach and cleanse it complete—
Then steam in proportion revives life and motion:
A free perspiration must soon then begin:
Then makes the steam hotter—throws on some cold water,
And with a clean towel rubs off the old skin.

When washed and dressed, it must be confessed,
We feel so much better than we could have thought:
The fever abated, the sense reinstated:
How simple the process! How easily taught!
This truth we have tested, and when we have rested,
Some food that is wholesome the stomach doth crave.
We need not be fearful, but eat and be cheerful,
And thankful we're sav'd from an untimely grave.
(Anonymous)[11]

The acrostic, popular in the antebellum period, was a verse or arrangement of words in which certain letters in each line, such as the first or last, spelled out a word or phrase.

TO DR. SAMUEL THOMSON
S AMUEL THOMSON, Nature's son,
A noble vict'ry thou has won;
M idst all the threats from min'ral hives,
U nletter'd Thomson's system thrives:—
E 'en spite of *lies,* which *quacks* do vend.
L obelia stands as man's best friend.

T hough quacks do *bleed* and *poison* men,
H eat you *restore,* with good *Cayenne*:—
O! how sublime, your native theme:—
M uch fame surrounds *Thomsonian* steam.
S cience, as taught by *learned* fools,
O n human lives doth sharp its tools;—
N or doth abate its cruel course.

B ut with the advance of Thomson's force,
O ft have learn'd quacks and foes oppress'd—
T heir forces join'd, your rights to wrest;
A nd laws obtain'd quite plain—direct—
N o Botanist shall debts collect,
I n vain have they their malice tried—
S amuel still lives—a healthy guide;—
T homsonian System's spreading wide.

(Stephen F. Fowler)[12]

Along with poetry, songs became a regular part of the genre of protest or reform literature. As early as the 1820s, "Go Call the Doctor, and Be Quick or Anti-Calomel" appeared in the newspaper *Athenian,* published in Athens, Georgia. The satire, sung to the tune of "Old Hundred," attacked the prevailing use by regulars of calomel and bloodletting. Four decades later, when Surgeon-General William Hammond struck calomel from the Union Supply Table, the song was resurrected. Retitled simply "Calomel," and with minor variations from the original, the song was added to the repertoire of the family singing group known as the Five Hutchinsons (Asa, Jesse, John, Judson, and Abby) who traveled the country and who even sang before President Lincoln at the White House. The song was especially popular in Cincinnati where regulars and reformers had squared off following Hammond's May 4, 1863 decision.

CALOMEL
Physicians of the highest rank—
To pay whose fees would need a bank—

Have pressed their science, art, and skill
Into a dose of calomel.

What'er the patient may complain—
Of head, or heart, or nerve, or brain,
Of fever high, or parts that swell—
The remedy is calomel.

When Mr. A. or B. is sick,
"Go for the doctor; and be quick."
The Doctor comes with right good-will,
And ne'er forgets his calomel.

He turns unto the patient's wife,
And asks for paper, spoon, and knife;
"I think your husband will do well
To take a dose of calomel."

He then deals out the fatal grain,
"This, ma'am, will surely ease the pain,
Once in three hours, at chime of bell,
Give him a dose of calomel"

The man grows worse quite fast indeed,
The council's called. They ride with speed.
They crowd around his bed, and tell
The man to take more calomel.

The man in death begins to groan,
The fatal job for him is done.
His falt'ring voice in death doth tell
His friends to shun all calomel.

Now, when I must yield up my breath,
Pray let me die a natural death,
And bid you all the long farewell
Without the use of calomel.[13]

At the Eclectic Medical Institute, faculty and students alike celebrated their mission in the "Song of the Reformers," written by the college's dean and sung to the tune of "The Star-Spangled Banner."

Come rouse up, Reformers! The night has gone by!

Through the blue vault of Heaven the sunlight is beaming,
The clouds have departed, and beneath a clear sky,
Our flag far and wide is now gallantly streaming.
We march as an army—united and true.
Then rouse up, Reformers! The night has gone by,
And our flag, far and wide, is now floating on high.

We battle against the dread armies of Death!
And to God alone look for the biddings of duty;
Our oracles are not a frail mortal's breadth—
We kneel before Nature and worship her beauty.
And we march to a victory, bloodless and blessed!
'Tis to conquer Disease and relieve the distressed.
Then rouse up, Reformers! The night has gone by,
And our flag, far and wide, is now floating on high.

We've broken our fetters—they are trampled in dust,
We've crushed every barrier in our career;
And conquer we will—and conquer we must!
For the might of Jehovah shall go with us here.
Then on! Like the Templar Knights, valiant of old,
Yet gentle and graceful, and winning as bold.
Cry onward! Reformers! The night has gone by,
And our flag, far and wide, is now floating on high.

Away with your systems of falsehood and wrong,
That only were made for the dullard and craven;
When we battle for truth we are mighty and strong,
And we dare to be free as the wild winds of Heaven!
Our watchword's Progression! Our day is before us;
And the Sun of Reform has but dawned on its glories!
Cry onward! Reformers! The night has gone by,
And our flag, far and wide, is now floating on high![14]

Homeopathic Literature

By 1860, fifty-two journals in the United States were devoted to homeopathy. Of that number, five were established in the 1830s, eleven in the 1840s, and thirty-six between 1850 and 1860. Approximately fifteen were directed principally to laymen and the public at large and intended to promote the spread of homeopathic principles. Although important, they were of little value to the educated physician. Among the most favored early journals were the *Quarterly Homeopathic Journal of Boston* edited by Gersdorff and Birnstill; the *North-Western Journal of Homeopathy* published in Chicago and edited by George E. Shipman; and the *American Journal of Homeopathy* published in New York and edited by S. R. Kirby, and known for its "fearless expression of opinion" and its motto, "The agitation of thought is the beginning of truth." Lesser known but still a good representation of homeopathy was the *American Magazine of Homeopathy* (later named the *Quarterly Homeopathic Magazine*), edited by Joseph H. Pulte and H. P. Gatchell. These journals, together with the *North American Journal of Homeopathy*, sponsored by Constantine Hering of Philadelphia and E. E. Marcy and J. W. Metcalf of New York, were loyal supporters of the so-called New Science and determined in their spirit of reform and in their opposition to Old School medicine.

To address the needs of the academically educated physician, the *Philadelphia Journal of Homeopathy* was established in 1852 by Johann Rademacher and Jacob F. Sheek, and edited by William A. Gardiner, M.D., professor of anatomy in the Homeopathic Medical College of Pennsylvania. Gardiner introduced the journal's first issue with a statement on "The Present Position and Prospects of Homeopathy," explaining that it was a matter of gratification that the reform practice of medicine had made "steady and unwavering" progress for more than a half century. As reform ideas fell upon the "thick darkness of allopathy," they had driven back the mists that had for centuries hidden the heart of healing. Redeemed from its abuses, medicine was again assuming its "true dignity among the positive sciences." The doctrines of Hahnemann, once sneered at and treated with ridicule, had now become recognized and propounded around the world. Enemies continued to show their opposition, but the stigma of "humbug" no longer received the anticipated response. While scores of allopathic physicians "traveled from house to house, to deal in slander and secret detraction," their best efforts had failed to accomplish the task.[15]

From the beginning, homeopathy's journals were subjected to a host of internal feuds ranging from divisions between academically trained homeopaths and laymen; rivalry between competing publishers and editors; hostility among German, French, and American-based theories; political jockeying between liberals and conservatives; and divisions between high and low dilutionists. Most of these journals, especially those intended for laymen, gave a disproportionate amount of space to diseases peculiar to women and children; among middle- and upper-class women, homeopathy was especially popular.

The quarterly, the *United States Journal of Homeopathy,* introduced in February 1860, promised adherence to only one therapeutic law, that of *similia similibus curantur,* and under no circumstance would admit that it was one of several laws of cure. Such admissions were for the eclectic but not the true homeopath. Instead, the editors promised to "exert themselves faithfully" to advance the new science. "Personal puffery, arrogant assumptions of professional superiority, and vindictive calumnies against individuals" would have no place in its pages.[16]

The editorial position taken by the *United States Journal of Homeopathy* was the exception rather than the rule since reform journals were most often the playground of brisk, ambitious, and confident editors only too willing to attack their opponents. The best example of this muscular journalism was John Fitzgibbon Geary of the *Philadelphia Journal of Homeopathy* who seemed at times willing to attack anyone when opportunity presented. An 1855 graduate of the Philadelphia College of Homeopathy, Geary was perceived by his detractors as an inexperienced physician (without a practice), who had yet to prove any medicines or perform any significant cures. With the ink scarcely dry on his diploma, he had taken pen in hand to criticize the two most notable homeopathic doctors in America. Over the course of his association with the journal, Geary accused Charles J. Hempel of "despicable jugglery" and "charlatanism"; called Adolph Lippe an "intellectual cripple"; described the American Provers Union a "star chamber" that was "debased in intrigue" and "stained with cowardice"; and described Constantine Hering as someone whose knowledge and judgment was "deformed by every imperfection."[17]

E. E. Marcy, editor of the *North American Journal of Homeopathy,* regretted the degree to which Geary had "repeatedly plunged into unnecessary and unprofitable personal controversies." Geary's iconoclasm, he felt, had rendered homeopathy "fearfully divided against itself."[18] According to Curt Pretsch, M.D., the presence of Geary on the editorial staff of the *Philadelphia Journal of Homeopathy* was a sign that homeopathy had entered an age of "rowdyism" and "loaferdom" with persons using their fists when they ought to be working cooperatively. As one of the representative children of the new age, Geary showed that he could "lick any homeopathic physician betwixt this and the moon." Thus, Geary had fought, cut, and shot his way through the pages of the *Philadelphia Journal of Homeopathy* "till nothing [was] left on the battle field but that pair of long ears" which adorned his head. For Pretsch, this young graduate was no more than a "medical dwarf," poking fun at those laborers who dared to translate homeopathic medicine from its original German into English.[19]

In his response, written under the *nom de plume* of "Hercules de Paidagogo, M.D.," Geary proceeded to live up to his reputation by correcting Pretsch's punctuation and misspellings and ridiculing the graduates of the "old degree shop" at Allentown whose president was Hering and which had taught its classes in the German language. Geary's scorn for Pretsch was but an ill-disguised effort to oppose the early influence of "vulgar" and "ignorant" lay homeopaths as well as the reign of "German doctoring" in the United States.[20] His article in the *Philadelphia Journal of Homeopathy* entitled "Our Literature—A Review," did not hesitate to criticize the "base coin" of German authors who published in support of homeopathic principles. Geary much preferred the French homeopaths to the German, and no doubt reflected the attitudes of most recent graduates of East Coast medical schools who were enamored with the work of the Paris Clinical School. Geary's adulation of Tessier's experiments with the victims of Asiatic cholera between 1832 and 1849 was a case in point. He found Tessier much more useful than the "bewildering speculations on the essence, or quintessence" popular among German writers. Tessier had built his foundation on "the actual observations and experiments of a skilful and thoroughly qualified physician at the bedside of his patients." Unlike German authors who had "entered our ranks as unqualified intruders," and made their reputations in the "early dawn of our day, before the full light exposed them as trespassers on our sacred grounds," Tessier and his colleagues were grappling with disease with "well-proved, well-tried and well-known" homeopathic remedies.[21] Reflecting this bias, the *Philadelphia Journal of Homeopathy* included in almost every issue hospital and dispensary reports listing the disease, and then categorizing patients as either cured, left improved, left unimproved, results unknown, or died. More often than not, these reports included statistics of both allopathic and homeopathic institutions.

Accused of focusing the journal's attention principally against German homeopathy, Gardiner defended his magazine and his associate editor, explaining that the journal's war was "not only with Germans," but with "men of all lands" who did injury to the New Science. The time had come, Gardiner wrote, when people needed to decide whether a "domestic physician" and a few bottles of "medicated globules" represented true homeopathy or simply "fanciful" fraud.[22] As for Hering, his "free and independent college" in Allentown was "contemptible" and his "ignorance of medical science," his "bait of free lectures," and his support of a "fictitious" college would remain in the editorial crosshairs of the journal's editors.[23]

* * *

A total of 198 botanic, Thomsonian, physio-medical, homeopathic, and eclectic journals were published between 1800 and 1860, a number that should stand as a significant statistic for students of medical history and American culture. To be sure, a large number of the journals were short-lived while others on the list represent merged or changed names. Nevertheless, a review of these journals suggests that the advocates of medical reform were highly erudite and by no means catered to an illiterate public or a narrow rung in the socio-economic ladder. Indeed, the very essence of rough-and-tumble Jacksonianism and its attributes of anti-elitism, anti-monopoly, and egalitarianism depended for the delivery of its message on an increasingly literate society.[24]

The image of reform medicine portrayed in the journal literature is that of a courageous group of healers emerging from the domination of the prior century's "system-builders" and seeking to distinguish themselves at the patient's bedside by utilizing a variety of path breaking new procedures built upon observation and experimentation. Wherever Old School influence prevailed, the reformers were there collectively to designate it as "Old Hunkerism."[25] No one idea, method, or belief dominated their thinking. Instead, medicine was perceived as being in a building phase, which meant drawing from the experiences, methods, and accomplishments in the collateral sciences of physics, chemistry, and physiology to construct a newer image of the art and science of medicine. The image of reform medicine evident in the literature was a reflection of the nineteenth century itself. Innovations in medical science were surely measures of the century's activity, but so also were the pretences that existed in bogus healers, harmful drugs, worthless therapies, incompetent practices, and race- and class-based patient care. All these images were little more than transparencies of the time.

Chapter 5. Reform Colleges

The determination of sectarian reformers to establish their own medical colleges reflected a clear expression of sectarian strength and regional pride. It also represented a determination to improve status and respectability by transforming their particular notions of medicine into an authentic science built on a combination of clinical practice and natural science, that is, the Baconian principles of observation and induction. It remains a question, however, as to whether these early reformers were truly Baconian in practice. The suspicion is that it was probably Francis Bacon's materialistic bias that caused many of the century's reformers to mouth his theory but repudiate his methodology. Just how diligent were the reformers to the practice of observing and recording; of controlled treatments; of deriving an hypothesis from collected data; and taking account of the interaction of mind and body? Given so many of reform medicine's a priori reasonings, it is doubtful that either the French Clinical School or German laboratory science played a large part in the sectarian side of the reform movement.[1]

In their search for a professional identity, reform doctors became vocal antagonists of existing medical colleges as they sought to convince supporters that they build and sustain a competing set of educational alternatives. Awake to the importance of instruction in the art and science of medicine, reformers of the botanic, Thomsonian, physio-medical, eclectic, and homeopathic persuasion organized departments, schools, infirmaries, and colleges to teach and perpetuate their partisan views. Most were short-lived but several were capable of sustaining themselves through the decades, consolidating and merging when necessary to maintain their critical mass, and fighting off the growing political power of regulars. Of the 50 schools and departments organized by sectarians (See *Appendix B*) between 1826 to 1860, twenty-four were located in the Northeast while seventeen formed in the Middle West. Of the remainder, nine organized in the South. The list by no means includes all reform medical schools; excluded are miscellaneous colleges with titles such as "anthropological," "fine forces," "health," "Hippocratean," "hygeia," "hydropathic," "hygeio-therapeutic," "liberal," and "magnetic" in their formal names or charters.

Eclecticism and the West

By the early decades of the nineteenth century, Ohio had become the western terminus for numerous schools, beliefs, reformers, and "isms." There the blend of Scottish empiricism and German romanticism took form. There, too, the American advocates of medical eclecticism first put their ideas to work, intending to develop a process for selecting the elements of truth among competing systems and blending them into a whole new philosophy. The West was the ideal location for the task of filtering out the best from conflicting philosophies and producing a new philosophy that reflected the optimism and independent spirit of the American character.

When it became clear that the Reform Medical College of New York would be unable to obtain a charter from the state legislature, Wooster Beach (1794–1868), along with Thomas Vaughan Morrow (1804–1850) and Ichabod Gibson Jones (1807–1857) prepared a circular letter to prominent Americans in the Ohio and Mississippi Valleys inquiring on a suitable location for a reformed medical school. A positive response from the Reverend Doctor Philander Chase, bishop of Ohio, resulted in the establishment of the Reformed Medical Department at Worthington College in Ohio. The department opened in 1831, holding two terms a year of five months each. First under the leadership of Dr. John J. Steele, a former regular, and later under the stewardship of Morrow, the school walked a tightrope between the animosity of regulars and the hostility of Samuel Thomson and his disciples. Both groups became bitter enemies of the school's faculty and students. In defense of the school's beliefs, Morrow published the *Western Medical Reformer* to support Beach's ideas of Reformed Medicine and his Reformed Medical Society of the United States.[2]

In his address to the faculty and students following his oath of office as president of Worthington College, Morrow acknowledged the melancholy state of the medical sciences and the task that lay ahead. Pointing out that no one had exerted "a more ruinous and paralyzing influence" than the "high authorities" of past ages, he dedicated himself and the faculty to disposing of "scholastic dogma" by giving their unequal attention to medical reformation. Mindful of the ravages brought by mineral drugs and the depletive instruments of orthodoxy, he urged his listeners to investigate the medicinal properties of the plants that abounded in the vegetable world, vowing that they represented "the polar star of our medical hopes."[3]

At the time of his induction into office, Morrow was only twenty-five years of age. Nevertheless, he provided much needed leadership to the school for ten years. As the first chartered sectarian medical school in the United States, Worthington College became the most prominent symbol of Reformed Medicine in the West. Its graduates were variously described as "Botanic," "Reformed," "American," and even "Beachite." The victim of a resurrection riot, the school closed March 20, 1840 by act of the Ohio Legislature.

Following the riot, Morrow moved with several of the faculty to Cincinnati where he focused his efforts on establishing the Reformed Medical School of Cincinnati (1842–45). When officially chartered in 1845, the name of the school was changed to the Eclectic Medical Institute (EMI), dedicated to the growing prospects of Reformed practice. Morrow, who became the school's first dean and professor of theory and practice, chose the term "eclectic" over other titles as a way to best describe the school's purpose and function. The term derived from a suggestion made by one of the school's trustees and seemed to resonate among reform-minded advocates; it quickly became the official acronym, replacing all other terms. Although the Thomsonians were adamant in their objections, the eclectic title became a household name for more than a century.

In 1849, T. V. Morrow and Ichabod G. Jones attempted to define the term "eclectic" and those who accepted its views. "The leading doctrine of the eclectic medical profession," they explained, "is that the investigation and practice of medicine should be entirely free and untrammeled; that no central body, no association, combination or conspiracy should have power to prescribe a certain standard of faith or medical creed which shall be received and forced upon every member of the profession by threats of professional disgrace and ruin. We recognize every enlightened, educated and honest physician as standing upon the same platform of professional respectability, and enjoying the same rights no matter what doctrines he may advocate in medicine, or what system of practice he may deem it his duty to adopt."[4] This statement of principle had been prompted by the position taken by the newly formed American Medical Association which came into existence in New York in 1846 and which insisted on a single view of medicine, buttressing its position with a Code of Ethics that excluded from fraternal courtesies all who were not in harmony with the conditions of the organization.

With the establishment of EMI, attention turned to the opening of other reform schools in New York, Pennsylvania, and Georgia. Arrangements were made for the sharing of faculty, the establishment of a consolidated *Union Medical Journal*, and the merger of several competing schools in western New York. None of these efforts proved successful, and by 1852, the hopes and promises for a more unified organization of eclectics fell into disarray. With the exception of EMI, eclecticism failed to build a nucleus for its style of medicine.[5]

EMI lasted from 1845 until the relinquishing of its charter in 1942. Over the course of its ninety-seven year history, it served as the mecca of eclectic schools from the perspective of research, the origination of medical theory, authorship of texts, political influence, numbers of graduates, and overall reputation. As the titular leader of eclecticism, it reflected both the strengths and weaknesses of this distinctive branch of American medicine. Its early years were rich in optimism, strong individualism, and raucous debate. But equally important was the school's highly visible move to a more narrowly defined botanical approach to therapeutics and, at the same time, the lip service the school's faculty gave to the broader intellectual aspects of eclecticism. This foreshadowing of the school's more restrictive view of medicine came by way of its misplaced allegiance to the so-called oleoresins that were the medicinal principles of plants precipitated by water from their alcoholic solutions. Manufactured for commercial use and introduced as resinoids into the vegetable materia medica by William S. Merrell, proprietor of Union Drug Store in Cincinnati, the concentrated fluid medicines soon became a distinctive attribute of EMI's academic teaching. The concentrated medicines were introduced as a cornerstone of eclectic medicine and touted as a competitor to the alkaloid pharmaceuticals of allopathic medicine, and of the triturations introduced by homeopathy.

Thinking that the resinoids would be a welcome stimulus to the needs of reform medicine, the eclectics found themselves quickly entrapped in the craze. Eventually, however, they became disenchanted with the mercenary aspects of eclectic pharmacy and, when the manufacturers of the concentrated medicines squared off with the larger drug manufacturers, they found themselves at a distinct disadvantage. Charges of adulterations, faulty manufacturing processes, and outright fraud were leveled at resinoid manufacturers who were accused of having tarnished the cause of eclectic reform efforts in their enthusiasm to sell their products. Eventually John M. Scudder, dean and owner of EMI from 1861 to 1894, condemned the concentrated medicines as nothing but "unmitigated humbug." Nevertheless, these medicines continued to be manufactured and to plague eclecticism's reputation well into the late nineteenth century.[6]

Among the eclectic colleges, of which there were sixty-nine (including name changes, mergers, etc.), twenty-six schools organized before 1860; thirty-two during the remainder of the century; and eleven in the early twentieth century. At the Metropolitan Medical College of the City of New York (1852–62), Penn Medical College (1853–81), and at the University of Nebraska (1883–87), the eclectics were part of a "mixed" educational system that included other medical philosophies as well. At the Metropolitan Medical College, the eclectics were joined by physiopaths (Independent Thomsonians) until the school's charter was revoked in 1862. Ultimately, the curriculum came under the influence of the more liberal eclectics. Penn Medical College, established by Dr. Joseph S. Longshore and named after William Penn, was founded on the principles of eclecticism, homeopathy, and the chrono-thermal system of Samuel Dickson of London. For a time, it was touted by the American Medical Association for having adopted a progressive curriculum that was graded. At the University of Nebraska, the state's legislature had authorized the establishment of three medical departments within the college: regular, eclectic, and homeopathic. The three departments were closed in 1887.

Other eclectic schools included the Botanic College of Medicine in New York City (1836–46) and the Eclectic Medical Institute of New York which became the Medical School of Fredonia (1847) and then moved to Syracuse in 1849 to become the Central Medical College of New York. It moved back to Rochester in 1850 and closed two years later. The Eclectic Medical College of New York City formed in 1866 and closed in 1913.

By 1915, the number of eclectic schools had declined to four, and by 1920, only the Eclectic Medical College of Cincinnati (formerly EMI) remained. The licensure scandals of the 1920s brought an end to whatever reputation remained for eclecticism.[7]

Botanic, Thomsonian, and Physio-Medical Colleges

Among the twenty-four botanically based schools, only the College of Medicine founded by Dr. Isaac S. Smith in 1836 in New York City attempted to steer an independent course. Smith's father, Elisha, had been the founder of the New York Association of Botanic Physicians and author of *The Botanic Physician* (1830). When Smith died, his cause was taken up by his son Isaac. Throughout its short history, the college remained unchartered and fraught with faculty dissension. Failing to receive recognition by the New York Board of Regents, it closed in 1846.

The remainder of the botanical schools—chartered and unchartered—were tied to the beliefs and practices of the Thomsonians. The oldest was the Botanico-Medical College and Infirmary of Columbus, Ohio, founded by Alva Curtis in 1836. The school, which eventually became the intellectual center of the "Independent" or so-called "New Light" Thomsonians, operated without a state charter for three years before incorporating as the Literary and Botanico-Medical Institute of Ohio. This was the first chartered Thomsonian medical college in the United States and the first to use the word *botanic* in its official name. In 1841, the school moved to Cincinnati where it became the University of the Literary and Botanico-Medical College of the State of Ohio with Curtis as chancellor. Over the ensuing years, the school went through numerous transformations until its charter expired in 1869.

Curtis's college was followed by a number of imitators, each founded on the principles established by Samuel Thomson but intended to ensure the perpetuation of his botanical system in a more orderly and structured manner. This meant no longer relying on the perpetuation of Thomsonism through the individual purchase of patent-rights or by franchised infirmaries, but by the establishment of programs offering both didactic and clinical experience on a medical college model. Colleges based on Thomsonism formed in Alabama, Georgia, Illinois, Indiana, Massachusetts, Ohio, Oklahoma, Pennsylvania, Tennessee, Texas, and Virginia. Some of these schools were blatantly fraudulent from the start while others, though high-minded, were never chartered. The majority succeeded in operating for a few years, and some for decades. The Southern Botanico-Medical College founded by Lanier Bankston in Forsyth, Georgia, in 1839, was the first sectarian medical school in the South; it lasted until 1884. Similarly, the Botanico-Medical College of Memphis, founded in 1847, continued until 1859 before coming under the influence of the eclectics. The Physopathic Medical College of Ohio organized in 1847 in Cincinnati and continued until 1880; and the Physio-Medical Institute of Cincinnati, organized in 1859 by William H. Cook, continued until 1885 when it moved to Chicago and became the Chicago Physio-Medical Institute, closing in 1911. The Physio-Medical College of Indiana was founded in 1873 by George Hasty and lasted until 1909 and the Curtis Physio-Medical Institute of Indiana lasted from 1881 to 1900.

Among the many factors that make Thomsonian schools interesting from an historical perspective were the chronic internal struggles over what constituted medical dogma and their disagreements as to Thomson's legitimate authority over the Friendly Botanic Society, publications, and schools. From the very beginning, the schools were the creation of individuals who rejected Thomson's authoritarianism and desired to exercise their reform beliefs beyond the narrow perspective of his six-step patented process. This meant expanding Thomson's original materia medica with additional herbals; refusing to purchase medicines and patent rights solely through authorized agents, infirmaries, and drug depots; expanding the theory and practice of herbal therapeutics; and credentialing and licensing medical doctors without Thomson's specific authorization. These schools stood as a challenge to Thomson's authority and to his self-help system of medicine. The moment of truth between Thomson and his disciples occurred in 1838 when the membership of his Friendly Botanic Society split between the adherents of strict Thomsonism and those who were inclined to a more liberal interpretation of his authority and ideas. The resulting schism not only destroyed the second nationally organized medical movement in the United States, it also precipitated an era of bad feelings within the botanically-based culture.

Once organized, the schools maintained very little direct contact with Thomson, whose death in 1843 caused a refocusing on more internal issues. Most were consumed by feuds between liberal and conservative wings within their ranks, making these colleges anything but placid learning environments for students. Time and time again their rancor caused splits and schisms among students and faculty; mass replacements of faculty by boards of trustees; the use of college journals to explain, denounce, and meddle in each other's teachings; suits and countersuits; occasional fist-fights between faculty; and the opening of competing schools and programs. Over time, the faculty in the colleges that were identified as botanico-medical turned increasingly liberal in their thinking and gravitated toward eclecticism; by contrast, those colleges that identified with the physio-medical name remained more entrenched in a purer form of vitalistic-based Thomsonian medicine.

Exemplary of the eclectic influence among the botanico-medical colleges was the renaming of the Southern Botanico-Medical College as the Reform Medical College of Georgia in 1854; the renaming of the New England Botanico-Medical College as the Worcester Medical College in 1851; and the renaming of the Botanico-Medical College of Memphis as the Eclectic Medical Institute of Memphis in 1859. In each instance, the hiring of botanics with eclectic tendencies forced changes in the nature and title of the institution. The College of Medicine and Surgery (physio-medical) of Chicago was absorbed by the College of Medicine and Surgery (eclectic) in 1911 and went over to the eclectics. This latter action officially ended the seventy-two year history of physio-medicalism in the United States.[8]

Homeopathic Colleges

Among the earliest homeopaths of German lineage, sectarianism was "neither dishonorable nor disgraceful." Indeed, it was "compatible with the highest degree of learning" and in the "preservation of its rights." True to Hahnemann's Protestant feelings, if sectarianism had not been part of medicine's overall history, the art and science of medicine would have remained "an incongruous mass of poorly ascertained facts." Since the earliest of periods in medical history, the progress of medical science was the work of acknowledged sectarians—Draco who founded the *Dogmatists*; Seraphion who originated the *Empirics*; Thermison who led the *Methodics*; Aretaeus who led the *Pneumatists*; and Archigenes who provided leadership for the *Eclectics*. These were followed by the *Chemists, Humoralists, Vitalists, Solidists,* and *Spiritualists*; and later by still other illustrious sectarians such as Friedrich Hoffmann, Johann Baptista Van Helmont, and Herman Boerhaave; then William Cullen, John Brown, and Thomas Sydenham. All of these individuals had founded or modified a system to their own liking, and influenced others who followed in their steps.[9]

Later homeopaths saw themselves as sectarian, not by choice, but because of persecution from Old School doctors whose bigotry and intolerance had forced them out of state and local societies, hospitals, and colleges. The Savannah Medical College in Georgia, for example, had imposed the following obligation on its candidates for the Doctor of Medicine.

> You hereby promise and declare, on the receipt of your Diploma, that you will maintain the honor, dignity, and respectability of the legitimate profession in which you have been educated, and that you will neither countenance nor affiliate with any system of irregular

> practice, nor engage either in the manufacture, sale, or recommendation of quack nostrums or patent medicines, nor countenance the practice of the senseless dogmas of hydropathy, homeopathy, or Thompsonianism (sic) under the penalty of having the degree conferred upon you, revoked by your alma mater.[10]

The reasoning behind this declaration was that Old School medical colleges had unwittingly become the source of homeopathy's earliest academically trained practitioners. Homeopaths enrolled as students in regular colleges and then, upon graduation, obtained postgraduate training in homeopathic therapeutics and materia medica through private instruction. Jefferson Medical College and the University of Pennsylvania educated an inordinate number of homeopathy's credentialed physicians. Silas S. Brooks graduated from Jefferson in 1846 and, after practicing Old School medicine for ten years, adopted homeopathy. The same was true of D. T. Trites and J. E. Houard in the class of 1842; of William P. Esrey and J. B. Gillman in the class of 1844; of G. H. Waters in 1845; J. R. Reading in 1847; J. I. Wright in 1851; and Pemberton Dudley and C. Karsner in 1859, to mention only a scattered few. Others such as H. N. Guernsey, William T. Helmuth, Charles F. Matlack, Joseph Griswold Loomis, matriculated at the University of Pennsylvania; Dr. William Ingalls (1842) from Brown University; John A. Tarbell (1843) from Bowdoin; and Dr. Hiram L. Chase (1846) and Josiah F. Flagg from Harvard Medical School. Other colleges that served as popular ports of entry into homeopathy included the College of Physicians and Surgeons of New York, the University of Vermont, and Rutgers Medical College, as well as the Central Medical College (eclectic) of New York, the Eclectic Medical College of Philadelphia, and the Eclectic Medical Institute of Cincinnati.[11]

In 1835, several early proponents of homeopathy in Pennsylvania organized the North American Academy of Homeopathic Medicine in Allentown, approximately fifty miles from Philadelphia. The intent was to supplement rather than replace the curriculum of the regular medical college with what amounted to postgraduate training. As instruction was in German, those that patronized the institution were few and it was not long before the school closed.

Sensing the need for a more organized and systematic approach to teaching the principles and practices of homeopathy, several Philadelphia homeopaths obtained a charter from the state in 1848 to organize the Homeopathic Medical College of Pennsylvania. By 1860, the college was in its twelfth session, with eighty matriculants and twenty-six graduates. The Western Homeopathic College organized in Cleveland, a city that competed with Buffalo, Toledo, Sandusky, Detroit, Milwaukee, and Chicago for the commerce of the Great Lakes. Founded in 1849, the college took pride in its accomplishments and quickly became representative of homeopathic reform in the

Middle West. The newly opened Homeopathic Medical College of Missouri in St. Louis, the geographical center of the republic, commenced its first annual course of lectures in October of 1859. New York Homeopathic College, founded in 1860, operated under the general supervision of the New York State Board of Regents. The college opened its doors at 116 East Twentieth Street and graduated its first class of twenty-seven students in 1861.

Homeopathy's strength came from three principal sources. The first stemmed from the fact that the earliest homeopathic physicians were educated as regulars and saw themselves not as sectarians but as having acquired an additional specialty in homeopathic principles. The second lay in the appeal of homeopathy to America's more affluent citizenry. Although there was the occasional Thomsonian or eclectic to be found among country's political, social, and economic elite, homeopathy claimed among its believers numerous senators and representatives, judges, teachers, industrialists, writers, poets, and religious thinkers. It also claimed a disproportionate number of women physicians when compared with the other medical schools. The final reason for homeopathy's strength was its tendency toward spirituality. There was an interconnection between life's physical and spiritual realms that gave homeopathy a dimension unlike most other reform groups. Homeopathy was different from the start, promoting an aura of spiritual and physiological superiority. It articulated a philosophy that made plausible not only a confidence in science and progress, but also a faith in the laws of nature, a metaphysical view of healing that included higher planes of reality, and a theoretical rationale for the primacy of spirit over matter. For those who saw themselves as society's "betters," homeopathy forged an effective alliance with unchurched religious thought that gave new meaning to holistic healing and man's capacity for inner harmony.[12]

National Colleges and Infirmaries

The Thomsonians, eclectics, and homeopaths applauded the establishment of colleges, but the sentiment was not always unanimous. In the early years, elements in all three groups feared that their colleges might not be capable of shouldering the cost of expensive equipment, the purchase of appropriate library materials, the availability of anatomical material, and the opportunity for clinical hospital experience. Hesitant to gamble with multiple schools, some urged the creation of a single national college that would teach the science of medicine according to their particular philosophy. Samuel Thomson feared the prospect of dozens of competing schools and infirmaries offering a questionable curriculum taught by uncertified teachers. After realizing that it would be nearly impossible to fend off attempts to organize schools and infirmaries, he agreed to support a single national infirmary provided that it be located in or near Baltimore and that all subsequent infirmaries would hold their charters by authority of that single national school. When the enabling legislation stalled in the 1832–33 session of the Maryland House of Delegates, it threw open the prospect of a more competitive free enterprise system across the country.[13]

Several decades later, a similar effort was undertaken by the faculty of the Eclectic Medical Institute of Cincinnati under the rubric of the "Free-School Movement." The school's dean, Joseph Rodes Buchanan (1814–1899), proposed a deceptively simple plan intended to make it one of the largest medical schools in the country where students enrolled in courses free of tuition and paid only for a matriculation fee, diploma, dissection, and special lectures. Beguiled by the dean's eloquence and intimidated by his threats, the faculty renounced their usual lecture fees and, in 1852, renamed the school the Central Free Medical College of America, intending by their new title to present themselves as a model of democratic medical education. Just as America had struck the first effective blow against Europe's class system, so it would now strike a blow against professional elitism by offering a cheaper route for young men to enter medicine. Behind the rhetoric was a more fundamental goal to place the college in undisputed control of eclectic medical education in the United States. Plans were promising as the faculty and dean anticipated enrollments of five to eight hundred students. The numbers never materialized and, instead, caused a lowering of the school's reputation and increased hostility from competing colleges forced to lower their own fees to remain competitive. In 1855, after several years of disappointing enrollments, the school quietly reversed its policy and returned to its former tuition-based system.[14]

Among American homeopaths, there was a similar call for a single national university, preferably located in the East. The initiative was the brainchild of a few well-educated homeopaths who feared the dilution of Hahnemann's principles if taught by inexperienced faculty outside the clinical advantages of a good metropolitan hospital. It was thought that, if diplomas were easily obtainable, the status of homeopathy would sink in the eyes of the public. Men unable to read, spell, or write, but who had obtained a medical degree, would drag the social position and income level of the profession to yet another low. "Make it impossible for the butcher in 1858 to be the 'M.D.' of 1859," demanded an anonymous critic writing in the *North American Journal of Homeopathy*.[15]

But efforts in all three reform groups failed to materialize beyond a few individual dreams. In each case, the call for a single national school or infirmary was met with harsh opposition from those who were convinced of the need to establish a regional identity for their particular medical philosophy. What better way than to build dozens of departments and free-standing schools in population centers.

Retrospective

Given the pattern of private choice that dominated medical practice in the early nineteenth century, and the significance that Americans placed on their freedoms as well as on the atrophy of Old World institutions and beliefs, it was natural for them to feel that out of their New World experiences a distinctive American practice might somehow emerge. The catalysts for this thinking came from both inside and outside regular medicine. Those on the inside who had been apprenticed or educated abroad and retained a heady opinion of their qualifications and professional authority, hoped to create a well-regulated and identifiable profession in America by attaching licensing authority to universities, and later, to their own medical societies or the state. Those on the outside who by dint of their own observations, experiences, and insight had succeeded as healers, looked similarly to the license authority vested in their proprietary medical colleges and, alternatively, to the authority of their societies and the state. The proliferation of medical schools, particularly those of a proprietary nature, gave added incentive to those who believed that a distinctive American School of medicine was possible. Supported by easily obtainable state charters, visionary reformers rose to the occasion with plans that were intended to capture the public's imagination. These plans, almost without exception, employed the uplifting language of anti-elitism, anti-monopoly, and anti-clericalism to justify the sectarian appetites of these medical protestants.

In looking at the schools geographically, the earliest and most long-lasting Thomsonian schools were founded in the South, drawing their strength from a society that was predominantly rural and a medical culture whose characteristics could best be described as folk-based, herbal, protestant, conservative, and highly independent. By contrast, the eclectic schools drew their support from rural and small-town America in the East and Midwest. Like the Thomsonian schools, the eclectic colleges were proprietary in nature and produced generalists rather than specialists. Over time, however, the Thomsonian schools gravitated to eclectic thinking and the leadership of the Eclectic Medical Institute of Cincinnati, the so-called "mother institute" of Reform Medicine. In part, the reason for this change was the more liberal accommodations made by the eclectics toward the Independent Thomsonians. Another was the success of William S. Merrell (1798–1880), an eclectic drug manufacturer, who introduced concentrated fluid extracts. Merrell was followed John Uri Lloyd (1849–1936) and his two brothers, Nelson Ashley (1851–1926) and Curtis Gates (1859–1926), owners of the Lloyd Brothers, Pharmacists Inc., and manufacturers of a line of botanical products known as "specific medicines."

Those homeopathic schools that organized in the first half of the nineteenth century were proprietary in nature and located in the eastern states of New York and

Pennsylvania, and in the Middle Western states of Ohio, Illinois, and Missouri. Unlike the Thomsonians, the homeopaths made few inroads into the South (except for New Orleans), preferring the more affluent urban areas. Nevertheless, like the eclectics, they showed immense pride in their colleges and used their considerable political influence to win the inclusion of their students and faculty in publicly funded hospitals, asylums, and dispensaries. And like both the Thomsonians and eclectics, they were able successfully to argue their cause before receptive legislators who, more often than not, voted to ensure their equal protection before the courts.

Typical of most medical schools of the day, financial problems and dissension were rife among sectarian faculty and between faculty and trustees. To be sure, sectarian schools were by no means alone in this characteristic. The professorial ranks of most medical schools seemed unusually full of those intending to "profess," with the expected result that many schools had the appearance of bear gardens. Debates between liberal and conservative factions over medical theory and practice; rivalry over student loyalty and editorial control of the school's journal; disagreements regarding fees and disbursement of tuition dollars; feuds over patient access; and competition for teaching chairs were just some of the many issues that hindered collegiality.

In the eastern states, there seemed to be a greater tolerance for diversity, a factor evident in the establishment of several schools offering a "mixed" system of education. These included the Albany Medical College, a regular school founded in 1838 and which openly filled some of its chairs with teachers who espoused homeopathic theory and practice; Metropolitan Medical College of the City of New York, organized in 1852, which included both eclectics and physiopaths as trustees and faculty; Penn Medical College in Philadelphia, chartered in 1853, which taught eclecticism, homeopathy, and the chrono-thermal system of medicine; and the New York Medical College and Hospital for Women, founded in 1866, which included both regulars and homeopaths on its teaching staff.

Unlike the Northeast and Eastern seaboard states, the Midwest was home to a myriad of competing schools, each set on establishing its own distinctive approach to healing. Both regulars and sectarians were zealous in their opinions, impetuous in their enthusiasms, boastful of their regional character, and anxious to build and sustain an indigenous medical tradition. One aberration occurred in 1849 when the faculty of the Eclectic Medical Institute (EMI) in Cincinnati invited Ohio homeopaths to select someone to teach the principles and practice of homeopathy in their curriculum. Since there were as yet no homeopathic colleges west of Pennsylvania, Dean Joseph R. Buchanan of EMI saw this offer as a means of quelling pressure for a separate homeopathic college in Ohio. However, much to the embarrassment of the EMI faculty, the school's token homeopath, Dr. Storm Rosa, turned out to be a very convincing teacher who took every opportunity to advance homeopathic ideas above all other methods of cure, including eclecticism. At the close of the 1849–50 session, the faculty voted to abolish the school's special relationship, explaining that the homeopathic system contained "practical errors, delusions and false philosophy."[16]

Measured against European experience, the achievement of freedom of choice in the selection of medical doctors in the United States was a triumph for the sectarians. Despite the semantic confusion created by regulars who claimed the high ground over irregular medicine, vindication came in the form of legislative action that leveled the medical market place and opened healthcare to free competition among the many sects. True, there were those who expressed contempt and scorn towards the beliefs of irregular healers, but few were willing to pass that same judgment on the patients who supported them. Most Americans, whether adhering to so-called orthodoxy or any of the dominant medical sects, accepted as axiomatic the competitive disarray of America's medical landscape. No clear definitions were established, no uniform orthodoxy mandated—only a diversity of beliefs and organizations. In the end, the sectarians wanted only the liberty of their convictions and the opportunity to establish a bond between themselves and the populace without legal or other forms of restriction, and to ensure unrestricted competition, allowing the winners and losers to be determined by individual choice in the market place. Medical freedom was the platform on which the sectarians most heartily came together. More than any other issue, it was the most uncontroversial. Here was the ideal issue on which they worked with a minimum of friction and a maximum of cooperation. Ironically, medical libertarians were more given to advocating their freedoms than sustaining them over time. Having staged a successful assault against organized medicine, they seemed oblivious to the fissures and internal tensions occurring in the structural foundations of their own schools.

The 1850s were a time of considerable anxiety among medicine's apostates. This was particularly evident among the Independent Thomsonians and physio-medicals who found themselves increasingly drawn to the siren appeals of the more liberal eclectics. The same proved true of certain homeopaths whose opposition to Hahnemann's more extreme theories of dynamization and psora had forced them into alliances with the more moderate eclectics. Generally, the eclectics had much to admire in homeopathy and viewed it, along with hydropathy, allopathy, and physio-medicalism as fully capable of curing disease. The question was whether one should choose one pathy exclusively, or alternatively, choose the best from each of the systems on a case-by-case basis. For W. Paine of Warren, Ohio, who had begun practice as a allopath before moving to eclecticism, it was "exclusivism in all its forms," that had been responsible for the high mortality among patients. Thus, the eclectic practice of medicine offered the solution.[17]

For more conservative homeopaths, any connection with eclecticism was a matter of considerable risk. "Among the homeopathic practitioners of the present day," observed Henry C. Preston in 1859, "we regret to notice a prevailing tendency of eclecticism which, if not checked or overcome, will, we fear, prove the utter downfall of our system." This dangerous tendency among colleagues came from accepting the proposition that there was good to be derived from every school or system of medicine. For Preston, this proposition went counter to his belief in the therapeutic law of similars.[18] The successful results of infinitesimal doses overshadowed "whether or not we are able to give a theory even for its modus operandi." Supporting purity in theory and in practice, he opposed the artificial distinctions made by others between rational and transcendental homeopathy as simply "nonsense." He saw no reason to use crude drug medicines, cathartics, and other compounds of the allopathic and antipathic schools, including so-called silver-coated pills of aloes and extract of Nux vomica. Preston was likewise unimpressed with the leaders in homeopathy who admitted to the eclectic affinity for finding something good in all systems. "To say that a man is eclectic seems to us very much like saying he is nowhere, or that he is like a ship at sea without a rudder, floating wherever the popular breeze or the prevailing hypothetical current may take him," Preston wrote. With such feelings, Preston had nothing good to say about the eclectics. "We never yet have seen an eclectic in medicine, or theology, that had any fixed ideas, or any very solid arguments on which to build his faith and principles." Essentially, the eclectic was nothing but "a weather-cock, revolving on a pivot . . . changing his position with the breath of every new-fangled theory."[19]

Chapter 6. Reform Societies

During the heady days of Jacksonian Democracy, state legislatures made preemptive strikes against the learned professions by loosening or removing licensure laws and allowing "the People" in their individual and collective wisdom to decide for themselves who to employ. Physicians whose medical credentials had been established through medical society or state certification were forced to compete in the market place with all other healers. In the absence of licensing it was difficult to tell one physician from another since all had equal access to the public and each strove in his own way to establish legitimacy. The terms "Orthodoxy," "Old School," and "Old Hunkerism" carried such negative connotations among the public at this time that many apprenticed and academically trained doctors preferred to be called "regulars" or even "allopaths." The latter was a title that originated with Samuel Hahnemann and used to show that medical orthodoxy was, like homeopathy, just one of many competing schools. Those who identified themselves as "Reformers" lost no opportunity to shackle regular doctors with the most rigid designations, hoping to force them into the backwaters of practice. By attacking regulars with such unmistaken sobriquets, and attributing to them bleeding and other depletive regimens, America's reformers hoped to claim "progress" and "science" as their own particular intellectual property.

The limitations placed on the licensing powers of medical societies in the early 1800s did not mean the end of these societies. To be sure, the revenue produced by the licensing boards became an important source of income to the societies and gave prestige and formality to their activities. Their authority as the recognized gatekeepers to the profession diminished, but voluntary medical societies continued to flourish. Actually, their role increased as they began the task of delineating and credentialing their members in ways that more accurately defined their real character. These associations were organized with a two-fold purpose in mind. First, they clarified the boundaries inside which their members sought professional legitimization. This included ensuring purity within their rank-in-file by a united stand on specific principles, beliefs, standards, and aspirations. In this regard, they served an important function as doctors faced off on such issues as bleeding and other depletive measures; fee bills; codes of ethics; education; consultation; patent medicines; published or oral testimonials; and quackery. Secondly, many of these state and regional organizations sought to project themselves on to a larger stage by becoming national in their breadth and scope. While the outcome of these efforts was mixed, those organizations that successfully made the transition from regional to national societies found themselves faced with a whole new set of challenges, not the least of which was who could most effectively influence national legislation.

For European intellectuals such as Alexis de Tocqueville, the existence of professional societies, institutes, and academies offered the promise of becoming instruments of democratic culture, striking a balance between the pronounced desire among American citizens to maintain their individualism and the recognition that without a multitude of associations, the power of government and of private individuals would increase exponentially at the expense of democracy. With the founding of the American Philosophical Society in 1743, followed by the American Academy of Arts in 1785, there emerged a claim, however modest at first, that the democracies might yet find scientific research, philosophic speculations, and the spirit of discovery to their liking. Through these agencies, Americans might plausibly overcome their suspicions of a too active intellect, especially if such agencies profited their communities with useful information and inventiveness. Not for contemplation, but for utility, would democratic society place its trust in professional organizations.[1]

Miscellaneous Medical Organizations

The calling of a national convention of regular doctors in New York in 1846 signaled the beginnings of the American Medical Association, but it by no means set a precedent. In fact, the scramble to legitimize the numerous assemblages of reform healers bent on pressing their particular view of medicine had been underway for several decades. Local and state reform medical societies began organizing as early as the 1820s and 1830s. In all, some 125 local and state reform medical societies had been established by the late 1840s.[2] By 1860, the number had swelled to over 200 (See *Appendix C*). Besides the hundred or more Friendly Botanic Societies of the Thomsonians, it included the Reformed Medical Society of the State of New York that organized on January 23, 1828 in Rochester and continued until 1863 when it merged with the Eclectic Medical Society of the State of New York; and the New York Association of Reformed Physicians, organized in 1828 by Dr. Elisha Smith of New York City and which looked regionally for its membership. It disbanded after Smith's death in 1831. There was also the Reformed Medical Society of the United States, organized in 1829 by Wooster Beach and his friends at the Reformed

Medical College of the City of New York and which looked nationally for its membership.[3] This was the first and oldest national medical association formed in the United States. In addition the Genesee Union Botanical Society formed in 1832; and the Medical Society of Botanic Physicians and Surgeons of the City of New York organized in 1835 with members including Isaac S. Smith, Abel Hanks, and Ives S. Barber. This latter society opened a college that continued until 1846.[4] There was also the Reform Medical Society organized in Conesus, New York, in 1832; and the Reformed Medical Association of Western New York formed at Dansville in Livinston County, New York.[5]

Beach's Reformed Medical Society of the United States never really developed as anticipated, particularly with the dissolution of his Reformed Medical College in 1838. Nevertheless, the society's early membership was national in scope and included Beach and Washington Starrett of New York; John J. Steele and Thompson Richardson of Pennsylvania; Thomas Vaughan Morrow of Kentucky; Amzi Sanborn of Maine; and S. A. Stanley of Connecticut. Beach served as president of the association, Steele as vice president, and Starrett as secretary. Other members of the society included J. F. Daniel Lobstein, George W. Chevers, John C. Kelly, A. Upham, James J. Vere, and Calvin Preston.[6]

In 1836, Morrow attempted to reactivate the Reformed Medical Society by bringing together the graduates of both the American Reformed School in New York and those of the Reformed Medical College at Worthington. However, the graduates of these two schools, who were variously designated as "Botanic," "Reformed," "American," and sometimes "Beachite," could arrive at no consensus as to their particular title or choice of designation. This lack of agreement spilled over into their organization, preventing it from coalescing around a common set of principles.[7]

Heartened by several successful state efforts to organize reform medical associations, Morrow made another attempt early in 1841 to bring together a national coalition of Reformed and botanic doctors. His motivation was primarily defensive, believing that, left in isolation, the dispersed reform groups would become easy prey to adverse medical legislation initiated by regulars. His objective was the formation of a "National Convention of the Reformed Brotherhood" with representation from every congressional district to authorize funding for a "National Reformed Medical Institution and Infirmary." Once again, sectional jealousies between the Independent Thomsonians and various Reformed (eclectic) schools of medicine worked against him.[8] In large measure, both the "National Convention of the Reformed Brotherhood" and the "National Reformed Medical Institution and Infirmary" were rejected by the general body of reformers who feared the imposition of such ambitious common cause efforts on their own regional societies and schools. The South's opposition came from Dr. Lanier Bankston of the Southern Botanico-Medical College (1839) at Forsyth, Georgia.[9] According to Alexander Wilder, the Thomsonians and Reformed physicians "entertained an unappeasable dislike for one another." Their differences and jealousies were such that fraternal courtesies were near impossible, turning the most innocuous issue into a viciousness that had few boundaries. Wilder considered these feuds worse than the persecutions originating from reform medicine's open adversaries.[10]

Friendly Botanic Societies

As early as the 1811, so-called "Friendly Botanic Societies" organized under the guidance and encouragement of itinerant healer Samuel Thomson of New Hampshire to communicate information among those individuals and families who had purchased a "right" to his proprietary course of medicine. The earliest were organized at Eastport, Kittery, Portland, and York in Maine; Bridgewater, Georgia, Jericho, and Woodstock in Vermont; Alstead, Deerfield, Eastham, Exeter, Pelham, Portsmouth, Richmond, Salisbury, Surry, and Walpole in New Hampshire; and Beverly, Boston, Charlestown, Eastham, Newburyport, Petersham, Royalston, Salem, Salisbury, South Reading, and Warwick in Massachusetts. These societies, whose members had adopted a constitution, rules, and regulations for securing, using, and protecting Thomson's patented therapeutic system (1813; 1823; 1836), were limited in size to about fifty members each. As these societies spread across New England, the Middle Atlantic, and the Middle West, differences arose between them and Thomson over the actual nature of their authority. Fearful that they were growing independent of his leadership, Thomson dissolved the societies and replaced them with a single national organization called the Friendly Botanic Society of the United States.

During the 1830s, Thomson appointed one to four agents in 91 towns in Connecticut, Massachusetts, Maine, New Hampshire, Rhode Island, and Vermont. Each of these towns had at least one branch of the Thomsonian Friendly Botanic Society. Outside of New England there were additional branch societies: New York (6); Pennsylvania (3); Indiana (8); Kentucky (1); Virginia (2); Tennessee (2); Ohio (2); North Carolina (1); South Carolina (1); Arkansas (1); Alabama (2); Georgia (2); Maryland (1); and Illinois (3). Having thus brought the societies under his personal control, Thomson then called for delegates to meet in Columbus, Ohio, in December 1832. The convention represented the second national meeting (following Beach's Reformed Medical Society of the United States which organized in 1829) of a medical organization in the United States, but the first really successful organization. A year later, the delegates adopted a constitution and placed the organization under Thomson's direct authority.[11]

Between 1832 and 1838, the society met each December to share knowledge of medicinal plants; discuss remedial procedures; trace the course of the Asiatic cholera; and hear from Samuel Thomson himself on the cause and future of his botanically-based medical system. Meeting first in Columbus, and later in Pittsburgh, Baltimore, Philadelphia, and other major cities, the conventions addressed several issues, including the establishment of a "National Thomsonian Infirmary;" certification of botanic practitioners; the propriety of a "test resolution" certifying loyalty to Thomson's system; the copyright to Thomson's *Guide to Health* (1822) and renewal of his patent; the hostility of regulars; the sale and use of authentic Thomsonian medicines; and the role of Thomson himself in the organization's future.[12]

In 1838 at Philadelphia, the organization split, with one group adhering to strict Thomsonism and the other, the so-called "New Lights" or "Independents," breaking from the dictatorial hold of Thomson over control of the convention and revisions to his medical system. Out of the schism emerged the Independent Thomsonian Botanic Society under the leadership of Alva Curtis, and the United States Thomsonian Society ("Old Lights") under the control of Samuel Thomson and his authorized agents.[13] The strict Thomsonians were near phobic in their fear of mongrelism, secretive in their meetings, and insistent that Thomsonism remain steadfastly opposed to the establishment of medical colleges. In 1840, the society died for lack of delegate support; its few remaining advocates carried on their activities within a decreasing number of state and county societies.[14]

By contrast, the members of the Independent Thomsonian Botanic Society concentrated their efforts on erecting infirmaries and medical colleges, and on electing boards of examiners before whom all applicants for general practice could appear. Unlike the strict Thomsonians, the Independents showed little concern with maintaining strict orthodoxy and were lax in defining the credentials of delegates to their national organization. As a result, their membership lists included a significant number of lay practitioners. The Independents also had a greater appreciation for individual and regional differences and more were open to new ideas. Over time, they moved closer and closer to the eclectics in their thinking and in their organization. Their initial challenge was building a consensus on the most appropriate name for their beliefs. Those in the South and West preferred the term "physiomedical," while those in the Northeast were enamored with the terms "physopathic," "physiopathic," or "physio-eclectic."[15]

As issues of sectionalism emerged among the Independents, editors Thomas Lapham and A. H. Platt of the *Poughkeepsie Thomsonian* proposed in 1841 that the Independent Thomsonian Botanic Society separate into two districts: a northern district to include Maine, New Hampshire, Vermont, Massachusetts, Rhode Island, Connecticut, New York, New Jersey, Pennsylvania, Delaware, Maryland, Michigan, Upper and Lower Canada, Nova Scotia, and New Brunswick; and a southern district consisting of Virginia, Ohio, Indiana, Illinois, Kentucky, Tennessee, North and South Carolina, Georgia, Alabama, Louisiana, Mississippi, Missouri, all the Northwest Territory, Texas, and the Spanish provinces. Although the proposed organization failed to materialize, delegates from Maine, New Hampshire, Vermont, Massachusetts, Connecticut and Rhode Island met in 1842 and drafted a constitution for a New England Thomsonian Society. Over the ensuing years, positive memories among the Independents of the earlier Thomsonian conventions spurred hopes that, despite the unfortunate schism of 1838, another national gathering of Thomson's disciples and other botanically-minded reformers might someday materialize.[16]

Legislation

In the meantime, the various organizations of botanic and reformed practitioners focused their efforts on repealing state legislation that blocked their right to practice. This cause brought them together despite their differences over the principles and practices of medicine. On the whole, the efforts succeeded as state after state passed bills for medical freedom of choice. Begun by Alabama, and followed by Indiana, Pennsylvania, Maine, and Connecticut, legislators began tearing down the barriers to patient choice.[17]

One of the few holdouts to the legislation was New York. Between 1813 and 1819, doctors in New York secured passage of several laws that incorporated county and state medical societies to regulate the practice of medicine and surgery and to examine all physicians to determine their qualifications for a certificate or a license to practice medicine in the state. Those not having such license were disqualified from using the courts to collect debts and were liable for prosecution if judged to be practicing without a license. Eclectic and botanic physicians were required to have studied with a regular physician for at least four years, and join a regular medical society, or face the prospect of not being recognized. The law did have an escape clause, permitting persons to practice without a license if they used roots, barks, or herbs; however, these healers were not entitled to any fee or payment for their services.[18]

Objecting to the malicious nature of the legislation, sectarian groups joined forces to fight for their interests. Together, they submitted petitions to the New York General Assembly from 1839 through 1844, and joined with reformers in other states to defend their common interests. In 1844, the Thomsonians, the more organized of the reform groups, presented to the New York Legislature a petition containing the signatures of forty thousand individuals requesting repeal of the laws. In addition, Reform doctors John C. Kelly and Isaac S. Smith spoke before the legislature in opposition to the laws. Influenced by this significant grassroots effort, the legislature repealed the law in 1844.[19]

Similar to the spirit of sectarianism in mid-nineteenth century religion, America's medical sectarians chose not to dwell publicly upon their differences but, instead, to work side by side in the political arena, furthering their common interests. To be sure, there were discordant notes in the midst of this harmony, but doctrinal laxity characterized their teachings and set them apart from the earlier eighteenth-century system-builders.

Although they professed all manner of heretical notions, they were zealous in their defense of what they considered to be the right of individual choice. This resulted in a plentitude of heretical notions, with their only agreement being the rejection of what they perceived to be the symbols of orthodoxy. Indeed, various "unions" or "accommodations" of Thomsonians and Grahamites, of homeopaths and hydropaths, and of Thomsonians and eclectics were openly discussed by parties within their respective organizations. No great amalgamation took place among the sectarian groups, but the fact that such a possibility was even considered gave credence to their willingness to embrace the common elements within sectarian medicine and to reject any authority beyond themselves.

American Institute of Homeopathy

Separate from the botanics, Thomsonians, and eclectics were the homeopaths who, failing to be recognized as a specialty within regular medicine, set out to form their own organizations for more effective communication and mutual protection. The American Institute of Homeopathy (A.I.H.) originated at a July 1843 meeting of the New York Homeopathic Physicians' Society which invited all homeopaths to meet in New York City to form a national society. The association, which held its first meeting at the Lyceum of Natural History in April 1844, became the third oldest national medical association in the United States, drawing its charter members from Illinois, Indiana, Kentucky, Massachusetts, Michigan, New York, Ohio, Pennsylvania, and Rhode Island.[20] The largest number came from Ohio (principally Cincinnati and Cleveland), followed by Pennsylvania, New York, and New Jersey.[21] Criteria for membership required applicants to have pursued a course of medical studies and to have obtained a certificate signed by three members of the association affirming good moral character, and qualification in the theory and practice of homeopathy. The association's earliest activities included a monthly journal, a volume on drug provings, a publication on topographical anatomy, and annual meetings of members.[22]

William A. Gardiner of the *North American Homeopathic Journal* urged all homeopaths to become active patrons of the Institute. "Let selfishness, indifference, and indolence . . . be abolished, or, rather, let them be banished; and let no duty be left undone," he urged readers.[23] In keeping with this advice, the A.I.H. recommended the formation of state and county societies; provided advice on their formation; and supervised their provings of medicines.[24] These societies consisted of academically trained physicians and laymen, the latter of whom served principally in small towns and rural districts. Their structure resembled the Friendly Botanic Society of the United States, and their activities including lobbying for equality before the law along with helping communities cope with cholera, yellow fever, and other epidemic diseases.

In 1853, the A.I.H. strengthened criteria for membership by requiring all applicants to provide the name of the medical college from which they had graduated. This had the effect of driving a wedge between academic homeopathy and its lay advocates, a division that would fester into the present day. That same year at their meeting in Cleveland, A.I.H. delegates appointed a committee to ascertain the names and residences of all homeopathic physicians in the United States and to make the report public at the next annual meeting. The delegates also established a Central Homeopathic Pharmacy under the control of the association.[25] When the A.I.H. met a year later at Albany, New York, the delegates reaffirmed the homeopathic law of similars, a higher standard of education for homeopathic physicians, and a determination to test and identify all potentially beneficial medicines.[26]

The A.I.H. was usually guarded in its public references to allopathic medicine. Since most of its members had been educated in regular schools, they considered themselves equal in education and status. Accordingly, the A.I.H. passed frequent resolutions urging dignity in speeches and writing, and refusing to resort to "blackguardism" and other actions unbecoming members of a scientific profession.[27] For example, in June 1858, in an address before the assembled delegates meeting in Brooklyn, Dr. Jabez Dake extended an olive branch to regular and eclectic medicine, noting that "the selfish and bitter manner" in which the different schools carried on their communication was "disgraceful to men, gentlemen, and Christians." While he could not control how regulars treated homeopaths, especially those opposed to high dilutions, he felt that homeopaths had much to learn from orthodox physicians. "We can never expect charitable and kindly treatment from others unless we exhibit it ourselves," Dake observed.[28]

American Medical Association

With twenty-nine regular medical schools issuing diplomas in 1846, with legislatures having decided to make no distinction between regular and irregular schools in licensing, and with Reformers (1829), Thomsonians (1832) and homeopaths (1844) having already formed national organizations, Samuel Jackson of the University of Pennsylvania complained that there was no common standard for the conferring of the Doctor of Medicine, much less credible standards for admission to practice. So serious had been the deterioration of the title "doctor" in the public's eye, that it ceased to be a title of distinction. Recognizing that the federal government lacked the power to interfere and that the states and territories could not provide uniform legislation, Jackson urged colleagues to undertake self-regulation. To achieve this, the medical community had to reform its ranks, formulate a code of ethics, institute positive regulations, elevate the moral and scientific tone of the profession, and return the title of Doctor of Medicine to its original high worth.[29]

The growing discontent among regulars about their fragile position led to a call by the New York State Medical Society for a National Medical Convention to be held in the spring of 1846 in the Medical Department of the University of the City of New York. The convention failed to obtain representation from half of the states and from a majority of the medical colleges, but it proudly claimed the presence of 119 delegates from fourteen states. This in turn led to a call for a broader assemblage the following year to look into such matters as standards of medical knowledge, the elevation of the science, and professional qualifications. Behind these high sounding words were heartfelt concerns about the excessively high numbers of practitioners, poor remuneration, poor medical education, and that quacks and empirics had captured the public's eye and pocketbook.[30]

Delegates to the second National Medical Convention met in the hall of the Academy of Natural Sciences in Philadelphia on May 5, 1847. Representatives from twenty-two states and the District of Columbia attended the meeting.[31] Among the convention's first chores was to approve the creation of standing committees on medical sciences, practical medicine, surgery, obstetrics, medical literature, medical education, publication, and arrangements. By resolution the delegates also created a committee on indigenous medical botany. As for the naming of their association, the delegates explored such titles as "The Medical Association of the United States of North America," "The Conventional Association of the United States," and "National Medical Association," and "American Medical Association." Eventually they settled on the American Medical Association (A.M.A.).[32]

Moderates within the association hoped for some type of accommodation with the sectarians, but the A.M.A. would have none of it. Instead, it chose to draw strict boundaries between the two schools. Its Code of Ethics, adopted in May 1847, included language that effectively excluded consultation between any sectarians and orthodox practitioners. The consultation clause quickly became the *cordon sanitaire* between regular and irregular medicine, aggravated by rhetoric that tended to exaggerate their respective differences. Symptomatic of this, at the 1855 meeting of the A.M.A. in Philadelphia, the delegates approved a resolution offered by J. L. Atlee, that formalized orthodox sentiment:

> Resolved, That any such unnatural union as the mingling of an exclusive system, such as Homeopathy with Scientific Medicine, in a School, setting aside all questions of its untruthfulness, cannot fail, by the destruction of union and confidence, and the production of confusion and disorder, unsettling and distracting the minds of the learners, to so far impair the usefulness of teaching as to render any

> School adopting such a policy unworthy the support of the profession.[33]

Not all regulars agreed with the position formulated by the national association. Perhaps the most significant communication on this matter came from Dr. James Jackson, professor of theory and practice at Harvard. Criticized by several of his professional colleagues for having consulted with a homeopathic member of the Massachusetts Medical Society, he responded that his conduct had been in accordance with the laws of the society. Although certainly not a proponent of homeopathy, he refused to persecute persons holding opinions different from his own. He considered it as wrong to refuse consultations with fellows of his own society who had adopted homeopathic principles as it was to refuse to consult with an advocate of the Brunonian system. Jackson was quick to point out that the Brunonians "did much positive harm to the sick, while homeopathy only fail[ed] to do them good." His rule was to meet with any fellow of the Massachusetts Medical Society "unless there is something objectionable in his character." More to the point, he considered many orthodox doctors more dangerous to their patients than homeopaths. "I cannot believe that the black sheep are found in one flock only," he concluded.[34]

Recognizing that the association lacked legislative powers, convention members nonetheless felt a strong sense of accomplishment in its work and in the future. At the beginning of the A.M.A.'s existence in 1846, only seven state medical societies and eleven local societies sent representatives to the convention in New York. The next year, sixteen state societies were represented at the Philadelphia meeting. By 1854, the number had increased to twenty-six state societies or associations, including the Society of Minnesota Territory and the Cherokee Nation Society, and more than one hundred county, district, and town societies.[35]

National Eclectic Medical Association

Hearing of the recent formation of the new American Medical Association, practitioners representing the different elements of Reformed medical practice met at the Eclectic Medical Institute in Cincinnati on May 25, 1848, to take up the issue of organizing a national association. Forty-three attended the convention, representing Illinois, Indiana, Iowa, Kentucky, Missouri, New York, Ohio, and Pennsylvania. The delegates met for three days and, before adjourning, adopted a permanent organization under the name of the American Eclectic Medical Association. Original members included T. V. Morrow, Wooster Beach, Joseph R. Buchanan, Lorenzo E. Jones, Ichabod Gibson Jones, John King, Orin Davis, Thomas Cooke, Benjamin L. Hill, and John H. Jordan. The association elected Morrow as president, and doctors John King and L. E. Jones as secretaries. The association, which also included Alva Curtis's Independent Thomsonians, urged the formation of state and local societies and the compilation of statistics to document the successes of Reformed medical practice. In May 1849, the convention met during the cholera epidemic and adopted a constitution and by-laws; it also changed its name to the National Eclectic Medical Association, with Morrow as its first president.[36]

For Morrow and members, it was the duty of the National Eclectic Medical Association to counteract the power and prestige of the A.M.A. and its designs on monopolizing medicine and medical practice. The challenge was never more clear. "The great struggle of the day in the medical profession is between the spirit of freedom on the one hand, which is seeking for truth in science, and the spirit of conservative despotism on the other, which aims to perpetuate its power and doctrines by organized combinations, and by discountenancing or suppressing every attempt at reform, whatever may be its merits or its source," explained Morrow.[37]

The eclectics were equally concerned with the efforts of homeopathy to expand into the West. The possibility of a homeopathic college in Cleveland had been discussed but no definitive action was taken by its supporters. To prevent this, the faculty and trustees of the Eclectic Medical Institute agreed to include the principles and practice of homeopathy in their instruction and invited the homeopathic physicians of the United States to nominate a professor to fill the chair. The appointment was given to Dr. Storm Rosa of Painesville, Ohio. In addition Dr. David Sheppard of Bainbridge, Ohio accepted the faculty's invitation to contribute a homeopathic column in the college's official organ, the *Eclectic Medical Journal.* Although the initiative collapsed following the 1849–50 session, the liberality of these two actions delayed by several years the eventual establishment of the first homeopathic college (Western College of Homeopathic Medicine) in the Middle West.[38] "Thus ended," wrote historian Harvey Wickes Felter, "the attempt to mix oil and water."[39]

In 1850, at the National Eclectic Medical Association's annual meeting held at Cincinnati, Joseph R. Buchanan was elected the association's new president. Unlike Morrow, Buchanan was not a strong advocate of the national organization, believing in his heart that regional conventions were more important. Nevertheless he established committees on theory and practice, obstetrics, surgery, physiology, materia medica, medical botany, chemistry, pharmacy, statistics, hydropathy, homeopathy, neurology, chrono-thermalism, and one that would study and compare the relative merits of the different systems of medicine. Buchanan was a strong supporter of Louis's numerical system and urged use of his methodology as a means of demonstrating the strength of the eclectic approach to therapeutics.[40]

Following Buchanan's presidency, the association was sustained by the efforts of Calvin Newton, the next president, and Thomas Cooke and others from New England

and the Middle States. At its annual meeting in New York in 1851, the association adopted a platform that supported vitalism and condemned all regimens that were depletive in nature, including bloodletting and the use of mercury and tartar emetic. The convention also recognized the merger of physiopathic and eclectic physicians under the name "Reform Medical Physicians" and renounced all other appellations. As a result of this action, numerous Independent Thomsonian groups, using the older titles of "physo," "physio," and "physio-medical" changed their names to conform with the new title.[41]

Regardless of pretenses, the annual meetings of the National Eclectic Medical Association were anything but cordial. Those in attendance sought to take advantage of their position by redressing old wounds, making accusations, and forcing votes on partisan issues. Topics turned on professional dissensions and jealousies, resolutions lodged against unchartered schools, unhealthy competition, free tuition strategies, and qualifications for membership. Despite the outward appearance of cooperation, the eclectics and Independent Thomsonians were never good bedfellows.

At the third annual meeting of the National Eclectic Medical Association in Rochester, New York, in May 1852, members traveled from Canada as well as from the eastern and middle states. They adopted the designation of "eclectic" and announced the association's determination to give the eclectic theory of medicine a scientific as well as a practical respectability, pulling it and its members away from the influence of the Thomsonians.

Three years later, the eclectic physicians of New York convened a two-day national convention in June 1855 at Fountain Hall in New York City. Their object was to prepare a constitution and platform of principles that would bring together under a single banner all medical reformers. Wooster Beach, chairman of the convention, failed to obtain consensus and the meeting ended with a committee of six appointed to draft a platform of principles and report their results at their next annual meeting of the National Eclectic Medical Association.

The following year, the National Eclectic Medical Association met at the Stuyvesant Institute in New York City with delegates from Ohio, Connecticut, Pennsylvania and several other states. Unfortunately, the proposed union between the Independent Thomsonians (physopaths) and eclectics in New York created apprehension among reformers in both the South and West who derisively regarded the union as "a conglomeration."[42] Before the convention adjourned, the delegates passed the following resolutions:

> 1st. Resolved, That we regard it as one of the most important duties of the medical profession, to investigate truth, from whatever source it may come, and in every proper mode to encourage the fullest and freest investigation by all.

> 2d. Resolved, That we regard all combinations to proscribe and degrade any portion of the medical profession, merely on account of a difference of opinion in matters of science, as a serious crime against the true interest of the profession, against the welfare of the community, and against the common rights of man.
>
> 3d. Resolved, That it is incumbent upon all medical reformers to regard all members of the profession in a spirit of liberality and courtesy; to abstain from all personal and disparaging remarks in reference to differences of doctrine, and to cultivate those amicable relations which admit of co-operation in the pursuit of truth.
>
> 4th. Resolved, That the great struggle of the present day in medical science is between the spirit of freedom on the one hand, which is seeking boldly for truth in science, and the spirit of conservative despotism on the other, which aims to perpetuate opinions by the force of organized combinations, and to discountenance or suppress every attempt at reform, whatever may be its merits or its source.
>
> 5th. Resolved, That we regard all medical reformers who are struggling for the improvement and the freedom of the profession, as engaged in a holy cause, and that we regard it as a duty of all such, whatever may be their differences of opinion upon minor points, to unite in the most cordial manner, as the American colonies united in their struggle for freedom.
>
> 6th. Resolved, That as the confederacy of the patriotic colonies which achieved the freedom of America resulted in the establishment of a national union of independent States, forming a true republic, so we hope that the confederacy of the medical reformers may not only achieve a revolution, but establish in the highest degree of freedom and harmony, the confederated republic of medical sciences.[43]

Notwithstanding its platform of principles, the National Eclectic Medical Association showed signs of distress. A combination of regional jealousies, national sectionalism, party spirit, and apprehension regarding the power and intrusiveness of the national association caused these two sectarian groups to maintain their separate identities. In reality, the National Eclectic Medical Association survived as long as it did because it accepted the individuality of its many parts. However, its annual meetings were discontinued after the eighth convention held in June 1857 at Cincinnati. So few attended the meeting that there was not even a notification canceling the 1858 meeting.

According to Alexander Wilder, the association "passed away unnoticed and hardly remembered."[44]

Baltimore Convention

Spurred by their victories in state legislatures, and motivated as well by the waning of strict Thomsonism, medical reformers of different stripes began talking once again about some form of reconciliation. In October 1852, reformers from across the United States agreed to meet in Baltimore with the intention of resolving the philosophical and sectional differences left after the 1838 schism. The convention elected Alva Curtis of Cincinnati as president and twenty-nine vice presidents (one from each state). Despite strong hopes for consensus building, the delegates became hopelessly divided over an appropriate name for their national organization. A slim majority urged the term "Reformed Medical Association of the United States," while others offered substitute names that included "Thomsonian," "Physiological Medical," "Physio-Medical," "Physopathic," "Antipathic," and "Physio-American." Eventually, the convention settled on Reformed Medical Association of the United States.

Before closing, the convention formulated a platform of principles that held forth the ideas of Reform Medicine. The two-day convention also established committees on medical journals, a platform of medical principles, the convening of a national convention, a committee on state medical reform, and a committee on concentrated medicines.[45]

In terms of principles, the convention approved the following:

1. The rejection of all dangerous and deleterious methods that tend to impair the vital powers.

2. In every case of disease or morbid action such remedies only are necessary as will aid, not retard, the recuperative efforts of the system; therefore depletive agents, or those which are permanently so, are not needed to cure disease.

3. While we rely almost entirely upon vegetable medicines in the treatment of disease, and believe that they are best adapted to restore the sick to a normal or healthy condition, we do not proscribe such mineral or animal preparations as are found to act in harmony with the laws of human economy.

4. We will be known and recognized by the name of Reformed Medical Physicians, renouncing all former distinctive appellations and unite on the foregoing broad platform of principles.[46]

Following the Baltimore meeting, reform societies from Maine to Georgia adopted the new title of "Reform" in their official name. In 1858, for example, the Botanic Medical Society of the State of New York changed its name to the New York State Association of Reformed Physicians. Other schools made similar changes. The Southern Botanico-Medical College of Macon became the Reform Medical College in 1856. Additionally, southerners formed the Southern Reform Medical Association. Much of this was evidence of movement among liberal Thomsonians toward more eclectic principles.[47]

Unfortunately for the Reform medical movement, only the southern states (Virginia, Georgia, Alabama, Mississippi, Arkansas, Tennessee, and Kentucky) seemed able to come together in harmony over matters of common concern. Recognizing their inability to bring about a "national" association, southerners urged that there be strong state associations as well as a "southern" association. Thus the Southern Reform Medical Association continued to meet until the outbreak of the Civil War. After the war, the surviving elements of reform medicine and their respective colleges coalesced around the "eclectics" and became known as the American Reformed School of Medical Practice in the South. By contrast, the botanic and eclectic schools in the Northeast remained factionalized and unyielding in their relations with one another.[48]

Chapter 7. Between the Abrahams

In the period marked at one end by the assassination of Abraham Lincoln and at the other by the publication of Abraham Flexner's *Medical Education in the United States and Canada* (1910), the nation's acceptance of medical sectarianism began to wane. The explosiveness of new medical technologies along with advances in physiological knowledge, the greater sharing of professional information, and the promotion of medical uniformity, combined with the organized attacks by the American Medical Association to reshape the nation's view of irregular medical groups. The unswerving confidence that society once held in the free market of medical theories and practices came under doubt as public opinion shifted the boundaries of acceptability between orthodox and irregular or sectarian therapies. The emergence of biomedicine constituted a radically different reality to the generation that had once placed its trust in multiple healing systems. The plausibility that the universe could be reduced to a single set of governing principles lost cachet as the sphere of scientific reductionism gained ascendancy over the unseen spiritual forces governing sectarian medicine's world view.

In this new era of medical empiricism, challenging new benchmarks were established for the education and the licensing of physicians. Having thrived in an age of unsettled standards, sectarian medicine faced the daunting challenge of growing beyond its fiery renunciations of mainstream medicine to build a permanent and defensible structure for its beliefs. The age of empiricism had arrived, and with it, the emergence of laboratory science, controlled clinical trials, pharmacology, and the proliferation of medical specialties. Medicine that was once speculative and built on *first principles* was now reined in by results that were both measurable and repeatable. Cryptic references to spirit-like activity and an overtly metaphysical view of the universe were replaced with an empirically-tested system of medicine. Healing had moved from heroic practices and an articulated philosophy that aligned the patient with providential laws and purposes to procedures based on physical examination by hand and ear, pathological anatomy, statistical analysis, and laboratory medicine.

The Physios

As noted in chapter 4, the garrulous followers of Samuel Thomson had split in 1838 into two competing groups: the strict Thomsonians and the Independents or "New Lights." Within a short few years, the strict Thomsonians melted into obscurity while the Independents positioned themselves within the broader landscape of medical education by establishing schools whose curricula, for the most part, followed the model set by medical orthodoxy. A total of fourteen schools, variously called Thomsonian, Independent Thomsonian, Botanico-Medical, or Physio-Medical, opened before 1860. This included one school that taught both Thomsonism and eclectic practice. Another ten schools organized during the second half of the century. While none of these schools could be deemed equivalent to any of the elite university-based regular schools, they were by no means without credibility. Proprietary (i.e., single ownership or joint-stock company) in their organizational and fiscal structure, they functioned like many regular schools by relying on a combination of tuition and fees to underwrite the salaries of their professors, almost all of whom supplemented their teaching with income from private practice. Proud of their sectarian identity and equally proud of their physician-patient focus, they laid claim to preserving the role and function of the family practitioner in an age of increasing specialism. In the absence of effective licensing or a consensus within the broader culture as to the appropriate standards for educating physicians, the proprietary school model offered blue-collar American medical students a relatively quick and inexpensive ticket into the profession.

The Independent Thomsonians were holdovers in the transition from the eighteenth-century system-builders to the Paris Clinical School, and from the French clinical tradition to modern bacteriology and German laboratory medicine. While better funded schools were coming to recognize the importance of laboratory facilities; building a firm connection between the medical department and the larger university; revolutionizing the teaching wards in hospitals; and increasing the number of faculty teaching basic medical science, the physios chose a much more cautious path. For them, laboratory medicine represented a choice and a direction that took the physician away from the patient and encouraged a professionalism that seemed alien to the personal side of medicine. Notwithstanding their public utterances, the physios were never at ease with the demands of the new age. Moreover, they had neither the financial power nor the intellectual force to manage the changes expected of them.

Few of the physio-medical colleges graduated more than a handful of students annually. Like other reform schools, they were principally didactic in their pedagogy, offering four to six lectures each day, except for Wednesdays and Saturdays when students attended clinics. While the physios extended to women the opportunity to participate in the role of healer, in truth, more women took advantage of the opportunity in the first half of the century than in the second half. As it turned out, women became the earliest casualties of medicine's increased standards.

The intellectual center for physio-medicalism was the Physio-Medical College of Indiana. The school garnered the title because of the strong theoretical grounding of its program and the reputation of its faculty, principally Joseph M. Thurston, author of *The Philosophy of Physiomedicalism. Its Theorem, Corollary, and Laws of Application for the Cure of Disease* (1900). Thurston, who held the chair of histology and pathology at the college, made vitalistic principles the bedrock of physio-medical theory. As an active participant in the regional meetings, he annually put forward resolutions advocating vitalism and condemning the materialistic philosophies of English naturalist Charles Darwin (1809–1882), German biologist and philosopher Ernst Haeckel (1834–1919), and English biologist Thomas Huxley (1825–1895).[1]

Given that vitalism was the first principle of physio-medical practice, its medicines were viewed as a form of matter acted on by the bioplasm (the form upon which the life and functional activity of the cell depended) and integrated into the organism as vital energy. In essence, the physician's responsibility was to imitate the efforts of vital force in treating disease. In choosing their medicines, the physios relied principally on lobelia, capsicum, and the vapor bath—all remedies touted by Samuel Thomson. Although they expanded upon Thomson's original materia medica, they remained well within the botanic framework of Thomsonian practice.[2]

Because of their emphasis on "sanative medicines" (those that supported the healing power of nature), the physios condemned all manner of "poisons" (i.e., opium, morphine, belladonna, aconite, alcohol, arsenic, mercury, strychnine, etc.) used by regulars in their daily practice. Their opposition also extended to Koch's Postulates and serum therapy. No amount of dilution could change an antitoxin's inherent virulency or convert it into a sanative agent. Rather than rely on an antitoxin immunization, the physios turned to capsicum and lobelia to assist the vital force in asserting itself over the organism and thus checking the toxins in the system; and instead of typical antiseptics such as bichloride of mercury or carbolic acid, they turned to poultices of lobelia seed and elm, hayseed and wood ashes, or charcoal and hop yeast.[3] As self-proclaimed "bug cranks," they held fast to the belief that bacteria were "a good thing to have in a wound" and that Edward Koch was nothing more than a "German Bacilli-Maniac." Bacteria were not pathogenic; rather, disease was the result of a depressed or lowered vital action in the living organism and thus furnished a culture medium for microorganisms which proceeded to lower the condition of the neighboring solids and fluids. But microorganisms were not themselves the cause of disease.[4]

While the early physios had access to a broad choice of botanical medicines prepared by regular pharmacies and wholesale botanic firms, the decline of Thomsonism meant a commensurate decline of this supportive drug industry. However grateful they were for these botanic preparations, the physios begrudged their lack of options and objected as well to the concentrated medicines of the eclectics. Unlike the eclectics and homeopaths, the physios opposed the use of alcohol in their medicines, preferring instead to use liquid syrups or water. Given the limitations placed on the preparation of their medicines, those physios practicing in the second half of the century were forced to depend on an ever narrowing list of eclectic and regular pharmaceutical preparations. As a result, it was not uncommon for physios to gather and prepare their own medicines.[5]

A major impediment to the future of physio-medicalism stemmed from the inability to establish and sustain its national organization. After the dissolution of the Reformed Medical Association of the United States that formed in the wake of the Baltimore Convention in 1852 and its replacement with two regional organizations known as the Middle States Reformed Medical Society and the Southern Reform Medical Association, efforts were undertaken in 1877 and 1879 to bring together botanic reformers in another national undertaking. Although some state societies responded positively to the invitation, most divided on the nature of representation and whether the invitation included "uncertified" individuals, including eclectics. The Indiana physios, for example, were intent on opening the proposed convention to *all* reformers, regardless of affiliation or credentials. Those who opposed an open convention feared that the meeting would be inundated with graduates of unchartered schools and nefarious diploma mills.[6]

As a result of this internecine bickering, plans were delayed until 1883 when forty-eight physios representing nine states met in Indianapolis and organized the American Association of Physio-Medical Physicians and Surgeons. Known affectionately as "The American," the association was soon consumed by controversy as members argued over the germ theory; debated the doctrine of vitalism; fought over the minutes of their meetings; lamented the lack of statistics to support their claims; discussed the avoidance of research and investigation; and worried over the incursion of "eclecto-allopathic" ideas into the organization. Despite these divisive issues, the truth of the matter was that the members of "The American" were more parochial than national in their interests; moreover, throughout the organization's brief history, it consisted of too many malcontents eager to fight and bully their opponents. The meetings themselves were unstructured, with the president of the association acting as discussion leader in what could only be described as a convention of extremely opinionated individuals. This lack of internal cohesion was a principal reason for the organization's demise. The last formal meeting of "The American" occurred in 1905.[7]

It became clear to the faculty of the remaining schools that their overtly metaphysical view of the causal forces underlying disease and their dogged insistence on a truly vegetable materia medica had limited the impact of their reform ideas to an ever narrowing corps of believers. In order to survive, they found themselves moving into the eclectics' camp and eventually coming under their direction. Over time, each of the schools with the word "botanico" in its title (i.e., Southern Botanico-Medical College; New England Botanico-Medical College; and The Botanico-Medical College of Mempis) was renamed and the word "eclectic" added. In each instance, the merger with eclectics forced changes in the philosophy and direction of the institutions.

Of the Independent Thomsonian schools that existed in the second half of the nineteenth century, both Alva Curtis's Physio-Medical College and William Nicely's Physio-Eclectic Medical College became out-and-out diploma mills conducting their affairs without trustees, faculty, or a charter, and offering students a "good diploma" for the price of fifty dollars. For William H. Cook (1832–99) who owned and managed the Physio-Medical Institute of Cincinnati, and who helped expose them to authorities, the good name of physio-medicalism had been sullied by these crooks and their deceptive practices.[8] Other schools designated as fraudulent included the Curtis Physio-Medical Institute of Marion, Indiana, incorporated in 1881, and the Twentieth Century Physio-Medical College of Guthrie, Oklahoma, incorporated in 1900.

By the time of Abraham Flexner's visits in 1909 to the 155 schools operating in North America, only one physio-medical college remained—the College of Medicine and Surgery, Physio-Medical, of Chicago. Flexner visited the school in April of that year and, after a "diligent search of the office desk and safe, failed to discover any credentials of students now in the school." With an attendance of thirty-three students and a teaching staff of forty-two, none of whom were fulltime, he found that the school survived on tuition revenues of less than $3,000 annually. As for clinical facilities, students had the opportunity to attend a total of 167 patients (half of whom were surgical) at a private hospital and 250 in its dispensary over the course of a year.[9] In 1911, the college was absorbed by the College of Medicine and Surgery (eclectic). This action officially ended the seventy-two year history of physio-medicalism in the United States.[10]

The Eclectics

Among the eclectic colleges, twenty-six (including two mixed systems) were organized before 1860; and forty-three (including one mixed system) were founded after 1860. Along with other proprietary schools—both regular and irregular—that served America's demand for family doctors in the last half of the century, the eclectics were forced to take their place in the backwaters of the nation's medical reform efforts. Far in advance were university-based schools such as Harvard, Yale, Columbia, Pennsylvania, Michigan, Syracuse, and Cornell that had begun to overhaul their programs utilizing the emerging laboratory medicine drawn from the German educational system. These were reforms that forward-looking presidents such as Charles Eliot at Harvard, Seth Low and Nicholas Murray Butler of Columbia, James Angell of Michigan, and William Pepper at Pennsylvania had heralded and under whose leadership emerged the modern university. Supported by a combination of public tax revenues, private endowments, student tuition and fees, these university-based medical schools were able to pay their faculty, build modern laboratories, purchase needed equipment, and affiliate with hospitals and dispensaries.[11]

Along with university-based medical schools that moved with dispatch to advance the ethos of research, leadership came from the A.M.A.'s Council of Medical Education, the Association of American Medical Colleges, as well as from private foundations, state licensing boards, and state boards of health. Added to this list were scientific societies such as the American Surgical Association (1880), the Association of American Physicians (1886), the American Physiological Society (1887), the American Association of Anatomists (1888), the Pediatric Society (1888), and the American Association of Pathologists and Bacteriologists (1900), whose membership played a key role in transforming academic medicine into a stronger pedagogy.

By the 1890s, only sixty of the approximately 158 medical schools in North America had some connection, however tenuous, to a university—a factor that became increasingly important when considering the cost of library collections and laboratory equipment, and the importance of the basic medical sciences (physics, chemistry, anatomy, zoology, physiology, and bacteriology) in the curriculum. As medicine was coming into its own as an applied science, schools had all the more reason to demand that students be trained in the "fundamentals" of the basic sciences. This new reality hit hardest among the proprietary schools whose financial stability depended upon the less expensive lecture mode of teaching.[12]

By 1890, twenty-three of the ninety-four regular medical schools still had no established requirements for matriculation. Of the nineteen homeopathic colleges and ten eclectic schools, only one required a grammar school education; the other nine required an examination, *or its equivalent*. One need emphasize that, until certification became a nationally accepted phenomenon requiring a standardized set of course requirements, the provision, *or its equivalent,* concealed a host of omissions and indiscretions. In fact, the actual admissions standards listed in school catalogs bore little resemblance to accepted practices. Numerous schools even allowed students to embark on their programs with the understanding that they would make up any deficiencies after admission.[13]

By 1893, the eclectics had moved forward with lengthened terms and three annual courses of lectures. These changes still lagged behind the 1894 recommendation of the Association of American Medical Colleges for a four-year program of at least four courses of lectures of not less than six months each.[14] In defense of their three-year terms, the eclectics argued that while the proposed new curricula and longer sessions would most certainly assist medical students qualifying for the more advanced specialties, the changes would inadvertently undermine the importance of the general practitioner and ultimately leave millions of families without adequate medical care. In essence, the eclectics hoped to avoid public criticism by establishing the legitimacy of what they believed was an alternative path to a medical degree that would ensure the future of the family practitioner. Notwithstanding this rationale, the eclectic schools that resisted change fell from sight. Some closed; others found themselves providing an increasingly marginalized education; and a few, like the Wisconsin Eclectic Medical College in Milwaukee, chose to move into the arena of outright fraud by offering diplomas for thirty-five dollars to all with aspirations of practicing medicine.[15]

During this period, the eclectic colleges were drawing their students from three principal sources. One was the sons and daughters of eclectic physicians and blue-collar families. These students were typically strong proponents of eclectic philosophy and entered the profession as family physicians. They joined their local and state societies and were members as well in the National Eclectic Medical Association; they stayed in close touch with former teachers and fellow graduates, subscribed to eclectic journals, and remained true to their eclectic affiliation.

A second source of students were those who, having received low grades and "honorable dismissals" (dismissal for academic reasons rather than behavior problems, cheating, etc.) from a regular medical college, transferred to eclectic schools in the hope of being given a "second chance." For them, eclectic medicine did not represent a belief system so much as an alternative point of entry into medicine. A perusal of admission documents at the Eclectic Medical Institute in Cincinnati indicates that these students were, at best, marginal, many of whom carried grades of C, D, and F into their programs and remained at some level of academic distress through the remainder of their education. Even though these students owed their medical degree to the forbearance of eclectic administrators, upon graduation, they almost always cut their ties with eclecticism. Few chose to support their alma mater or show any allegiance with the philosophy or with their fellow graduates.[16]

The third source of students, sometimes representing more than half of each graduating class, and clearly the most eager, bright, and anxious to excel, were Orthodox Jews. These students were not adherents to eclectic philosophy; rather they had matriculated in eclectic schools because of selective admissions policies and "quotas" erected to prevent their entrance into mainstream medical schools. These were the sons of orthodox Jews whose families had migrated from Eastern Europe and who found themselves barred from regular medical schools in the Northeast. Without question, they were among the brightest students in the eclectic colleges and earned some of the highest scores on state licensure tests. Nevertheless, like the "second chance" students, they were anxious to divest themselves of any association with eclecticism following their graduation obligations. Most returned to the East Coast where they quickly mainstreamed into regular medicine, disowned any eclectic affiliation, made no effort to identify with their fellow graduates or with eclectic philosophy, and refused to provide their alma mater with financial support.[17]

The motivation of these three groups of students suggest that eclectic education was being perpetuated under a mixed set of reasons, only one of which was genuinely supportive of eclectic philosophy. Lacking public revenues to support their schools, and dependent upon the good will of alumni and friends, the eclectic schools found themselves estranged from a large percentage of their alumni. The actions of these graduates left the colleges politically weak and financially starved. Each had been motivated to attend eclectic colleges for reasons other than an adherence to eclectic philosophy. No school, least of all those whose financial futures depended upon faithful alumni and a healthy endowments, could survive under these circumstances.

The National Eclectic Medical Association, organized in 1849, had little of the power flexed by its nemesis, the American Medical Association. Consisting of a loose confederation of local and state societies, it represented between eight and ten thousand eclectics across the country. In truth, however, the societies had been overrun by interlopers of all types. They became a "catch-all" for all types of healers and diploma-mill graduates seeking some semblance of legitimacy. True eclectics felt dirtied by their presence but did little to eject them.

The lack of strong local, state, and national organizations weighed heavily in the eclectics' inability to establish the legitimacy of what they thought important in medicine, medical education, and the nation's health care. At the forefront of the new reform was the leadership of the nation's premier universities who focused their energies on the adoption of German-based pedagogy; the replacement of student tuition- and fee-based structures with tax-supported revenues; strengthening clinical arrangements with hospitals; demanding stronger premedical academic competencies; and insisting on graded and lengthened curricula. While the American Medical Association and its membership seized control of state examining boards and took pleasure in claiming responsibility for tighter standards, the eclectics found themselves fighting a rearguard action by continuing to defend minimal standards and the diminished status of the family practitioner.

Overwhelmed by the movement to higher standards, the eclectics grudgingly began to blend their pedagogy with that of regular medicine. This included greater attention to research and scientific medicine, graded courses, additional curricula, lengthened terms, and more clinical experience. Nevertheless, as proprietary schools dependent upon tuition and fees, they were obliged to temper their reforms with available resources. This caused them to lag behind more aggressive university-based schools and to find excuses for delaying implementation of generally accepted reforms. For a nation on its way to becoming a world power, the eclectics came to be perceived as living in the past rather than preparing students for the future. There is little question that the proponents of true eclecticism had become lethargic. Clearly, the reform spirit of eclecticism's halycon years had long passed and the newer forces of industrialism, urbanization, immigration, and educational reform were feeding on energies that had earlier formed the basis of their inner strength and stamina.

When the American Medical Association revised its Code of Ethics in 1901, it offered in a spirit of good will and liberality to accept the eclectics as bona fide members provided they drop their sectarian designation. For hardcore eclectics the offer was interpreted as a deceptive method for destroying sectarianism once and for all. "How peaceful the regular lion will look, after swallowing the innocent eclectic and homeopathic lambs," remarked Rolla Thomas, dean of the Eclectic Medical College in Cincinnati.[18] Nevertheless, for many eclectics, including those student groups who had little allegiance with eclectic philosophy, the offer was accepted as a matter of expediency.

The eclectics were hard-pressed to ignore the implications of their declining numbers. By 1902 there were only ten colleges still in existence and only the Eclectic Medical Institute of Cincinnati, founded in 1845, continued into the second half of the century. All the others had organized between 1865 and 1901. By the time of Flexner's visits, only eight eclectic schools remained: the Eclectic Medical Institute (1845) of Cincinnati; the Eclectic Medical College of the City of New York (1865); Lincoln Medical College (1889) in Nebraska; California Medical College (1879) in San Francisco; American Medical College (1873) in St. Louis; Georgia College of Eclectic Medicine and Surgery (1866) in the Hospital Medical College (1908) of Atlanta; and the Western Eclectic College of Medicine (1898) in Kansas City, Kansas.

Flexner's comments on each of these remaining schools was both explicit and compelling.

1. *California Medical College*—Organized in Oakland in 1879, it had "a roving and precarious existence," moving to San Francisco in 1887 and then reorganizing in Los Angeles in 1907. The school occupied "a few neglected rooms on the second floor of a fifty-foot frame building" with equipment that was "dirty and disorderly beyond description." Its anatomy program consisted of a "box of bones" and the "dried-up filthy fragments of a single cadaver." Its chemical laboratory consisted of a "few bottles of reagents," and its pathology equipment consisted of a single microscope and "a few unlabeled" specimens. Flexner concluded that the school "is a disgrace to the state whose laws permit its existence."[19]

2. *Georgia College of Eclectic Medicine and Surgery*—Organized in 1877, it occupied a building which, with respect to filth, "has few equals, but no superiors, among medical schools." Its anatomy room contained a single foul cadaver while its

chemical laboratory consisted of a few old tables, a number of nondescript bottles and no water or drains. Its pathological laboratory was supported with three microscopes and a few dirty slides. The school was without clinical facilities and "nothing more disgraceful calling itself a medical school can be found anywhere."[20]

3. *Hospital Medical College*—Organized in 1908 "on four weeks' notice" by secessionists from the Georgia College of Eclectic Medicine and Surgery, it had resources in the amount of $3,950 and occupied several rooms at the rear of a private infirmary. Flexner could find little in the way of equipment that belonged to the school.[21]

4. *Western Eclectic College of Medicine and Surgery*—Organized as a stock company in 1898 in Kansas City, Kansas, it operated on approximately $1,600 in tuition and fees each year. Its laboratory facilities were "indescribably dirty and disorderly," containing three microscopes, a few bacteriological stains, meager chemistry equipment, and no running water. All laboratory work was conducted by one teacher who divided his time with the two local osteopathic and homeopathic schools. Although Flexner noted that the school's catalog indicated that clinics were held weekly at the Kansas City Missouri Hospital, the statement was vigorously denied by the hospital's superintendent.[22]

5. *American Medical College*—Organized in 1873 in St. Louis, it operated on an estimated $3,800 in tuition and fees. According to Flexner, its equipment for anatomy, chemistry, pathology and bacteriology was "meager" and "there is no suggestion of use." It offered a weekly clinic at the City Hospital, and at its dispensary, "almost every day some one comes."[23]

6. *Lincoln Medical College*—Organized in 1890, it was nominally the medical department of Cotner University. Forty-two students were in attendance and its available resources from tuition and fees amounted to $3,800 annually. According to Flexner there were virtually no laboratory facilites beyond a "separate room set aside for dissecting." Moreover there were no clinical opportunities for students, not even a dispensary.[24]

7. *Eclectic Medical College*—Organized in 1865 in New York City, it had an attendance of 96 students and no full-time instructors. Flexner noted that its chemical laboratory was adequate for teaching but its other facilities were not up to standard. The school contained a "fair-sized library" of older texts and clinical facilities were provided twice weekly at Sydenham Hospital which had eighty free beds.[25]

8. *Eclectic Medical Institute*—Chartered in 1845, it required a four-year high school education, or its equivalent, for Ohio students but students from other states were

> not held to the same standard. Its attendance was 86 students with no fulltime instructors. Flexner noted that a new building had been provided for its laboratory facilities and that it contained a good dissecting-room; meager equipment for histology, pathology, and bacteriology; a small museum and library; and that its course of instruction was not graded. As for clinical facilities, it adjoined Seton Hospital and had access to the institution's 60 beds ("of which not over 24 are usable") and that the school's authorities did not know whether their students attended public clinics at the city hospital.[26]

Of the eight eclectic schools, Flexner found nothing even remotely resembling what they described in their catalogs. They talked of having laboratories, "not because they appreciate their place or significance, but because it pays them to defer thus far to the spirit of the times." Indeed, the schools were "utter failures" in making good on their own tenets. With the exception of the Eclectic Medical Institute of Cincinnati, laboratory facilities were nearly nonexistent. Five of the schools were "without exception filthy and almost bare," and of the eight, none provided adequate clinical opportunities for their students. "All of this is criminally inadequate, yet it is the best that the eclectics offer," Flexner concluded. To their detriment, all were dependent on tuition and fees and only three—the New York, Cincinnati, and Atlanta schools—enjoyed revenues in excess of $5,000 annually. Their combined enrollments had decreased from 1,014 in 1904 to a mere 84 in 1909.[27]

In the aftermath of Flexner's polemical report, the older generation of eclectics became introspective and truculent, drifting increasingly into a more contemptuous attitude toward change, defensive when it came to the role of the family practitioner, and comfortable in their musings about their illustrative past. Rather than surrender to regular medicine's lexicon of germ theory, serotherapy, and scientific reductionism, they held firm to vitalistic principles, opposed the use of coal-tar preparations, showed a decided preference for general practice, advocated conservation in gynecology and surgery, and pushed specific diagnosis and specific medication as the distinctive elements of their practice. The younger eclectics, on the other hand, continued to downplay their differences with mainstream medicine thereby avoiding the stigma of sectarianism that the public had concluded was no longer justified.[28]

Failing to provide its students with needed laboratories and instruction, the Eclectic Medical College of the City of New York closed in 1913, while the Georgia College of Eclectic Medicine and Surgery in Atlanta closed a year later. In the Far West, the California Eclectic Medical College closed its doors in 1915, while in the Midwest the Western Eclectic College of Medicine and Surgery was reorganized as the Kansas City College of Medicine and Surgery in 1915 and then suspended operations in 1918. Lincoln Medical College in Nebraska was renamed the Cotner University Medical

College in 1911 and then resumed its older title in 1915 before closing permanently in 1918. The American Medical College of St. Louis dropped its eclectic affiliation in 1910 and absorbed Barnes Medical College to become the Medical Department of the National University of Arts and Sciences which suspended operations in 1918.

Following licensure scandals in the 1920s involving eclectic examining boards in Arkansas, Kansas, and Connecticut, the eclectics fell into even greater disfavor. These, along with a host of diploma-mill trials and other scandals, including published reports on the percentage of eclectics failing state licensing exams, sullied what was left of their reputation. One by one, the last of the proprietary schools closed, leaving only the Eclectic Medical Institute of Cincinnati which succeeded in obtaining a "Class B" status from the Council on Medical Education of the American Medical Association. Although the school gave up its proprietary status, it too, would close its doors following the July 1, 1938 decision of the Council on Medical Education and Hospitals to carry no sectarian schools on its approved list.[29]

As for the National Eclectic Medical Association, it continued to function as a "knife and fork" society into the 1960s. The last record of its quarterly journal was the September-December issue in 1965.

The Homeopaths

Like the eclectics, there were a greater number of homeopathic schools organized after the Civil War than before. Although only nine (including one mixed system) were founded before 1860, fifty-seven schools (including two mixed-systems) were organized in the last half of the nineteenth century.

Unlike other sectarians, the clear majority of homeopaths in the first half of the century came from the ranks of regulars. Some had been in active practice for years before switching their allegiance over to homeopathy; others took their degrees from regular medical schools while faculty turned a blind eye to their homeopathic intentions. These experiences gave American homeopaths a unique perspective as well as options unavailable to most other irregulars. It is also important to understand that these early disciples of Hahnemann never intended to break away from regular medicine. Instead, they hoped homeopathy would eventually be recognized as a specialization. But when homeopaths turned to the dynamization of inert substances undergoing succussion or trituration, touted the immaterial powers of infinitesimal doses, and hypothesized on more spiritual and metaphysical views of healing, relations soured with their regular colleagues. As the oracular and mystical elements within homeopathy rose in importance, particularly those ideas and practices inspired by Emmanuel Swedenborg, homeopaths were shunned by mainstream doctors and ejected from their allopathic societies, thus forcing them to build their own parallel organizations.

Through the first half of the nineteenth century, American homeopathy projected two competing concepts of medicine. One was in consequence of the Paris Clinical School and evinced a non-ideological confidence in clinical record-keeping, empirical research, clinical anatomy, and an ever present confidence in the scientific method. The other was a more eccentric, religious disposition, that mingled homeopathy with liberal Christianity and tinkered with various fringe systems such as Isopathy, Baunscheidtism, Hydropathy, Mesmerism, and Grahamism, to mention only a few. For this latter group, homeopathy had transformed itself into *Hahnemannianism*, a term that acquired special meaning among the more visionary followers of Samuel Hahnemann who rejected pathology and physiology for a more eccentric, religious, and meandering spiritualism.[30]

For Flexner, the idea that homeopaths could accept the teaching of anatomy, pathology, bacteriology, physiology and clinical microscopy as the foundation blocks of modern medical education, and at the same time, assert certain a priori notions as first principles in some grandiose scheme was a wholly "self-contradictory" and incompatible proposition. Scientific medicine "brushes aside all historic dogma," whether from Hahnemann, Rush, or any other medical prophet. "The tendency to build a system out of a few partially apprehended facts, deductive inference filling in the rest, has not indeed been limited to medicine, but it has nowhere else had more calamitous consequences," Flexner wrote.[31]

> One may begin with science and work through the entire medical curriculum consistently, exposing everything to the same sort of test; or one may begin with a dogmatic assertion and resolutely refuse to entertain anything at variance with it. But one cannot do both. One cannot simultaneously assert science and dogma; one cannot travel half the road under the former banner, in the hope of taking up the latter, too, at the middle of the march. Science, once embraced, will conquer the whole.[32]

To his credit, Flexner praised homeopathy for its role in "discrediting" allopathic medicine when it was itself little more than a sect. Now, however, scientific medicine had brushed aside all of historical dogma, including allopathy. As William Osler once remarked, "A new school of practitioners has arisen which cares nothing for homeopathy and less for so-called allopathy. It seeks to study, rationally and scientifically, the actions of drugs, old and new."[33]

Over the course of the nineteenth century, sixty-four homeopathic schools were established to educate students and foster a sense of collective identity. By far, the majority of them were proprietary in nature, reflecting the impatience of American society for meeting the needs of a market-driven educational system; a smaller number were affiliated with stated-funded or private universities. Approximately a third of the schools were founded in Maryland, Massachusetts, New York, Pennsylvania, and the District of Columbia. The remaining two-thirds opened in California, Colorado, Illinois, Iowa, Kentucky, Michigan, Minnesota, Missouri, and Ohio. By 1900, only twenty-two schools remained with a combined enrollment of about 2,000 students.

The ridicule that came from the writings of regulars such as Oliver Wendell Holmes, John Forbes, Worthington Hooker, and James Y. Simpson in the second half of the nineteenth century did much to discredit the doctrine of infinitesimals and force academic homeopaths to abandon the more transcendental aspects of their medicine for a more laboratory-based system. Grudgingly, homeopaths admitted that their system had ignored too many of the advances in pathology and physiology and had lost sight of regular medicine's notable achievements in clinical therapeutics. By the 1870s, homeopaths were not only joining regulars in seeking additional training in Germany but there was a marked similarity in the curriculum of both regular and homeopathic schools. It appeared evident that the faculty in these schools were intent on supporting new research and building a professional identity unconnected with homeopathy's earlier dogmas. Leaders such as William Tod Helmuth, president of the Homeopathic Medical Society of New York State, went on record embracing a more catholic definition of homeopathy, including a commitment to laboratory science, advocating the mixture of homeopathic and regular therapies, and acknowledging the need for a more unified scientific practice of medicine.[34]

As increased numbers of homeopathic schools turned to more liberal interpretations of Hahnemann's principles, a divide occurred between the "purists" or high-potency Hahnemannians, and the "mixers" or low-potency wing often seen as more sympathetic with regulars and eclectics. The delicate relationship between these two contending groups had been maintained into the late 1870s but threatened to break apart local and state societies as well as create a schism within the American Institute of Homeopathy. Indicative of this was the establishment of the International Hahnemannian Association (1881) designed to preserve pure homeopathy against the incursion of more liberal views. The association's set of defining resolutions spoke volumes on the issues separating the two groups.

> Whereas, We believe the *Organon of the Healing Art* as promulgated by Samuel Hahnemann to be the only reliable guide in therapeutics; and
>
> Whereas, This clearly teaches that homeopathy consists in the law of similars, the single remedy, and the minimum dose of the dynamized drug, not singly, but collectively; and

> Whereas, A number of professed homeopathists not only repudiate these tenets, but violate them in practice; and
>
> Whereas, An effort has been made on the part of such physicians to unite the homeopathic with the allopathic school; therefore
>
> Resolved, That the time has fully come when legitimate Hahnemannian homeopathy should free itself from all such innovations, hurtful alike to its reputation as a science and fatal to the best interests of the sick.
>
> Resolved, That the mixing or alternating of two or more medicines displays on the part of the prescriber a lack of skill, besides being a species of empiricism, inexcusable and non-homeopathic.
>
> Resolved, That in non-surgical cases we regard medicated topical appliances and mechanical appliances as relics of the defunct customs of past ages, unscientific, non-homeopathic and often injurious.
>
> Resolved, That as "the best dose of medicine is ever the smallest," we cannot recognize as homeopathic the treatment of any physician who administers medicine in such quantities as to suppress symptoms by their primary or toxical action.
>
> Resolved, That we have no sympathy in common with those physicians who would engraft on to homeopathy the crude ideas and doses of the eclectics, and we will not hold ourselves responsible for their "fatal errors" and failures in practice.
>
> Resolved, That as some self-styled homeopathists have take occasion to traduce Hahnemann as a "fanatic," "dishonest" and "visionary," and his teachings as "not being the standard of the homeopathy of to-day," that we denounce all such as being traitors to our cause and recreant to its best interests.[35]

These resolutions became a clarion call for Hahnemannians to wrest control of their schools and societies; insist on practices that reinforced the true principles of Hahnemann, including the universality of the law of similars; and ensure that homeopathy represented a distinct school, not just a specialty within mainstream medicine.

When the American Medical Association revised its Constitution and Code of Ethics, giving members greater leeway in matters of consultation and admitting into membership eclectics and homeopaths willing to forgo their sectarian affiliations, the strategy succeeded in ending much of organized viciousness that had dominated the organization's past relationship with sectarians. But, more importantly, it diluted homeopathic identity as the public, including America's influential social elites, turned away from unconventional practices and to the acceptance of more rigorous medical standards. In effect, a migration took place within the liberal wing of homeopathy as they took the opportunity to mainstream into regular medicine. In the wake of tightened standards, licensing legislation, greater A.M.A. oversight, and a wholesale change in public opinion, homeopathy faced one of two options: either to withdraw into isolation to protect its remaining tenets, or join the "melting-pot" of schools moving resolutely into the camp of modern medicine. For the liberal wing of homeopathy, there seemed to be only one option available.[36]

By the turn of the century, few of homeopathy's colleges continued to teach Hahnemann's original principles. A search of school catalogs found only two schools offering lectures on Hahnemann's *Organon of the Rational Art of Healing* and only one school had it taught by a fulltime faculty member. In other words, the anchor of homeopathic instruction had been replaced by a variety of new texts, few of which were homeopathic in content. Neither faculty nor students had remained loyal to the principles of Hahnemann. Most had concluded that Hahnemann's critique of orthodox medicine and his principles of reform were no longer relevant by modern standards; that the homeopathic materia medica lacked scientific verification; that provings lacked completeness; that homeopathic repertories were unreliable; and that all had been trumped by the newer advances in medical science. Indeed, it was not uncommon to find faculty and students talking about coal tar derivatives, antitoxins, serum treatments, hypodermic medication, drug combinations, and an assortment of palliative treatments.

In was in this context that Flexner made his visits to the fifteen remaining homeopathic colleges in 1909. He found that only five required more than a high school education for admission; the remaining eleven had admission standards that, like the eclectics, were best defined by the words "or its equivalent." As for laboratories, he concluded that although homeopathic faculty agreed on their importance, they seemed to have taken "no active part" in their development. And with the exception of Boston University, there seemed to be little or no evidence of research being carried out at any of the schools. In the state universities of Iowa and Michigan which offered both regular and homeopathic instruction, and where the basic sciences were provided by the regular department, homeopathic students found themselves at a marked disadvantage because of their lower admission standards and, therefore, lack of adequate academic preparation. Of all the schools, only Boston University, the New York Homeopathic College, and Hahnemann of Philadelphia possessed the necessary equipment to teach the fundamental branches of science. The remaining schools had little to offer in the way of equipment and facilities beyond dissection and elementary chemistry. In San Francisco Hahnemann, no experimental physiology was taught because the faculty "doesn't believe in it."[37]

Six of the homeopathic schools came in for special criticism. Southwestern in Louisville, Pulte in Cincinnati, Atlantic in Baltimore, and the Detroit and Kansas City schools were categorized as "utterly hopeless" due to the "total unfitness of their managers for any sort of educational responsibility." The six were "hopelessly poor," operating on between $1,500 and $4,000 annually. Over and over again, Flexner used phrases such as "poor record-keeping," "blot on the state," "scant and dirty," "woe-begone," and "without merit" to describe these weaker schools.[38]

In the decade following the publication of Flexner's *Medical Education in the United States and Canada,* the number of homeopathic schools declined. In 1912, the Detroit Homeopathic closed while the College of Homeopathic Medicine in the State University of Iowa merged with the regular medical department. Within a year, Hering Medical College closed, as did the Kansas City Hahnemann Medical College and the Homeopathic Medical College of Missouri. By 1923, only Hahnemann Medical College and Hospital of Philadelphia and New York Homeopathic Medical College and Flower Hospital continued operations. But the financial weakness of these remaining schools combined with the reduction of students, forced American homeopaths to question their future as a distinct sect.

In the years that followed the publication of Flexner's report, homeopathic doctors and the homeopathic laity began debating the causes that lay behind the disintegration of their educational system and the options that remained. Leaders from the liberal wing of the movement thought the time was long overdue for homeopathy to surrender its sectarian label and merge into regular medicine. For this group, homeopathy had run its course and the reasons for its separate existence were no longer justified. Indeed, both regular medicine and "low potency" homeopathy had changed dramatically over the course of their history—to the degree that their remaining differences were minimal. A second group advocated the closing of all but the strongest schools which, if strategically located, could be supported at a level that would transform them into models of homeopathic education and research. Finally, there were those who were convinced that homeopathy should divest itself of its colleges and, instead, establish postgraduate schools attached to hospitals, dispensaries, and laboratories and staffed by paid teachers and clinicians. The supporters of this last option blamed the colleges and their faculties for destroying the authenticity of academic homeopathy; nevertheless, they carried the hope that eventually it would find a place as a specialty within regular medicine.[39]

The failure of homeopathy to be recognized as a specialty in regular medicine and the concomitant rise in power of the laity whose lot had been cast with the more esoteric and "high potency" beliefs of Hahnemann, resulted in homeopathy's rejection of the reductionist biomedical paradigm and its gradual transformation into a faith-based system of healing.

* * *

The dream of a uniquely "American Practice" of medicine died slowly, brought about by an increasing number of clinicians who favored therapies based on empirically based laboratory and clinical research; the freeing of medical schools from their over dependence on student fees; higher salaried professorships; the support of governmental and philanthropic agencies for regular medicine; and the identification of several model university-centered and hospital-based medical schools. The catalyst for this mind-change came from the nearly 700 American doctors who studied in Paris between 1820 and the Civil War, acquiring an interest in clinical pathology; and the approximately 15,000 American doctors who augmented their medical education with additional laboratory and clinical training in Germany between 1870 and 1914. With these experiences came educational reform, the abatement of substandard schools, the building of research laboratories on American soil, and higher licensing standards.[40]

When assessing what the Thomsonians, eclectics, homeopaths, and physio-medicals accomplished, it is important to recognize that they represented a uniquely American ritual, tantamount to asserting that the principles of sectarian belief were not only different from medical orthodoxy, but that the diversity of medicine could survive and prosper within American society. It was clear from the early national period onward that every medical sect saw itself as the logical culmination of native experience and was particularly annoyed when European notions, whether by happenstance or design, slipped into their beliefs and practices. But what they hoped above all else was that no one medical approach, no one theory, and no one group could ever become exclusively dominant. Reflective of America's Protestant tradition, medical sectarians viewed the care and treatment of the sick as the responsibility of all, vindicating the principle of individual free will and voluntarism. These sectarians prospered in the first half of the nineteenth century, driven in large measure by the compatibility that their beliefs had with the culture's spirit of individualism, its love affair with voluntary associations, and its belief in community. Sectarianism in its many manifestations was among the irrepressible energies of the age.

After 1860, medical sectarianism had to confront the forces of a new age—industrialism, urbanization, an armamentarium of new healing weapons, and the rising expectations of the profession. Whereas the social landscape of the 1830s and 40s had barely comprehended how medicine would play out its part other than continued expansion into the far-reaching hinterland and an aversion to any legal restraints on the marketplace, the second half of the nineteenth century ushered in a more profound appreciation for the ideals and traditions of the learned profession. Using the inductive method, the object was to teach medicine not as a system of insulated rules or a priori principles but as the outcome of observations and experiments, where patience, utility, and science were understood to be the underpinnings of sound clinical judgment. One can hardly be astonished that doctors educated in Europe would argue the superiority of their training over the provincial inferiority of instruction received at home. Patriotic indignation against things European no longer inflamed the public as it had in earlier years. Moving from a democratic era where no single school could pretend to be the official orthodoxy, and where the courts and legislatures had invoked the concept of laissez faire, it now became obvious that an organized profession built on clinical and laboratory science was infinitely better and more reliable than the charms of unchurched and unorthodox dissenters.

Notes

Introduction

1 Paul Johnson, *Intellectuals* (New York: Harper Perennial, 1990 [1988]), 2, 342.
2 Jefferson to Dr. Caspar Wistar, Jr., June 21, 1807, in Paul L. Ford (ed.), *The Writings of Thomas Jefferson* (10 volumes; New York: G. P. Putnam's Sons, 1892–99), IX, 81–85.
3 William G. Rothstein, *American Physicians in the Nineteenth Century: From Sects to Science* (Baltimore: Johns Hopkins University Press, 1985), 7.
4 Abraham Flexner, *Medical Education in the United States and Canada: A Report to the Carnegie Foundation on the Advancement of Teaching* (New York: Carnegie Foundation, 1910), 156.

Chapter 1

1 Lester S. King, *Medical World of the Eighteenth Century* (Huntington, NY: Robert E. Krieger Publishing, 1971), 62–63.
2 John Brown, *Locke and Sydenham* (Edinburgh: Edmonston and Douglas, 1866), 279–81.
3 Jeffrey Boss, "The Medical Philosophy of Francis Bacon (1561–1626)," *Medical Hypotheses*, 4 (1978), 208–20.
4 J. C. Reeve, "Some of the Latest Systems of Medicine," *Transactions of the Annual Meeting of the Ohio State Medical Society* (1885), 34.
5 King, *Medical World of the Eighteenth Century*, 140–42; Guenter B. Risse, "Doctor William Cullen, Physician, Edinburgh: A Consultation Practice in the Eighteenth Century," *Bulletin of the History of Medicine*, XLVIII (1974), 348–49; Ester Fischer-Homberger, "Eighteenth-Century Nosology and Its Survivors," *Medical History*, XIV (1970), 397–402; Edward Berdoe, *The Origins and Growth of the Healing Art* (London: Swan Sonnerschein and Co., 1893), 426.
6 Samuel Jackson, *A Discourse Commemorative of Nathaniel Chapman, M.D., Late Professor of the Theory and Practice of Medicine and of Clinical Medicine. Delivered Before the Trustees,*

the Medical Faculty, and Students of the University of Pennsylvania, October 13, 1854 (Philadelphia: T. K. and P. G. Collins, 1854), 17.

7 Reeve, "Some of the Latest Systems in Medicine," 37–39; Guenter B. Risse, "The Brunonian System of Medicine: Its Theoretical and Practical Implications," *Clio Medica*, V (1970), 45–51.

8 Reeve, "Some of the Latest Systems in Medicine," 40–42.

9 Reeve, "Some of the Latest Systems in Medicine," 43; Alfred S. Taylor, "On Poisoning by Tartarized Antimony," *Guy's Hospital Reports*, III (1857), 391–92; Thomas Marryat, *The Art of Healing, Or a New Practice of Physic* (London: M. Swinney, 1777). See also John S. Haller, Jr., "The History of Tartar Emetic in the Nineteenth Century Materia Medica," *Bulletin of the History of Medicine*, XLIV (1975), 235–57.

10 Carroll Dunham, "Freedom of Medical Opinion and Action: A Vital Necessity, and a Great Responsibility," *North American Journal of Homeopathy*, XIX (1870), 116.

11 Daniel Drake quoted in [Editor], "Something Worth Noticing," *Thomsonian Recorder*, II (1833), 14. See also John S. Haller, Jr., "Samson of the Materia Medica: Medical Theory and the Use and Abuse of Calomel in Nineteenth Century America," *Pharmacy in History*, XIII (1971), 22–34; 67–76.

12 Ralph St. J. Perry, "Arsenic—The Multipotent Drug," *American Journal of Clinical Medicine*, XIX (1912), 54–55; S. O. Habershon, "On the Medical Preparations of Arsenic," *Guy's Hospital Reports*, X (1864), 72; Lloyd Bullock, "On the Best Preparation of Arsenic for Internal Administration," *Lancet*, II (1850), 674–75; Stewart Lockie, "On the Use of Arsenic as a Blood and Cardiac Tonic," *British Medical Journal*, II (1875), 828–30. See also John S. Haller, Jr., "Therapeutic Mule: The Use of Arsenic in the Nineteenth Century Materia Medica," *Pharmacy in History*, XVII (1975), 87–100.

13 Henry Wilkins, *An Inaugural Dissertation on the Theory and Practice of Emetics* (Philadelphia: Parry Hall, 1793), 1–16.

14 Robert Chevallier Cream, *Inaugural Dissertation on the Chemical History and Physiological and Therapeutical Action of Tartarized Antimony* (Edinburgh: s.n., 1835), 25.

15 L. C. Boisliniere, "Pustular Eruption of the Skin From the Internal Use of Tartar Emetic," *St. Louis Medical and Surgical Journal*, XIV (1856), 20–21.

16 A. W. Haggis, "Fundamental Errors in the Early History of Cinchona," *Bulletin of the History of Medicine*, X (1941), 417–59; 568–92; Dale C. Smith, "Quinine and Fever: The Development of the Effective Dosage," *Journal of the History of Medicine and the Allied Sciences*, XXI (1976), 343–67.

17 Oliver W. Holmes, *Currents and Counter-Currents in Medical Science* (Boston: Tichnor and Fields, 1860), 27.

18 Perry Miller, *Errand Into the Wilderness* (New York: Harper and Row, 1956).

19 Alexander Wilder, *History of Medicine. A Brief Outline of Medical History and Sects of Physicians, From the Earliest Historic Period; With an Extended Account of the New Schools of the Healing Art in the Nineteenth Century, and Especially a History of the American Eclectic Practice of Medicine, Never Before Published* (New Sharon, Maine: New England Eclectic Publishing Company, 1901), 407–08.

20 Wilder, *History of Medicine*, 406–07.

21 Wilder, *History of Medicine*, 415–16.

22 Sydney Smith, *The Works of the Reverend Sydney Smith* (Boston: Sampson and Company, 1856), 141.

23 Quoted in Perry Miller, *The Life of the Mind in America from the Revolution to the Civil War* (New York: Harcourt, Brace and World, Inc., 1965), 284.

24 Thomas Jefferson to Dr. Caspar Wistar, Jr., June 21, 1807, in Paul L. Ford (ed.), *The Writings of Thomas Jefferson* (10 vols.; New York: G. P. Putnam's Sons, 1892–99), IX, 81–85.

25 Quoted in Wilder, *History of Medicine*, 413.

26 Quoted in Alexander Wilder, "Eclectic Medicine: Its History and Scientific Basis," *Transactions of the National Eclectic Medical Association*, XXI (1894), 56.

27 John S. Haller, Jr., *American Medicine in Transition, 1840–1910* (Urbana: University of Illinois Press, 1980), Chapter 1; John S. Haller, Jr., "The Negro and the Southern Physician: A Study of Medical and Racial Attitudes, 1800–1860," *Medical History*, XVI (1972), 238–53.

28 Jackson, *A Discourse Commemorative of Nathaniel Chapman*, 18–19.

29 Wilder, *History of Medicine,* 410.

30 Wilder, *History of Medicine*, viii.

31 Quoted in *Journal of the American Institute of Homeopathy,* 56 (1963), 202.

32 Quoted in Wilder, *History of Medicine*, 404.

33 John Harley Warner, *The Therapeutic Perspective: Medical Practice, Knowledge, and Identity in America, 1820–1885* (Cambridge: Harvard University Press, 1986), 42–43. See also Richard H. Shryock, "Empiricism vs. Rationalism in American Medicine, 1650–1950," *Proceedings of the American Antiquarian Society,* XCIX (1969), 99–150.

Chapter 2

1 Alexander Wilder, *History of Medicine. A Brief Outline of Medical History and Sects of Physicians, from the Earliest Historic Period; With an Extended Account of the New Schools of the Healing Art in the Nineteenth Century, and Especially a History of the American Eclectic Practice of Medicine, Never Before Published* (New Sharon, Maine: New England Eclectic Publishing Company, 1901), 212–13.

2 Morris Fishbein, "The End of Eclecticism," *American Mercury*, VIII (July, 1926), 327.

3 See George Boas, *French Philosophies of the Romantic Period* (Baltimore: Johns Hopkins University Press, 1925); and W. V. Brewer, *Victor Cousin as a Comparative Educator* (New York: Teachers College Press, 1971).

4 Victor Cousin, *Exposition of Eclecticism* (Edinburgh: Thomas Clark, 1839), 40–42.

5 John I. Brooks, *Academic Philosophy and the Human Sciences in Nineteenth-Century France* (Newark, New Jersey: University of Delaware Press, 1998), 47–49. Cousin's opponents were Pierre Leroux whose *Refutation of Eclecticism* (1838), Félix Ravaisson-Mollien whose *Report on Philosophy in France in the Nineteenth Century* (1867), and Auguste Comte whose *Der Positivismus* (1894) set the stage for eclecticism's gradual replacement as the state

philosophy of France. See also Ralph Barton Perry, *Philosophy of the Recent Past* (New York: Charles Scribner's Sons, 1926), 102–07.

6 Brooks, *Academic Philosophy and the Human Sciences in Nineteenth-Century France*, 50–55.

7 Cousin, *Exposition of Eclecticism*, 42–43.

8 Erwin H. Ackerknecht, *Medicine at the Paris Hospital, 1794–1848* (Baltimore: Johns Hopkins University Press, 1967), 101.

9 See A. F. Chomel, *Des Fièvres et des Maladies Pestilentielles* (Paris: Crochard, 1821).

10 Quoted in Ackerknecht, *Medicine at the Paris Hospital,* 102–04. See also Pierre Charles Alexander Louis, *Examen de l'Examen de M. Broussais Relativement à la Phthisie et l'Affection Typhoide* (Paris: Baillière, 1834).

11 Ackerknecht, *Medicine at the Paris Hospital*, 105–06; Harris L. Coulter, *Divided Legacy: A History of the Schism in Medical Thought. Volume II. Progress and Regress: J. B. Van Helmont to Claude Bernard* (Washington, DC: Wehawken Book Co., 1977), 534.

12 Ackerknecht, *Medicine at the Paris Hospital*, 107–11.

13 Ackerknecht, *Medicine at the Paris Hospital*, 111–12.

14 See A. Trousseau and H. Pidoux, *Treatise on Therapeutics* (9th ed.; three volumes; New York: William Wood and Company, 1880).

15 John Harley Warner, *Against The Spirit of the System: The French Impulse in Nineteenth Century American Medicine* (New Jersey: Princeton University Press, 1998), 4.

16 Godeloieve van Heteren, "Students Facing Boundaries: The Shift of Nineteenth-Century British Student Travel to German Universities and the Flexible Boundaries of a Medical Education System," in Vivian Nutton and Roy Porter (eds.), *The History of Medical Education in Britain* (Amsterdam: Rodopi, 1995), 280–340.

17 Wilder, *History of Medicine*, vii.

18 Quoted in Wilder, *History of Medicine*, ix.

19 John Forbes, *Of Nature and Art in the Cure of Disease* (New York: Samuel S. and William Wood, 1858), 2, 17.

20 Forbes, *Of Nature and Art in the Cure of Disease*, 159.

21 Forbes, *Of Nature and Art in the Cure of Disease*, 216, 236.

22 Marshall Hall, *Principles of the Theory and Practice of Medicine* (1st American edition, revised and enlarged; Boston: Charles C. Little and James Brown, 1839).

23 Wilder, *History of Medicine*, 286.

24 John Hughes Bennett, *Clinical Lectures on the Principles and Practice of Medicine* (3rd ed.; Edinburgh, Adam and Charles Black, 1859), 4–6.

25 Bennett, *Clinical Lectures on the Principles and Practice of Medicine*, 9.

26 William Pulteney Alison, "Reflections on the Results of Experience as to the Symptoms of Internal Inflammations, and the Effects of Bloodletting, During the Last Forty Years," *Edinburgh Medical Journal*, I (1855–56), 771–74.

27 Ludlam, "Reviews and Bibliographical Notices," *North American Journal of Homeopathy*, IX (1860), 319–22.

28 See John S. Haller, Jr., *Medical Protestants: The Eclectics in American Medicine, 1825–1939* (Carbondale: Southern Illinois University Press, 1994), 150–51; 237.

29 Woodbridge Riley, *American Thought: From Puritanism to Pragmatism and Beyond* (Gloucester, MA: Peter Smith, 1959 [1915]), 392–93.

30 Charles Crowe, *George Ripley: Transcendentalist and Utopian Socialist* (Athens: University of Georgia Press, 1967), 69.

31 Crowe, *George Ripley*, 70.

32 Quoted in Riley, *American Thought: From Puritanism to Pragmatism and Beyond*, 391.

33 Ralph Waldo Emerson, "The American Scholar," in *Nature, Addresses, and Lectures* (Boston: Houghton, Mifflin, 1887), 71.

34 Ralph Waldo Emerson, "Self Reliance," in *Essays, First and Second Series* (New York: T. Crowell, 1951), 42–43.

35 Ralph Waldo Emerson, "Man the Reformer," in *Nature, Addresses, and Lectures*, 200.

36 Quoted in Winthrop S. Hudson, *Religion in America: An Historical Account of the Development of American Religious Life* (New York: Charles Scribner's Sons, 1965), 181.

37 Lowell quoted in Robert E. Spiller, et al., *Literary History of the United States* (3rd ed.: New York: McMillan Publishing Co., Inc., 1963), 358.

38 Riley, *American Thought: From Puritanism to Pragmatism and Beyond*, 390.

39 Russell M. Jones, "An American Medical Student in Paris, 1831–1833," *Harvard Library Bulletin*, XV (1967), 59–81; James Jackson, *A Memoir of James Jackson, Jr. With Extracts from his Letters to his Father and Medical Cases Collected by Him* (Boston: Hilliard, Gray, 1835); Elisha Bartlett, *An Essay on the Philosophy of Medical Science* (Philadelphia: Lea and Blanchard 1844); Erwin H. Ackerknecht, "Elisha Bartlett and the Philosophy of the Paris Clinical School," *Bulletin of the History of Medicine*, XXIV (1950), 43–60; J. Chalmers DaCosta, "The French School of Surgery in the Reign of Louis Philippe," *Annals of Medical History*, IV (1922), 77–79; George Rosen, "The Philosophy of Ideology and the Emergence of Modern Medicine in France," *Bulletin of the History of Medicine*, XX (1946), 328–39; Richard H. Shryock, *The Development of Modern Medicine: An Interpretation of the Social and Scientific Factors Involved* (Madison, WI: University of Wisconsin Press, 1979).

40 Jones, "An American Medical Student in Paris, 1831–1833," 61–62. See also Oliver W. Holmes, *The Position and Prospects of the Medical Student. An Address Delivered Before the Boylston Medical Society of Harvard University, January 12, 1844* (Boston: John Putnam, 1844).

41 Shryock, *The Development of Modern Medicine: An Interpretation of the Social and Scientific Factors Involved*, 171, 193; John Harley Warner, "American Doctors in London During the Age of Paris Medicine," in Vivian Nutton and Roy Porter (eds.), *The History of Medical Education in Britain* (Amsterdam: Rodopi, 1995), 341–65.

42 Warner, *Against the Spirit of System: The French Impulse in Nineteenth-Century American Medicine*, 4–5.

43 John Harley Warner, "The Selective Transport of Medical Knowledge: Antebellum American Physicians and Parisian Medical Therapeutics," *Bulletin of the History of Medicine*, 59 (1985), 213–19.

44 Warner, "The Selective Transport of Medical Knowledge," 222.

45 John Harley Warner, "The Idea of Science in English Medicine: The 'Decline of Science' and the Rhetoric of Reform, 1815–45," in Roger French and Andrew Wear (eds.), *British Medicine in an Age of Reform* (London and New York, Routledge, 1991), 136–64.

46 Morris Fishbein, "The End of Eclecticism," *American* Mercury, VIII (July, 1926), 328.

47 James C. Whorton, *Nature Cures: The History of Alternative Medicine in America* (New York: Cambridge University Press, 2002), 47.

48 Michael A. Flannery, "The Medicine and Medicinal Plants of C. S. Rafinesque," *Economic Botany*, LII (1998), 27–43.

49 Wilder, "Eclectic Medicine: Its History and Scientific Basis," *Transactions,* National Eclectic Medical Association, XXI (1894), 58; Flannery, "The Medicine and Medicinal Plants of C. S. Rafinesque," 31–40. See also Richard E. Call, *The Life and Writings of Rafinesque* (Louisville: J. P. Morton, 1895); and T. J. Fitzpatrick, Rafinesque: A Sketch of His Life (Des Moines: Historical Department of Iowa, 1911); and Alex Berman and Michael A. Flannery, *America's Botanico-Medical Movements: Vox Populi* (New York: Haworth Press, 2001), 59–60, 62.

50 Flannery, "For 'a Voluptuous Glow of Health and Vigor': Medical Botany in Kentucky, 1792–1910," *Journal of the Kentucky Academy of Science*, XL (1999), 15–30.

51 Wilder, "Eclectic Medicine: Its History and Scientific Basis," 59.

52 Packard quoted in Flannery, "For 'a Voluptuous Glow of Health and Vigor,'" 8.

53 Wilder, "Eclectic Medicine: Its History and Scientific Basis," 61.

54 H. E. Firth, "The Origin of the American Eclectic Practice of Medicine, and Its Early History in the State of New York," *Transactions of the Eclectic Medical Society of New York*, X (1878), 172–73.

55 Firth, "The Origin of the American Eclectic Practice of Medicine," 174.

56 Quoted in Wilder, "Eclecticism in Medicine as Defined by Eclectic Writers," 98.

57 Quoted in Wilder, "Eclecticism in Medicine as Defined by Eclectic Writers," 97–98.

58 Firth, "The Origin of the American Eclectic Practice of Medicine," 174–75.

59 "An Earnest Appeal," *Eclectic Medical Journal*, I (1850), 39.

60 Quoted in Wilder, *History of Medicine*, 562.

61 Quoted in Wilder, *History of Medicine*, 562.

62 Alexander Wilder, "Eclectic Medicine: Its History and Scientific Basis," *Transactions of the National Eclectic Medical Association,* XXI (1894), 57.

63 Wilder, "Eclecticism in Medicine as Defined by Eclectic Writers," 97.

64 Wilder, "Eclectic Medicine: Its History and Scientific Basis," 59.

65 John Dill Robertson, "Are we Americans?" *Transactions of the National Eclectic Medical Association*, XXXI (1902–1903), 64–67.

66 William H. Cook, "Eclecticism," *Physio-Medical Recorder*, XXX (1866), 136–37.

67 Cook, "Eclecticism," 146–47.

68 Cook, "Eclecticism," 150.

69 Cook, "Eclecticism," 137.

70 James McClintock, *Annual Lecture. Introductory Lecture Delivered in the Castleton Medical College, March 8, 1842* (Castleton, Vermont: Robinson and Southmayd, 1842), 5–6.

71 McClintock, *Annual Lecture*, 6.

72 James McClintock, *An Introductory Lecture, Delivered in the Castleton Medical College, on the 10th April, 1843* (Albany: C. Van Benthuysen, 1843), 1–28.

73 McClintock, *Annual Lecture,* 16.

74 Wilder, *History of Medicine*, 642.

75 Wilder, *History of Medicine*, 642.

76 James McClintock, *Introductory Lecture to Session of 1860 and 1861 in the Eclectic Medical College of Philadelphia on Wednesday, at 7 1/2 o'clock, P.M., October 24, 1860* (Philadelphia: William S. Young, 1860), 4.

77 McClintock, *Introductory Lecture*, 5.

78 Wilder quoted in "The World's Medical Congress of Eclectic Physicians and Surgeons," *Transactions of the National Eclectic Medical Association,* XXI (1894), 54.

79 Stuart Close, "Eclecticism, Homeopathy and the Medical Millennium," *Homeopathic Recorder,* 42 (1927), 392.

Chapter 3

1 Woodbridge Riley, *American Thought: From Puritanism to Pragmatism and Beyond* (Gloucester, MA: Peter Smith, 1959 [1915]), 390; Gilbert Seldes, *The Stammering Century* (New York: Harper and Row, 1965 [1928], 4.

2 Logie Barrow, "Why Were Most Medical Heretics at Their Most Confident Around the 1840s? (The Other Side of Mid-Victorian Medicine)," in Roger French and Andrew Wear, *British Medicine in An Age of Reform* (London: Routledge, 1991), 165.

3 Elisha Bartlett, "The Head and the Heart, or the Relative Importance of Intellectual and Moral Education, a Lecture Delivered Before the American Institute of Instruction, In Lowell, August, 1838," in *A Brief Memoir of Dr. Elisha Bartlett With Selections From His Writings and a Bibliography of the Same* (Providence: Sidney S. Rider, 1878), 29–30.

4 Elisha Bartlett, *An Inquiry into the Degree of Certainty in Medicine; and into the Nature and Extent of Its Power Over Disease* (Philadelphia: Lea and Blanchard, 1848), 9.

5 Bartlett, *An Inquiry into the Degree of Certainty in Medicine*, 17.

6 Bartlett, *An Inquiry into the Degree of Certainty in Medicine*, 30–36.

7 James H. Cassedy, *American Medicine and Statistical Thinking, 1800–1860* (Cambridge, Massachusetts: Harvard University Press, 1984), 67.

8 John Ware, *Discourses on Medical Education and on the Medical Profession* (Boston: James Munroe, 1847), 102.

9 Ware, *Discourses on Medical Education and on the Medical Profession*, 105.

10 Ware, *Discourses on Medical Education and on the Medical Profession*, 35, 37.

11 Ware, *Discourses on Medical Education and on the Medical Profession*, 47.

12 Samuel Jackson, *An Introductory Lecture to the Institutes of Medicine* (Philadelphia: Printed for the Class by William Sharpless, 1830), 5, 8–9, 12.

13 Jackson, *An Introductory Lecture to the Institutes of Medicine* (1830), 30–31, 33. See also Richard H. Shryock, "Empiricism vs. Rationalism in American Medicine, 1650–1950," *Proceedings of the American Antiquarian Society*, LXXIX (1968), 99–150.

14 Jackson also included the homeopaths in this group. See Samuel Jackson, *The Principles of Medicine, Founded on the Structure and Functions of the Animal Organization* (Philadelphia: Carey and Lea, 1832), xix.

15 Jackson, *The Principles of Medicine*, xv–xvi.

16 Jackson, *The Principles of Medicine*, xvi–xvii, xx.

17 Samuel Jackson, *A Lecture on Medical Education, Introductory to the Course of the Institutes of Medicine, in the University of Pennsylvania, for the Session 1833–34* (Philadelphia: The Class, 1833), 8. This lecture was especially popular among homeopaths. See also I. G. Rosenstein, *Theory and Practice of Homeopathy First Part, Containing a Theory of Homeopathy, with Dietetic Rules, etc.* (Louisville: Henkle and Logan, 1840), 21.

18 Jackson, *A Lecture on Medical Education*, (1833) 11–16.

19 Jackson, *A Lecture on Medical Education*, (1833), 10–11.

20 Jackson, *A Lecture on Medical Education*, (1833), 18.

21 Jackson, *A Lecture on Medical Education*, (1833) 24, 26.

22 Jackson, *A Lecture on Medical Education*, (1833), 26–28.

23 Samuel Jackson, *A Lecture Introductory to the Course of Institutes of Medicine, in the University of Pennsylvania, for the Session of 1835–36* (Philadelphia: Thomas H. Town, 1835), 9.

24 Jackson, *A Lecture Introductory to the Course of Institutes of Medicine* (1835), 18.

25 See John S. Haller, *The People's Doctors: Samuel Thomson and the American Botanical Movement, 1790–1860* (Carbondale: Southern Illinois University Press, 2000).

26 Samuel Thomson, *New Guide to Health, or Botanic Family Physician Containing a Complete System of Practice Upon a Plan Entirely New: With a Description of the Vegetables Made Use of, and Directions for Preparing and Administering Them to Cure Disease: To Which is Added a Description of Several Cases of Disease Attended by the Author, with the Mode of Treatment and Cure* (9th ed.; Columbus, OH: Jarvis Pike and Company, 1833), 7–8.

27 Samuel Thomson, "A Chapter of Life; Or, Concise Physiological Hints of the Laws of Animalization," *Thomsonian Recorder* I (1833), 212–13.

28 Samuel Thomson, *New Guide to Health*, 4–5.

29 Alexander Wilder, *History of Medicine. A Brief Outline of Medical History and Sects of Physicians, From the Earliest Historic Period; With an Extended Account of the New Schools of the Healing Art in the Nineteenth Century, and Especially a History of the American Eclectic Practice of Medicine, Never Before Published* (New Sharon, Maine: New England Eclectic Publishing Company, 1901), 462.

30 Quoted in Wilder, *History of Medicine*, 498.

31 Alexander Wilder, "Eclecticism in Medicine as Defined by Eclectic Writers," *Transactions*, National Eclectic Medical Association, XXVIII (1901), 97.

32 Benjamin Waterhouse, "The Eclectic—No.5," *Thomsonian Recorder*, I (1833), 418–19.

33 Benjamin Waterhouse, "The Eclectic—No. 1," *Thomsonian Recorder*, I (1833), 109–10.

34 Samuel Robinson, *A Course of Fifteen Lectures, On Medical Botany, Denominated Thomson's New Theory of Medical Practice; in Which the Various Theories that have Preceded it are Reviewed and Compared* (Columbus, OH: Horton Howard, 1829), 19, 190.

35 Robinson, *A Course of Fifteen Lectures*, 19.

36 Robinson, *A Course of Fifteen Lectures*, 151.

37 Robinson, *A Course of Fifteen Lectures*, 142–43, 176.

38 Alex Berman, "A Striving for Scientific Respectability: Some American Botanics and the Nineteenth-Century Plant Materia Medica," *Bulletin of the History of Medicine*, XXX (1956), 10–11.

39 Wilder, "Eclectic Medicine: Its History and Scientific Basis," 60.

40 Wilder, *History of Medicine*, 533–34.

41 Samuel Hahnemann, "On the Present Want of Foreign Medicines," in R. E. Dudgeon, *The Lesser Writings of Samuel Hahnemann* (New York: William Radde, 1852), 486.

42 Samuel Hahnemann, *Organon of Homeopathic Medicine* (Allentown, PA: Academical Bookstore, 1836), 10–19.

43 Hahnemann, *Organon of Homeopathic Medicine,* 80–81.

44 William A. Gardiner, "Progressive Homeopathy," *The Philadelphia Journal of Homeopathy,* I (1852), 236.

45 James Y. Simpson, *Homeopathy: Its Tenets and Tendencies, Theoretical, Theological, and Therapeutical* (Philadelphia: Lindsay and Blakiston, 1854), 55.

46 Samuel Hahnemann, *The Chronic Diseases: Their Specific Nature and Homeopathic Treatment* (5 vols.; New York; William Radde, 1845–46), V, v–vi.

47 Samuel Hahnemann, "Remarks on the Extreme Attenuation of Homeopathic Medicines," in R. E. Dudgeon, *The Lesser Writings of Samuel Hahnemann* (New York: William Radde, 1852), 765.

48 Samuel Hahnemann, "How can Small Doses of Such Very Attenuated Medicines as Homeopathy Employs Still Possess Great Power?" in Dudgeon, *The Lesser Writings of Samuel Hahnemann*, 733.

49 I. G. Rosenstein, *Theory and Practice of Homeopathy First Part, Containing a Theory of Homeopathy, with Dietetic Rules, etc.* (Louisville: Henkle and Logan, 1840), 92–93, 104.

50 "The Hahnemannian Institute," *The Philadelphia Journal of Homeopathy,* II (1853–54), 628–30.

51 Charles J. Hempel, *Homeopathy, a Principle in Nature. Its Scientific Universality Unfolded: Its Development and Philosophy Explained; And Its Applicability to the Treatment of Diseases Shown* (New York: C. T. Hurlburt, 1860), 1860), 225, 237–38.

52 Quoted in James Y. Simpson, *Homeopathy: Its Tenets and Tendencies, Theoretical, Theological, and Therapeutical* (Philadelphia: Lindsay and Blakiston, 1854), 36, 39.

53 Quoted in Simpson, *Homeopathy: Its Tenets and Tendencies, Theoretical, Theological, and Therapeutical*, 42.

54 E. M. Hale, "New Homeopathic Provings," *American Homeopathic Observer*, I (1864), 7–8; Charles F. Millspaugh, *American Medicinal Plants: An Illustrated and Descriptive Guide to the American Plants Used as Homoeopthic Remedies: Their History, Preparation, Chemistry and Physiological Effects* (2 vols.; New York: Boericke and Tafel, 1887).

55 "Historical and Statistical Report of Homeopathy in the United States of America," *Transactions of the World's Homeopathic Convention, Held at Philadelphia, Under the Auspices of the American Institute of Homeopathy, at Its Twenty-Ninth Session, June 26–July*

1, 1876. Vol. II. History of Homeopathy (Philadelphia: Sherman and Company, 1880), 435–37,

56 "Homeopathy in the United States," *Transactions of the World's Homeopathic Convention, Held at Philadelphia, Under the Auspices of the American Institute of Homeopathy, at Its Twenty-Ninth Session, June 26–July 1, 1876. Vol. II. History of Homeopathy* (Philadelphia: Sherman and Company, 1880), 434.

57 "Historical and Statistical Report of Homeopathy in the United States of America," 436.

58 E. E. Marcy, *Homeopathy and Allopathy: Reply to An Examination of the Doctrines and Evidences of Homeopathy, by Worthington Hooker, M.D.* (New York: William Radde, 1852), 63–65.

59 I. G. Rosenstein, *Theory and Practice of Homeopathy. First Part, Containing a Theory of Homeopathy, with Dietetic Rules, etc.* (Louisville: Henkle and Logan, 1840), 111–16.

60 George B. Peck, "1851—Homeopathy—1901," *North American Journal of Homeopathy*, L (1902), 60–62.

61 "Celebration of the Centennial Birthday of Dr. Samuel Hahnemann in Boston," *North American Journal of Homeopathy*, IV (1855), 150–52.

62 J. P. Dake, "Pseudo-Homeopathists," *The Philadelphia Journal of Homeopathy,* I (1852), 62–64.

63 Hahnemann, *Organon of Homeopathic Medicine,* 210–11.

64 Wilder, *History of Medicine,* 246.

65 Sidney E. Ahlstrom, *A Religious History of the American People* (2 vols.; Garden City, New York: Image Books, 1975), I, 584–89.

66 Robert C. Fuller, *Alternative Medicine and American Religious Life* (New York: Oxford University Press, 1989), 38–65.

67 See Ashley Paschal, Justin McNabney and Bryan Hanson, "The Prescribing Habits and Materia Medica of Dr. William D. Hutchings," *Pharmacy in History,* XLVII (2005), 94–111.

68 William A. Gardiner, "The Present Position and Prospects of Homeopathy," *Philadelphia Journal of Homeopathy*, I (1852), 45.

69 William A. Gardiner, "The Value of Allopathic Testimony," *Philadelphia Journal of Homeopathy*, I (1852), 91.

70 Abraham Flexner, *Medical Education in the United States and Canada; A Report to the Carnegie Foundation on the Advancement of Teaching* (New York: Carnegie Foundation, 1910), 156.

71 William A. Gardiner, "The Present Position and Prospects of Homeopathy," *The Philadelphia Journal of Homeopathy,* I (1852), 45.

72 Girtanner quoted in William A. Gardiner, "The Present Position and Prospects of Homeopathy," *The Philadelphia Journal of Homeopathy,* I (1852), 45.

Chapter 4

1 Carl Bode, *Antebellum Culture* (Carbondale: Southern Illinois University Press, 1959), 119–20.

2 Orville A. Roorbach, *Bibliotheca Americana. Catalogue of American Publications, Including Reprints and Original Works, from 1820 to 1852, Inclusive. Together with a List of Periodicals Published in the United States* (New York: P. Smith, 1939 [1852]).

3 Oliver Wendell Holmes, "The Young Practitioner," *Medical Essays, 1842–1882* (Boston: Houghton Mifflin, 1883), 379.

4 Carl Bode, *The Half-World of American Culture* (Carbondale: Southern Illinois University Press, 1965), 66–84. See also Carl Bode, *The American Lyceum: Town Meeting of the Mind* (Carbondale: Southern Illinois University Press, 1968).

5 I. G. Rosenstein, *Theory and Practice of Homeopathy. First Part, Containing a Theory of Homeopathy, with Dietetic Rules, etc.* (Louisville: Henkle and Logan, 1840), 181–83.

6 "Pathies," *New England Botanic Medical and Surgical Journal*, III (1849), 319.

7 Samuel Thomson, "Botanic Directions," in Cyrus Thomson (comp.), *Learned Quackery Exposed; Or, Theory According to Art, as Exemplified in the Practice of the honorable Doctors of the Present Day* (Syracuse: Lathrop and Dean, Printers, 1843), 50–52.

8 A. A. Clark, "Dr. Thomson's Materia Medica," *The Southern Botanic Journal*, I (1838), 409–10.

9 Samuel Thomson, "Three Crafts," in Thomson, *Learned Quackery Exposed; Or, Theory According to Art, as Exemplified in the Practice of the Honorable Doctors of the Present Day*, 12–15.

10 Richard J. Duke, "The Deeds of Allopathy," *Botanico-Medical Recorder*, XV (1847), 118.

11 Anonymous, "To Physicians," *Thomsonian Recorder*, III (1835), 240.

12 Stephen F. Fowler, "To Dr. Samuel Thomson," *Thomsonian Manual*, III (1837), 1.

13 "The Death-Knell of Calomel," *Physio-Medical Recorder*, XXVIII (1864), 89–90. See also Allen G. Debus, *Drug Store Cabaret* (Madison, WI: American Institute of the History of Pharmacy, 1991), 14–15; Philip D. Jordan, *Singin' Yankees* (Minneapolis: University of Minnesota Press, 1946). See also Michael A. Flannery, "Another House Divided: Union Medical Service and Sectarians during the Civil War," *Journal of the History of Medicine*, LIV (1999), 478–510.

14 "New Year's Night in the Eclectic," *Western Medical Reformer*, VII (1847), 167–78.

15 William A. Gardiner, "The Present Position and Prospects of Homeopathy," *The Philadelphia Journal of Homeopathy*, I (1852), 44–45.

16 [Editor], "Introduction," *United States Journal of Homeopathy*, I (1860), 3–4, 7.

17 J. F. Geary, "Our Literature," *The Philadelphia Journal of Homeopathy*, IV (1855), 530; J. F. Geary, "Our Literature—A Review," *The Philadelphia Journal of Homeopathy*, IV (1855) 327, 394, 396, 407;

18 [Editor], "Bibliographical Notices," *North American Journal of Homeopathy*, IV (1856), 575–76.

19 C. Pretsch, "A Reviewer Reviewed," *Philadelphia Journal of Homeopathy*, IV (1855), 461–62.

20 Hercules de Paidagogo, M.D., "A Letter to Dr. C. Pretsch," *Philadelphia Journal of Homeopathy*, V (1855), 477.

21 Geary, "Our Literature—A Review," 481–82.

22 "Editorial," *Philadelphia Journal of Homeopathy*, IV (1855), 573.

23 "Editorial," *Philadelphia Journal of Homeopathy*, IV (1855), 510.

24 Among the best scholarship on this topic are James H. Cassedy, "The Flourishing and Character of Early American Medical Journalism, 1797–1860," *Journal of the History of Medicine,* 38 (1983), 135–50; Michael A. Flannery, "The Early Botanical Medical Movement as a Reflection of Life, Liberty, and Literacy in Jacksonian America," *Journal of the Medical Library Association,* XC (2002), 442–54; Myrl Ebert, "The Rise and Development of the American Medical Periodical, 1797–1850," *Bulletin of the Medical Library Association,* 40 (1952), 243–76; John Shaw Billings, "The Medical Journals of the United States," *Boston Medical and Surgical Journal,* 100 (1879), 1–14; Henry B. Shafer, "Early Medical Magazines in America," *Annals of Medical History,* 7 (1935), 480–91; Frank Luther Mott, *A History of American Magazines* (Cambridge: Harvard University Press, 1938–68); L. W. Levine, *Highbrow/Lowbrow: The Emergence of Cultural Hierarchy in America* (Cambridge, MA: Harvard University Press, 1988); H. J. Graff, *The Labyrinths of Literacy: Reflections on Literacy Past and Present* (Pittsburgh, PA: University of Pittsburgh Press, 1995); and H. McMullen, *American Libraries Before 1876* (Westport, CT: Greenwood Press, 2000).

25 "An Earnest Appeal," *Eclectic Medical Journal*, I (1850), 39.

Chapter 5

1 Jeffrey Boss, "The Medical Philosophy of Francis Bacon (1561–1626)," *Medical Hypotheses,* 4 (1978), 208–20. See also Francis Bacon, *The Advancement of Learning* (London: Athlone Press, 1975).

2 Alexander Wilder, *History of Medicine. A Brief Outline of Medical History and Sects of Physicians, From the Earliest Historic Period; With an Extended Account of the New Schools of the Healing Art in the Nineteenth Century, and Especially a History of the American Eclectic Practice of Medicine, Never Before Published* (New Sharon, Maine: New England Eclectic Publishing Company, 1901), 483–87.

3 Thomas V. Morrow, "Address," *Reformed Medical Journal,* I (1832), 113–17.

4 Quoted in Alexander Wilder, "Eclecticism in Medicine Defined by Eclectic Writers," *Transactions of the National Eclectic Medical Association* (1901), 99–100.

5 Wilder, *History of Medicine*, 582–83.

6 John S. Haller, Jr., *Medical Protestants: The Eclectics in American Medicine, 1825–1939* (Carbondale: Southern Illinois University Press, 1994), 175.

7 Morris Fishbein, "The End of Eclecticism," *American* Mercury, VIII (July, 1926), 329–30. In the 1920s, the Kansas City College of Medicine and Surgery claimed to be eclectic but was disowned by the National Eclectic Association as a diploma-mill.

8 See John S. Haller, Jr., *Kindly Medicine: Physio-Medicalism in America, 1836–1911* (Kent, OH: Kent State University Press, 1997).

9 William Tod Helmuth, "Sectarianism in Medicine," Lloyd Library and Museum, Cincinnati, Special Collections, Box 38, Folder 1,100, p. 107.

10 Quoted in "A Dreadful Blow to Homeopathy," *North American Journal of Homeopathy*, IX (1860), 160.

11 The percentages of each class in the 1840s and 1850s who turned to homeopathy would make for a genuinely important piece of research. Who were their teachers and did they have a role in these decisions? How many at the time of their matriculation were already intending to practice homeopathy as distinct from those who graduated and then turned to homeopathy? The answers to these questions are significant in understanding the impact of homeopathy. Similar questions apply to those who turned to eclecticism, physio-medicalism, and hydropathy.

12 See John S. Haller, Jr., *The History of American Homeopathy: The Academic Years, 1820–1935* (Binghamton, NY: Haworth Press, 2005).

13 John S. Haller, Jr., *The People's Doctors: Samuel Thomson and the American Botanical Movement, 1790–1860* (Carbondale: Southern Illinois University Press, 2000), 90–96.

14 Haller, *Medical Protestants: The Eclectics in American Medicine, 1825–1939*, 103–07.

15 An American Physician, "Homeopathic Medical Education—Present and Future," *North American Journal of Homeopathy*, VIII (1859), 52–54.

16 Quoted in D. H. Beckwith, "The History of the Western College of Homeopathic Medicine from 1850 to 1860," *Cleveland Homeopathic Reporter*, I (1900), 9.

17 W. Paine, "Eclecticism and Homeopathy," *Eclectic Medical Journal*, II (1852), 208–09.

18 Henry C. Preston, "Observations Upon the Use of High Potencies," *North American Journal of Homeopathy*, VII (1859), 281.

19 Preston, "Our Journal," *North American Journal of Homeopathy*, VII (1859), 392–93.

Chapter 6

1 Alexis de Tocqueville, *Democracy in America* (New York: Anchor Books, 1969), 459–61, 513–17.

2 See Joseph M. Toner, "Address," *Transactions of the American Medical Association*, 25 (1874), 71–72; Stanford E. Chaille, "State Medicine and State Medical Societies," *Transactions of the American Medical Association,* 30 (1879), facing p. 320.

3 Alexander Wilder, *History of Medicine. A Brief Outline of Medical History and Sects of Physicians, From the Earliest Historic Period; With an Extended Account of the New Schools of the Healing Art in the Nineteenth Century, and Especially a History of the American Eclectic Practice of Medicine, Never Before Published* (New Sharon, Maine: New England Eclectic Publishing Company, 1901), 468; H. E. Firth, "The Origin of the American Eclectic Practice of Medicine, and Its Early History in the State of New York," *Transactions of the Eclectic Medical Society of New York,* X (1878), 180.

4 Firth, "The Origin of the American Eclectic Practice of Medicine," 182.

5 Firth, "The Origin of the American Eclectic Practice of Medicine," 183.

6 Firth, "The Origin of the American Eclectic Practice of Medicine," 180–81; Harvey Wickes Felter, *History of the Eclectic Medical Institute. Cincinnati, Ohio 1845–1902* (Cincinnati, OH: Alumnal Association of the Eclectic Medical Institute, 1902), 7.

7 Wilder, *History of Medicine*, 572–73.

8 Wilder, *History of Medicine*, 538–41.

9 Wilder, *History of Medicine*, 542–43.

10 Wilder, *History of Medicine*, 598.

11 John S. Haller, Jr., *The People's Doctors: Samuel Thomson and the American Botanical Movement, 1790–1860* (Carbondale: Southern Illinois University, 2000), 42–43, 144.

12 Wilder, *History of Medicine*, 489–90.

13 Wilder, *History of Medicine*, 493–94.

14 Haller, *The People's Doctors*, 163–85.

15 Haller, *The People's Doctors*, 163–85.

16 Haller, *The People's Doctors*, 244–45.

17 Alexander Wilder, "Eclectic Medicine in the Eastern States," *Transactions of the National Eclectic Medical Association* (1892–93), 477.

18 Firth, "The Origin of the American Eclectic Practice of Medicine," 176.

19 Firth, "The Origin of the American Eclectic Practice of Medicine," 178–79.

20 "The American Institute of Homeopathy," *North American Journal of Homeopathy*, XVI (1867), 145; "American Institute of Homeopathy," *Transactions of the American Institute of Homeopathy*, (1880), 679.

21 "Proceedings of the American Institute of Homeopathy," *Philadelphia Journal of Homeopathy*, II (1853), 267–68.

22 "Medical News," *Philadelphia Journal of Homeopathy*, I (1852), 95–96.

23 [William A. Gardiner, M.D.], "The American Institute of Homeopathy," *Philadelphia Journal of Homeopathy*, I (1853), 523–24.

24 "Historical and Statistical Report of Homeopathy in the United States of America," *Transactions of the World's Homeopathic Convention. Volume II. History of Homeopathy*, 438.

25 "Proceedings of the American Institute of Homeopathy," *North American Homeopathic Journal*, III (1853), 412, 416; "Proceedings of the American Institute of Homeopathy," *Philadelphia Journal of Homeopathy*, II (1853), 290.

26 "Proceedings of the Eleventh Annual Session of the American Institute of Homeopathy," *Philadelphia Journal of Homeopathy*, III (1854), 248.

27 "Illinois State Homeopathic Medical Association," *North American Journal of Homeopathy*, XIII (1864), 131–32.

28 Quoted in "Proceedings of the Fifteenth Annual Meeting of the American Institute of Homeopathy," *North American Journal of Homeopathy*, VII (1859), 502.

29 Samuel Jackson, *An Introductory Address, Delivered Before the Medical Class of the University of Pennsylvania* (Philadelphia: William S. Young, 1846), 12–13.

30 Jackson, *An Introductory Address, Delivered Before the Medical Class of the University of Pennsylvania*, 10–11.

31 "Minutes of the Proceedings," *Proceedings of the National Medical Conventions, Held in New York, May, 1846, and in Philadelphia, May, 1847* (Philadelphia: American Medical Association, 1847), 23–33.

32 "Minutes of the Proceedings," 42, 50–51.

33 Quoted in John Fitzgibbon Geary, "Remarks on a Resolution," *Philadelphia Journal of Homeopathy*, IV (1855), 106.

34 Quoted in Henry I. Bowditch, "The Past, Present, and Future Treatment of Homeopathy, Eclecticism, and Kindred Delusions," *Transactions of the Rhode Island Medical Society*, III (1877), 295–96.

35 "American Medical Association," *New Jersey Medical Reporter*, VIII (1855), 230–31.

36 Wilder, *History of Medicine*, 575–76.

37 Quoted in Wilder, "Eclecticism in Medicine as Defined by Eclectic Writers," 100.

38 John S. Haller, Jr. *Medical Protestants: The Eclectics in American Medicine, 1825–1939* (Carbondale: Southern Illinois University Press, 1994), 101–03.

39 Felter, *History of the Eclectic Medical Institute*, 30.

40 [Editor], "A National Convention," *American Medical and Surgical Journal*, I (1851), 127; Haller, *Medical Protestants*, 159–60.

41 [Editor], "A National Convention," 127; [Editor], "National Eclectic Medical Association," *American Medical and Surgical Reporter*, I (1851), 97–98.

42 Quoted in Firth, "The Origin of the American Eclectic Practice of Medicine," 188.

43 Firth, "The Origin of the American Eclectic Practice of Medicine," 189.

44 Wilder, *History of Medicine*, 619.

45 Firth, "The Origin of the American Eclectic Practice of Medicine," 184.

46 Quoted in Firth, "The Origin of the American Eclectic Practice of Medicine," 184–85.

47 Wilder, *History of Medicine*, 587–89.

48 Wilder, *History of Medicine*, 591.

Chapter 7

1 "The Indiana Physio-Medical Association," *Physio-Medical Record* IX (1906), 111.

2 Joseph M. Thurston, *The Philosophy of Physiomedicalism: Its Theroem, Corollary, and Laws of Application for the Cure of Disease* (Richmond, Indiana: Nocholson Printing and Mfg. Co., 1900), 218, 317, 324; William H. Cook, *The Physio-Medical Dispensatory: A Treatise on Therapeutics, Materia Medica, and Pharmacy, in Accordance with the Principles of Physiological Medication* (Cincinnati: By Author, 1869), 7.

3 Roger T. Farley, "Physio-Medicalism Antitoxin," *Physio-Medical Record*, V (1902), 152–55; George Hasty, "New Cures," *Physio-Medical Journal*, XX (1894), 428–30; See also William Bulloch, *The History of Bacteriology* (London: Oxford University Press, 1938).

4 F. O. Broady, "Are Bacteria Pathogenic?" *Sanative Medicine*, IV (1894), 125–38.; Hermance, "The Germ Theory of Disease—Is It True or False?" *Physio-Medical Journal*, XXI (1895), 94–101; "The Bacteriological Craze," *Sanative Medicine*, IV (1894), 167: "At It Again," *Physio-Medical Journal*, VIII (1882), 253–54.

5 A. H. Baird, "Alcohol," *Physio-Medical Journal* VIII (1882), 310–11; G. H. Mayhugh, "In Memorium," *Sanative Medicine*, I (1892), 214.

6 William H. Cook and H. E. Hoke, "A National P.-M Convention," *Cincinnati Medical Gazette and Recorder*, XLIV (1880), 184–86. See also John S. Haller, Jr., *Kindly Medicine: Physio-Medicalism in America, 1836–1911* (Kent, OH: Kent State University Press, 1997), 118–21.

7 "Proceedings of the American Association of Physio-Medical Physicians and Surgeons," *Physio-Medical Journal*, XV (1890), 359; "The National Association of Physio-Medical Physicians and Surgeons," *Physio-Medical Record*, VI 1903), 111–12; "An Ass in the Profession," *Physio-Medical Journal*, XVII (1891), 406; J. Ben Nichols, "Physio-Medicalism," *Medical News*, LV (1895), 152.

8 William H. Cook, "Diplomas Honorable and Dishonorable," *Cincinnati Medical Gazette: A Journal of Medical Reform,* I (1877), 370–71. William H. Cook, "A Champion of Corruption," *Cincinnati Medical Gazette and Recorder,* LV (1881), 34–35.

9 Abraham Flexner, *Medical Education in the United States and Canada: A Report to the Carnegie Foundation for the Advancement of Teaching* (New York: The Carnegie Foundation, 1910), 213.

10 See John S. Haller, Jr., *Kindly Medicine: Physio-Medicalism in America, 1836–1911* (Kent, OH: Kent State University Press, 1997).

11 Martin Kaufman, *American Medical Education: The Formative Years, 1765–1910* (Westport, CT: Greenwood Press, 1976), 127–28; Kenneth M. Ludmerer, *Learning to Heal: The Development of American Medical Education* (New York: Basic Books, 1985), 72–149; John M. Dodson, "The Modern University School—Its Purposes and Methods," *Journal of the American Medical Association,* XXXIX (1902), 521; Thomas N. Bonner, "The German Model of Training Physicians in the United States, 1870–1914: How Closely Was It Followed?" *Bulletin of the History of Medicine,* LXIV (1990), 31.

12 Thomas N. Bonner, *American Doctors and German Universities: A Chapter in International Intellectual Relations, 1870–1914* (Lincoln: University of Nebraska Press, 1963), 23; James H. Means, *The Association of American Physicians: Its First 75 Years* (New York: McGraw Hill, 1961); Robert P. Hudson, "Abraham Flexner in Perspective: American Medical Education, 1865–1910," *Bulletin of the History of Medicine,* XLVI (1972), 554.

13 J. E. Emerson, "The Requirements for Preliminary Education in the Medical Colleges of the United States and Canada," *Journal of the American Medical Association,* XIV (1890), 271–72; N. S. Davis, "Requirements for Admission to Medical Schools," *Journal of the American Medical Association,* XLI (1903), 409–10; George H. Simmons, "Medical Education and Preliminary Requirements," *Journal of the American Medical Association,* XLII (1904), 1208; Flexner, *Medical Education in the United States and Canada,* 30–32.

14 "Medical Education in the United States," *Journal of the American Medical Association,* XXII (1894), 394; Dean F. Smiley, "History of the Association of American Medical Colleges," *Journal of Medical Education,* XXXII (1957), 513–16.

15 John Uri Lloyd, "The Crisis Is Upon Us," *Eclectic Medical Journal,* LXXVIII (1918), 499–504; Martin Kaufman, "American Medical Diploma Mills," *Medical Faculty Bulletin,* Tulane University, XXVI (1967), 56.

16 "Eclectic Medical College Files," *Lloyd Library and Museum,* Student Matriculation Files, box 6.

17 Leon Sokoloff, "The Rise and Decline of the Jewish Quota in Medical School Admissions," *Bulletin of the New York Academy of Medicine,* LXVIII (1992), 506; Marcia Graham Synnott, *The Half-Opened Door; Discrimination and Admissions at Harvard, Yale, and Princeton, 1900–1970* (Westport, CT: Greenwood Press, 1979), 44–45; Harold S. Wechsler, *The Qualified Student; A History of Selective College Admission in America* (New York: Wiley, 1977), x.

18 Rolla L. Thomas, "Eclecticism," *Eclectic Medical Journal,* LXIV (1904), 228; Herbert T. Webster, "The Merger Proposition," *Eclectic Medical Journal,* LXVI (1906), 323.

19 Flexner, *Medical Education in the United States and Canada,* 192.

20 Flexner, *Medical Education in the United States and Canada,* 204–05.

21 Flexner, *Medical Education in the United States and Canada,* 205.

22 Flexner, *Medical Education in the United States and Canada,* 227.

23 Flexner, *Medical Education in the United States and Canada,* 257.

24 Flexner, *Medical Education in the United States and Canada,* 260.

25 Flexner, *Medical Education in the United States and Canada,* 271–72.

26 Flexner, *Medical Education in the United States and Canada,* 283–84.

27 Flexner, *Medical Education in the United States and Canada,* 162–63.

28 William E. Bloyer, "The 'Standard' and Other Dictionary Definitions of Eclectic Medicine," *Transactions,* National Eclectic Medical Association, XXIII (1895–96), 217–18.

29 R. O. Hoffman, "The Future of Eclecticism," *National Eclectic Medical Association Quarterly,* XXIX (1938), 201; Bryan H. Nellans, "Dean's Report," Minutes of the Board of Trustees, May 20, 1939, Lloyd Library and Museum, Cincinnati.

30 John S. Haller, *The History of American Homeopathy: The Academic Years, 1820–1935* (New York: Haworth Press, 2005), 73, 264.

31 Flexner, *Medical Education in the United States and Canada,* 157.

32 Flexner, *Medical Education in the United States and Canada,* 161.

33 Osler quoted in Flexner, *Medical Education in the United States and Canada,* 162.

34 William Tod Helmuth, "Sectarianism in Medicine," Lloyd Library and Museum, Cincinnati, Special Collections, Box 38, Folder 1,100, pp. 105–06.

35 Quoted in William Harvey King, *History of Homeopathy and Its Institutions in America: Their Founders, Benefactors, Faculties, Officers, Hospitals, Alumni, etc., With a Record of Achievement of Its Representatives in the World of Medicine* (4 vols; New York: Lewis Publishing, 1905), II, 423.

36 Flexner, *Medical Education in the United States and Canada,* 161.

37 Flexner, *Medical Education in the United States and Canada,* 159–60.

38 Flexner, *Medical Education in the United States and Canada,* 160–61.

39 R. F. Rabe, "Some Causes of Disintegration," *Homeopathic Recorder,* XXXVII (1922), 427–28; R. F. Rabe, "Homeopathy—A Review of Its Condition and Prospects," *Homeopathic Recorder,* XXXV (1920), 237–38. See also Haller, *The History of American Homeopathy: The Academic Years, 1820–1935,* 289–98.

40 Ronald L. Numbers and John Harley Warner, "The Maturation of American Medical Science," in Judith Walzer Leavitt and Ronald L. Numbers (eds.), *Sickness and Health in America; Readings in the History of Medicine and Public Health* (2nd ed., revised, Madison: University of Wisconsin Press, 1985), 113–25.

ILLUSTRATIONS

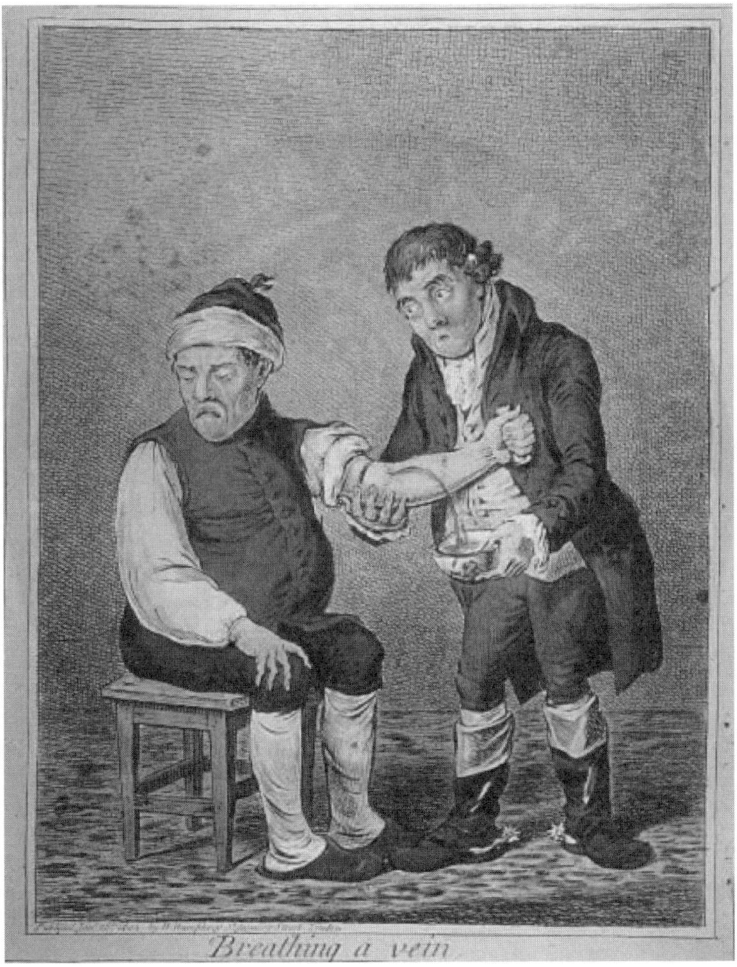

Fig. 1. Breathing a vein (1804). Courtesy of the National Library of Medicine.

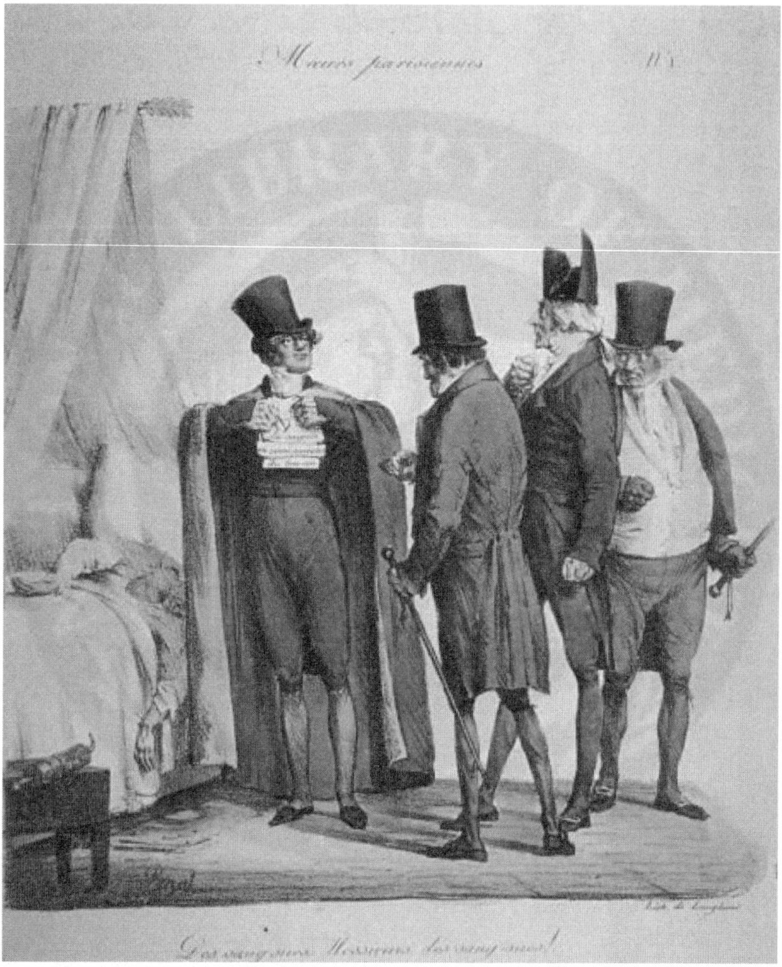

Fig. 2. Des sang-sues; Messueurs, des sang-sues! . . . Courtesy of the National Library of Medicine.

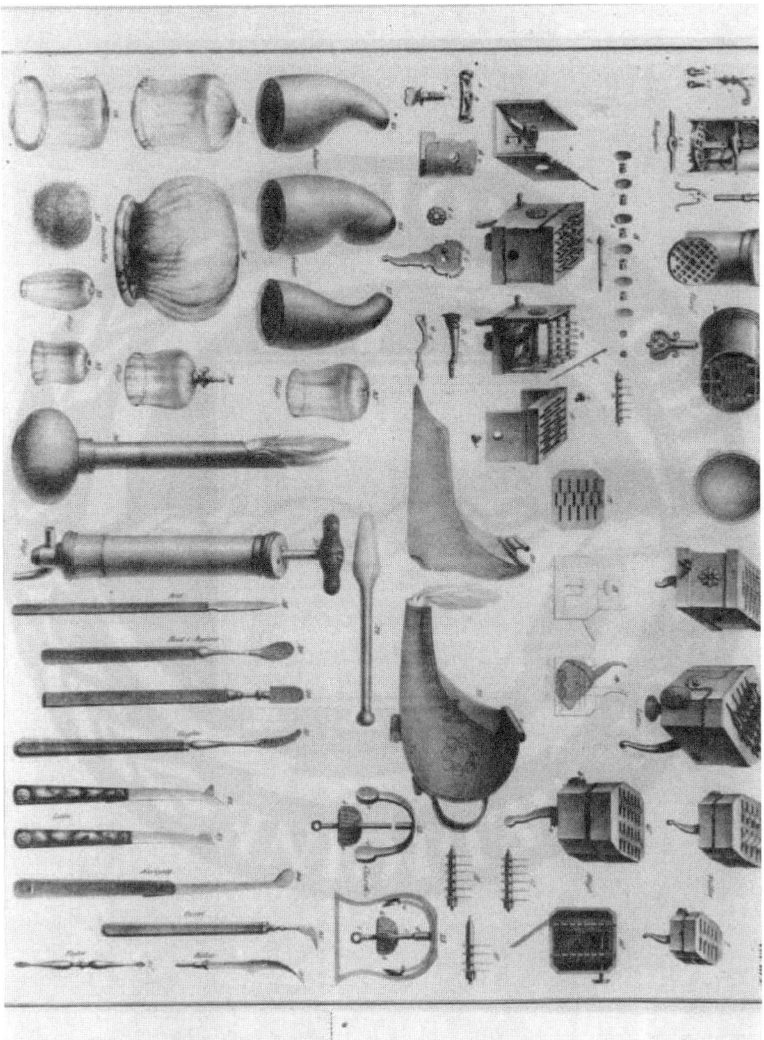

Fig. 3. Various types of bloodletting instruments 1 (1838). Courtesy of the National Library of Medicine.

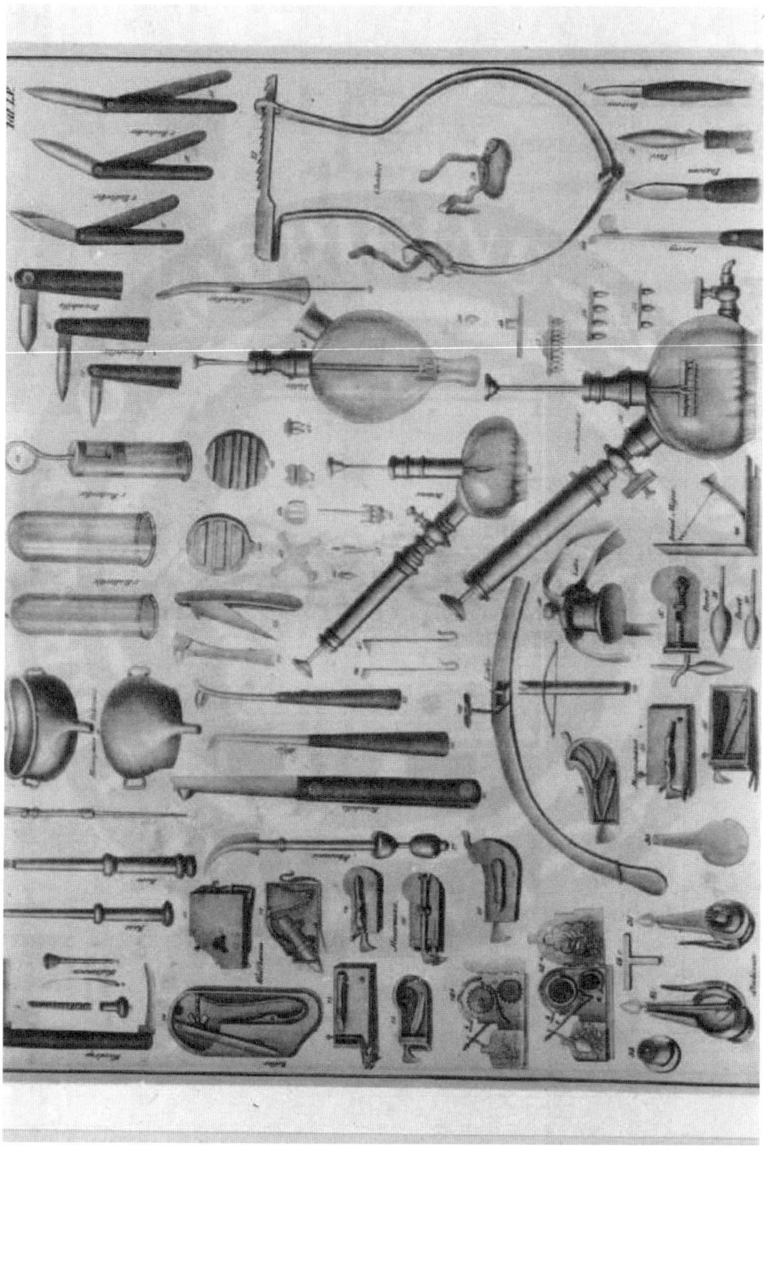

Fig. 4. Various types of bloodletting instruments 2 (1838). Courtesy of the National Library of Medicine.

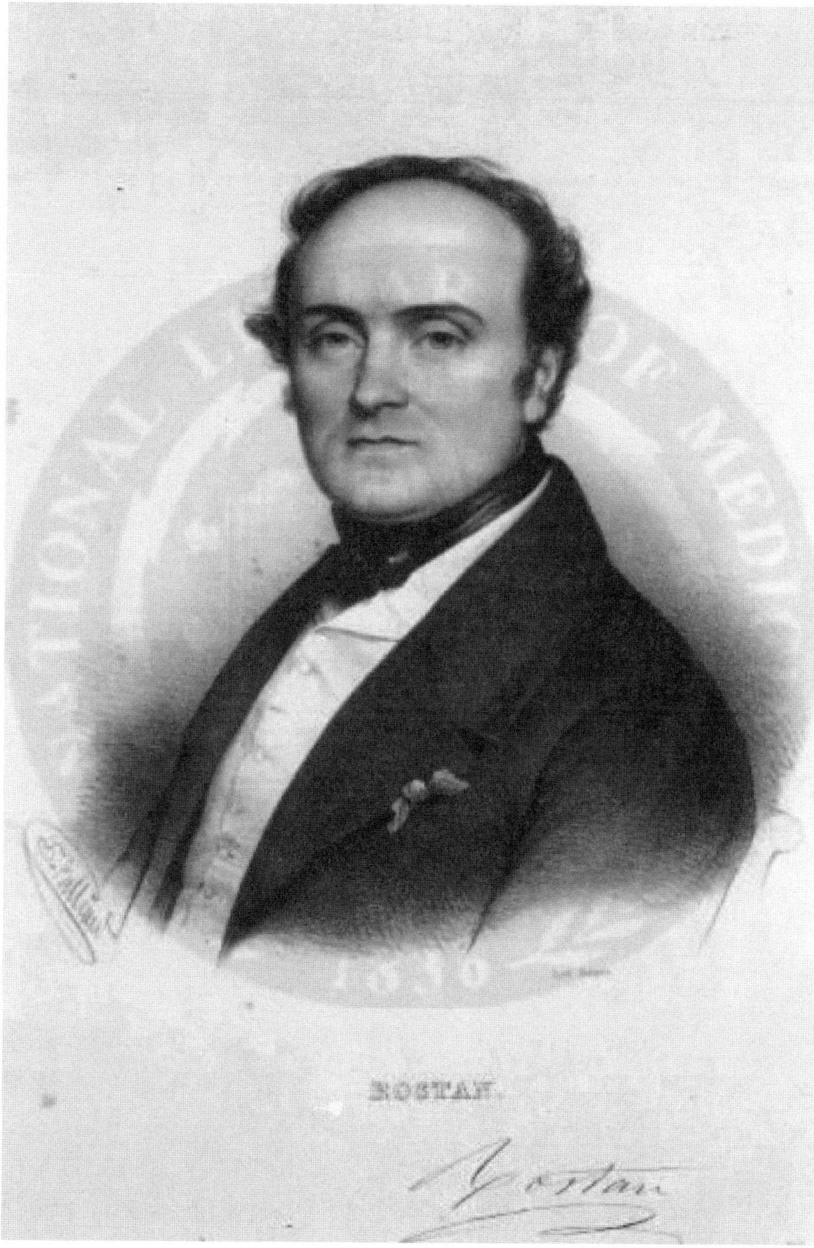

Fig. 5. Léon Rostan (1790–1866). Courtesy of the National Library of Medicine.

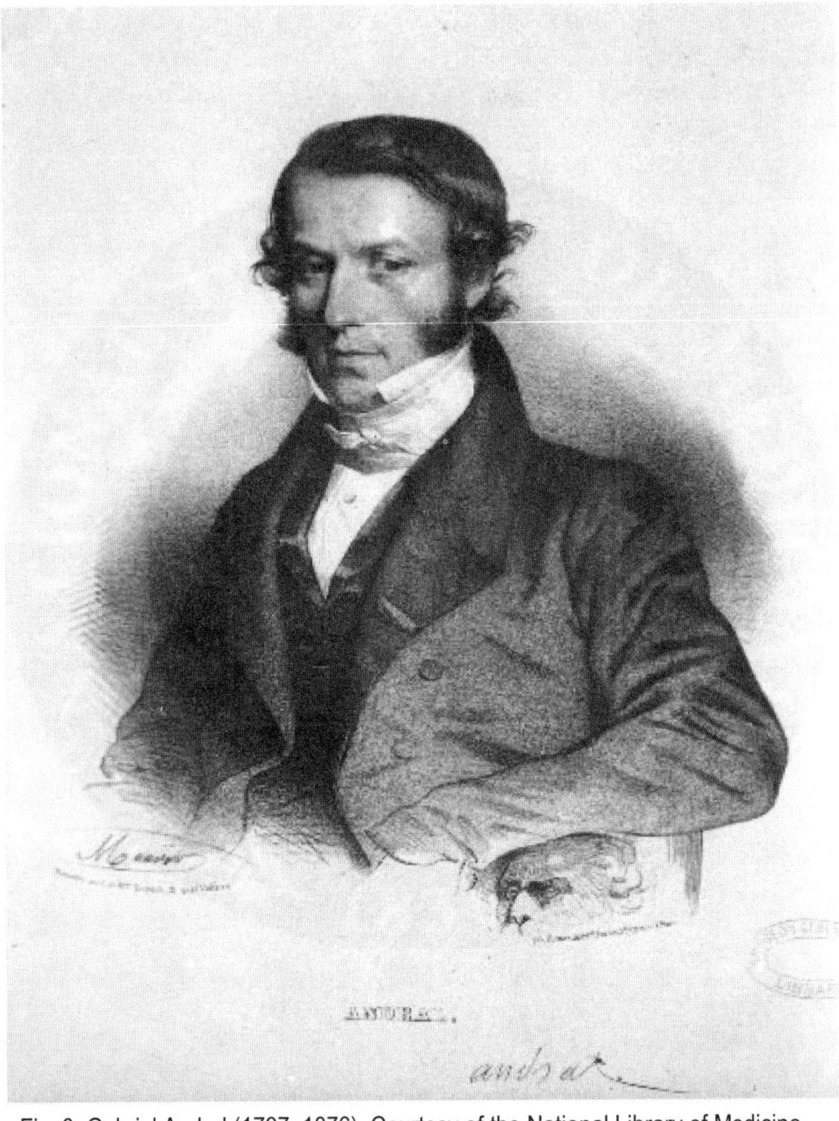

Fig. 6. Gabriel Andral (1797–1876). Courtesy of the National Library of Medicine.

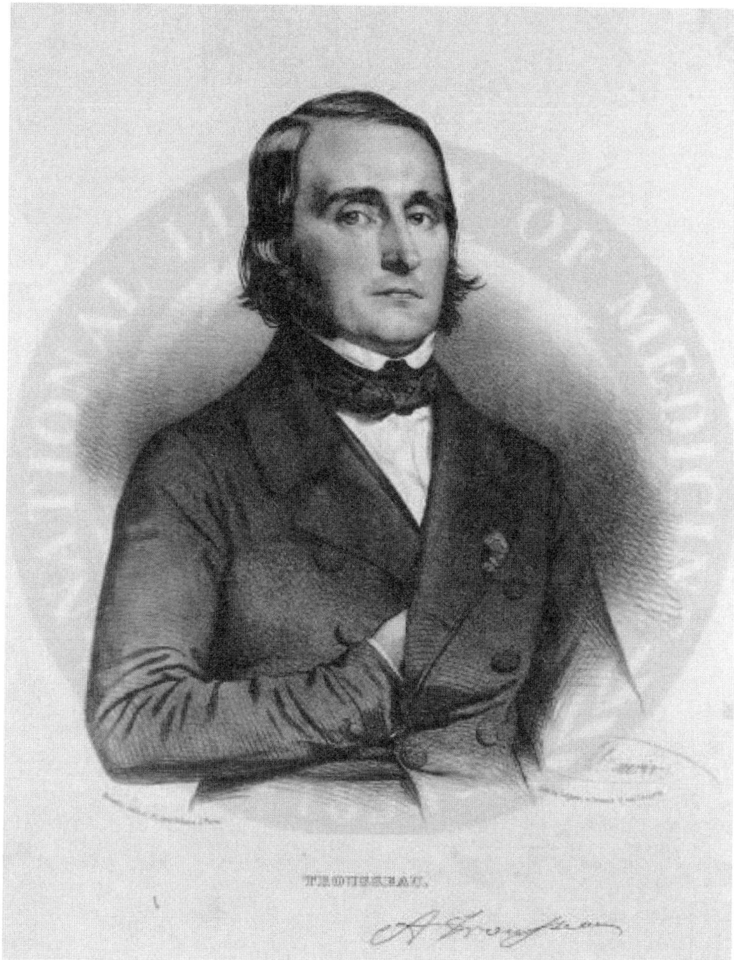

Fig. 7. Armand Trousseau (1801–1867). Courtesy of the National Library of Medicine.

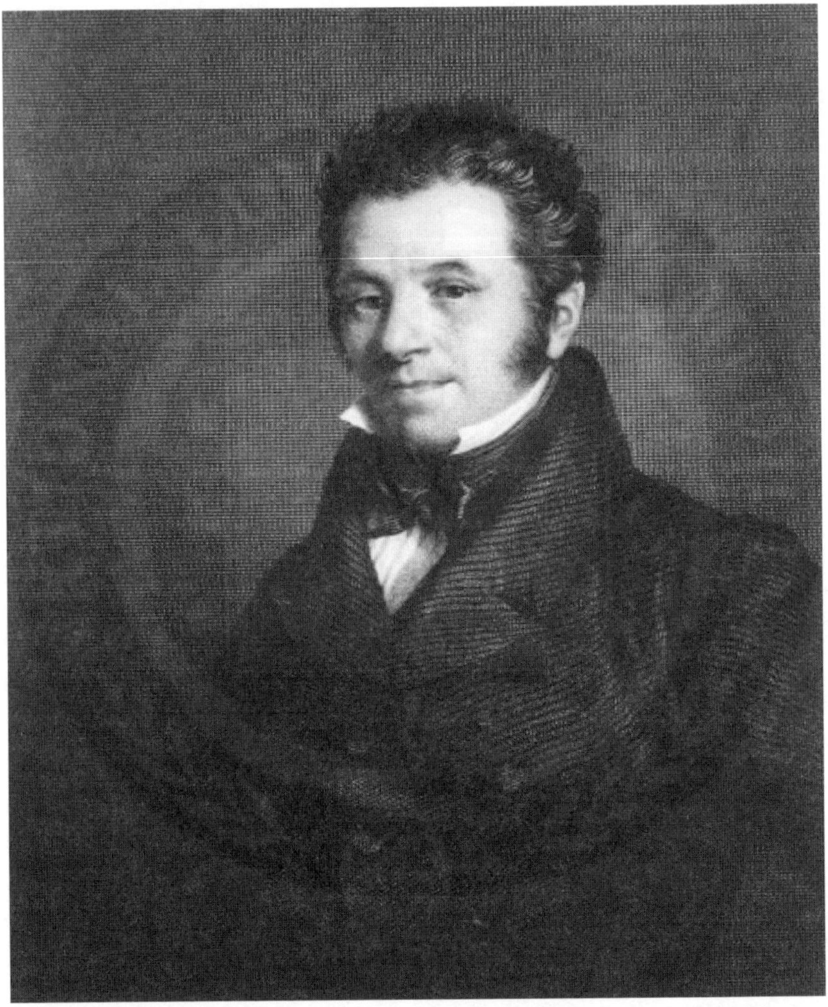

Fig. 8. Marshall Hall (1790–1857). Courtesy of the National Library of Medicine.

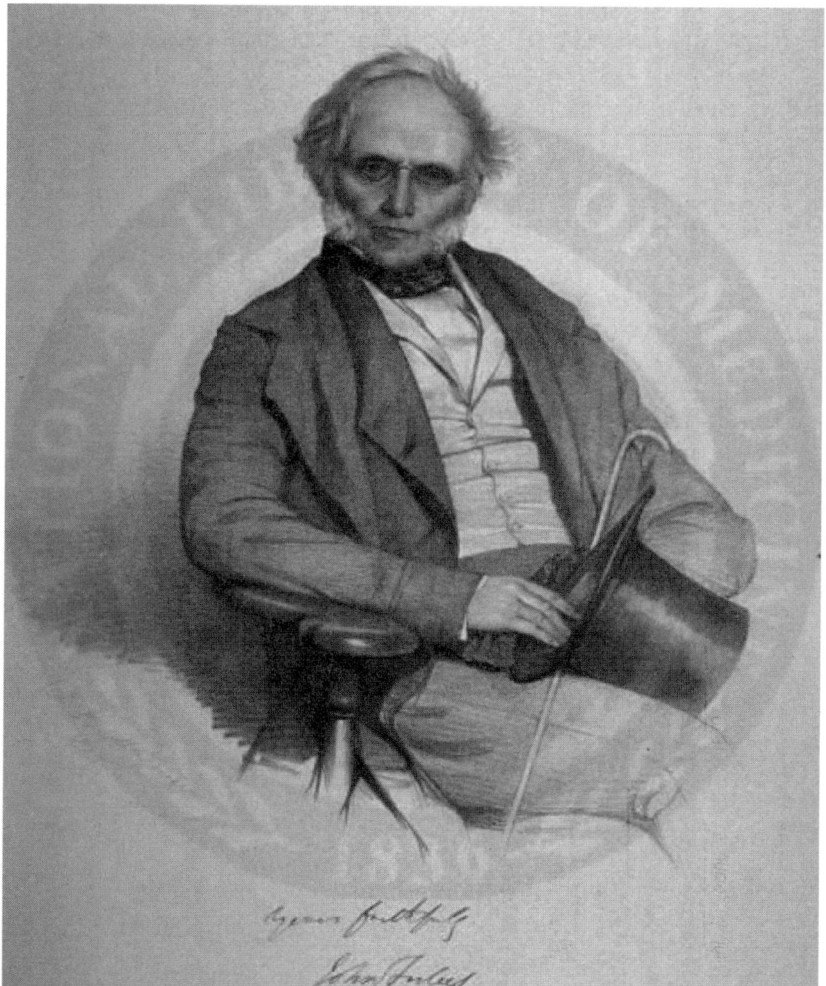

Fig. 9. Sir John Forbes (1787–1861). Courtesy of the National Library of Medicine.

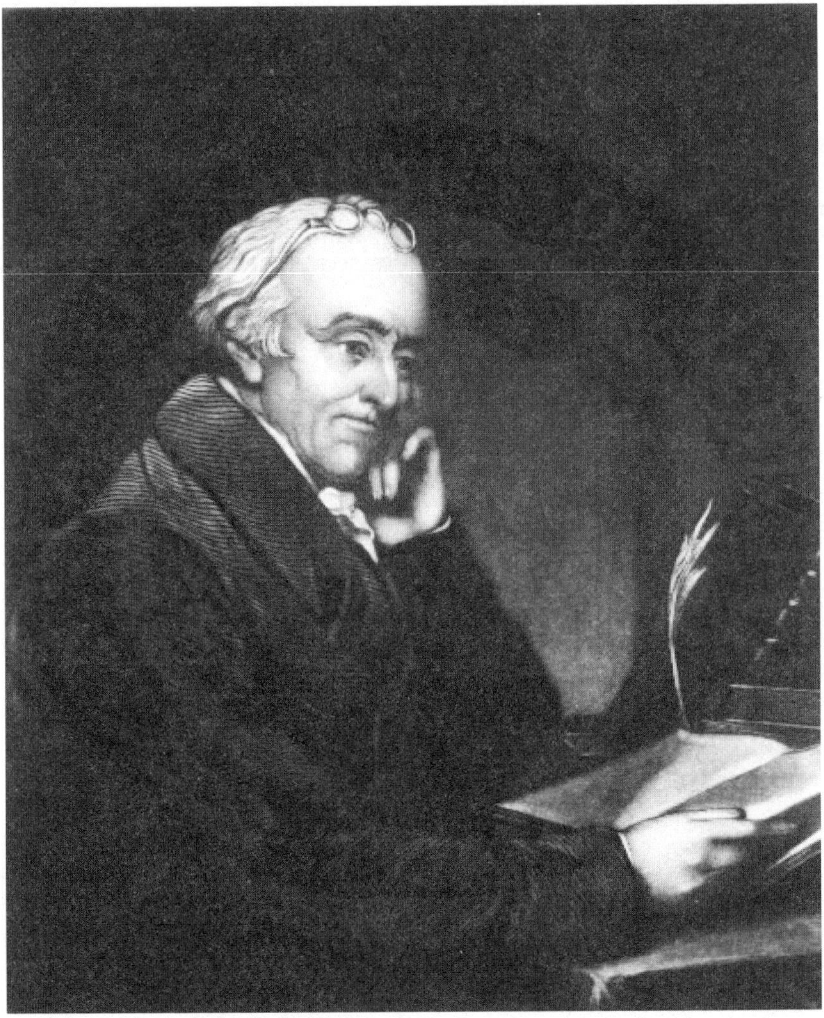

Fig. 10. Benjamin Rush (1745–1813). Courtesy of the National Library of Medicine.

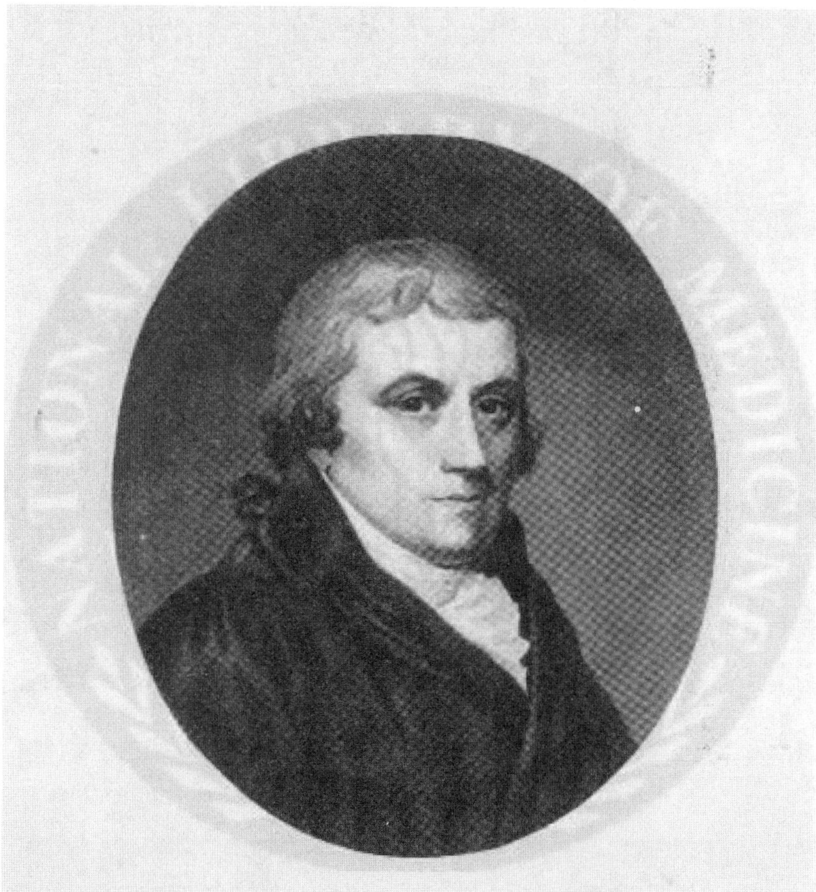

Fig. 11. Benjamin Waterhouse (1754–1846). Courtesy of the National Library of Medicine.

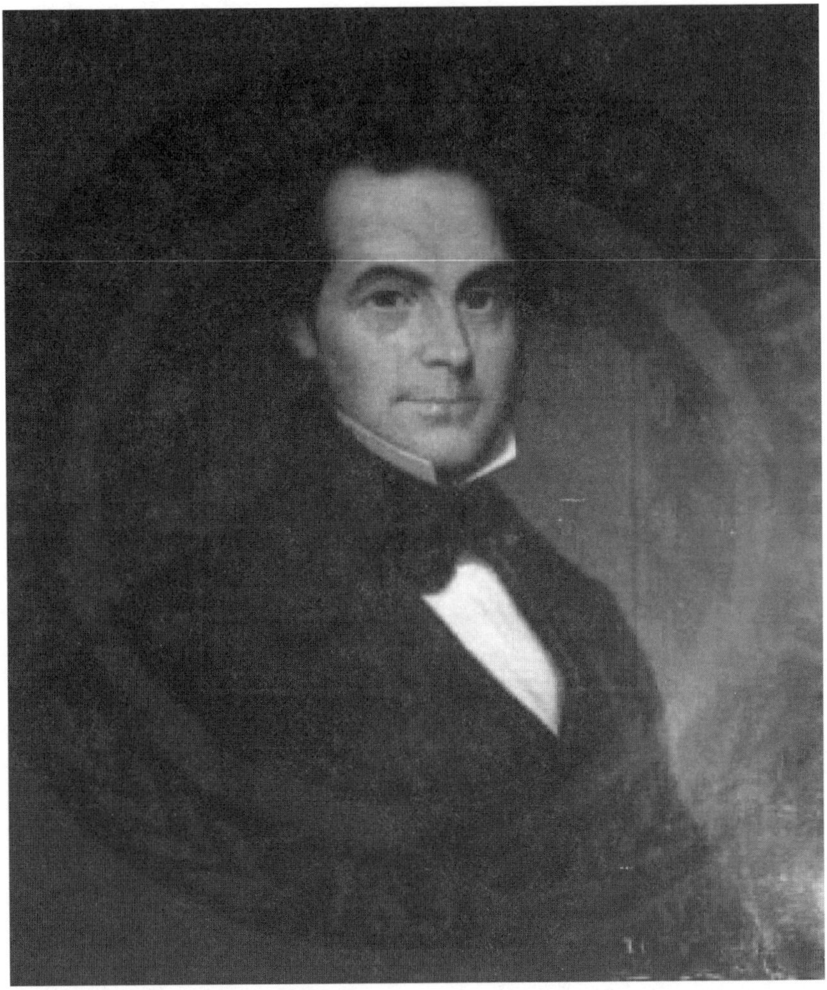

Fig. 12. Elisha Bartlett (1805–1855). Courtesy of the National Library of Medicine.

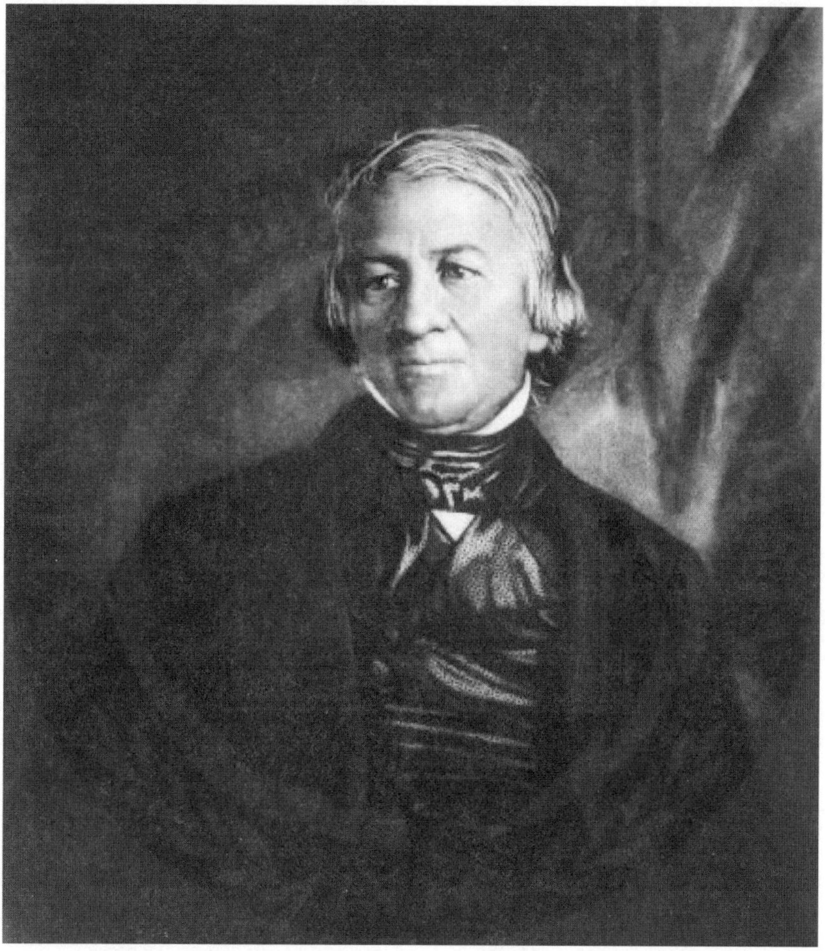

Fig. 13. Samuel Jackson (1787–1872). Courtesy of the National Library of Medicine.

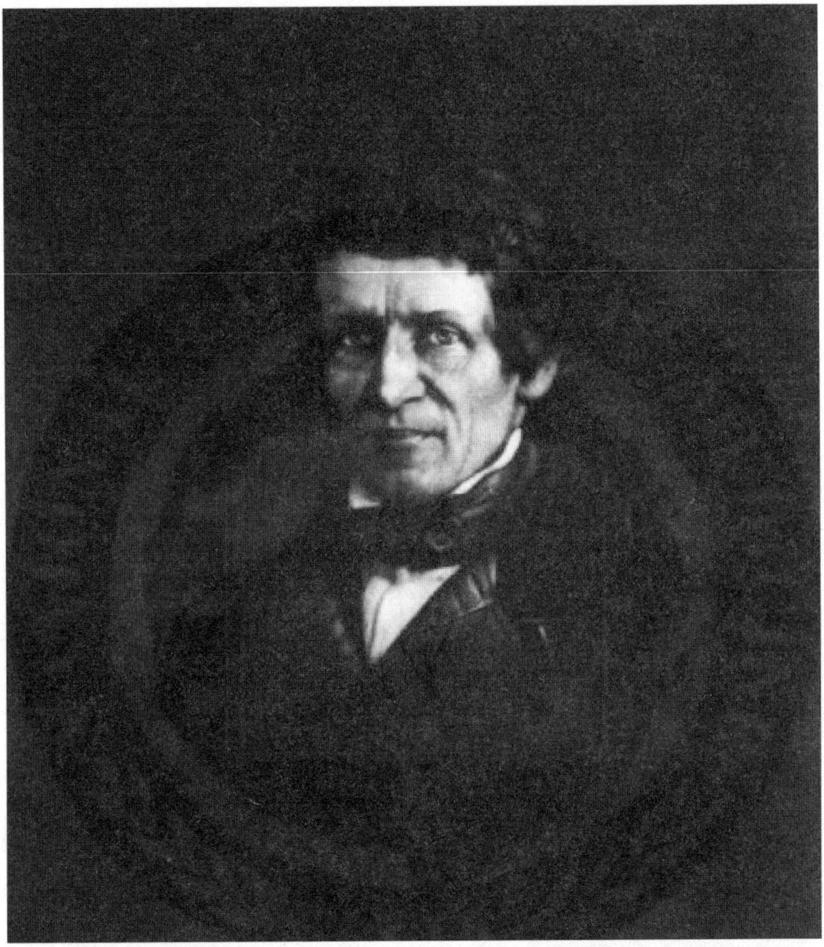

Fig. 14. George McClellan (1796–1847). Courtesy of the National Library of Medicine.

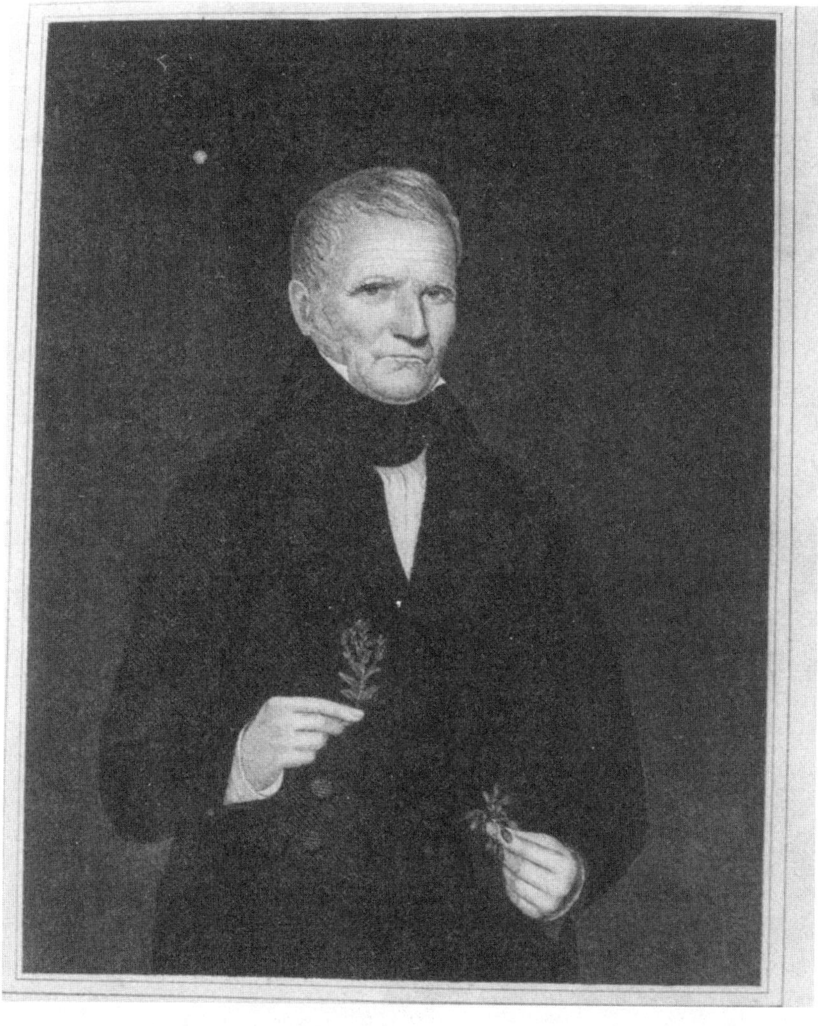

Fig. 15. Samuel Thomson (1769–1843) holding his lobelia plant. Courtesy of the Lloyd Library and Museum, Cincinnati.

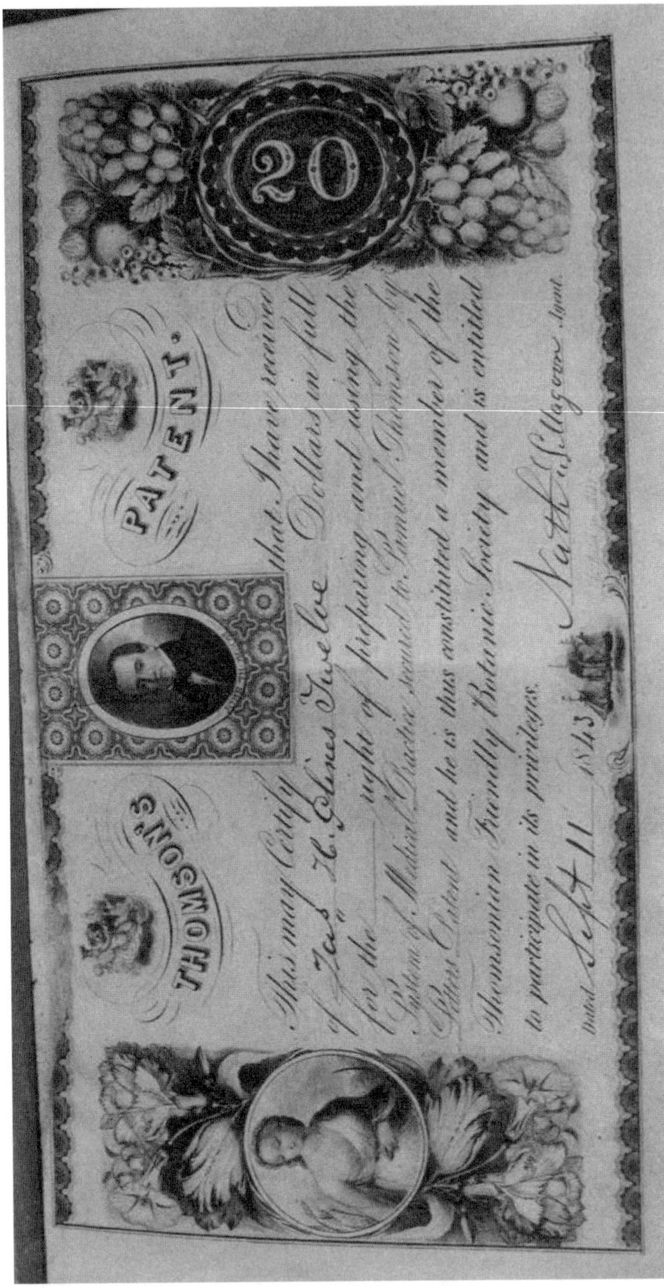

Fig. 16. Patent authorizing use of Samuel Thomson's system of medicine, 1843. Courtesy of the Lloyd Library and Museum, Cincinnati.

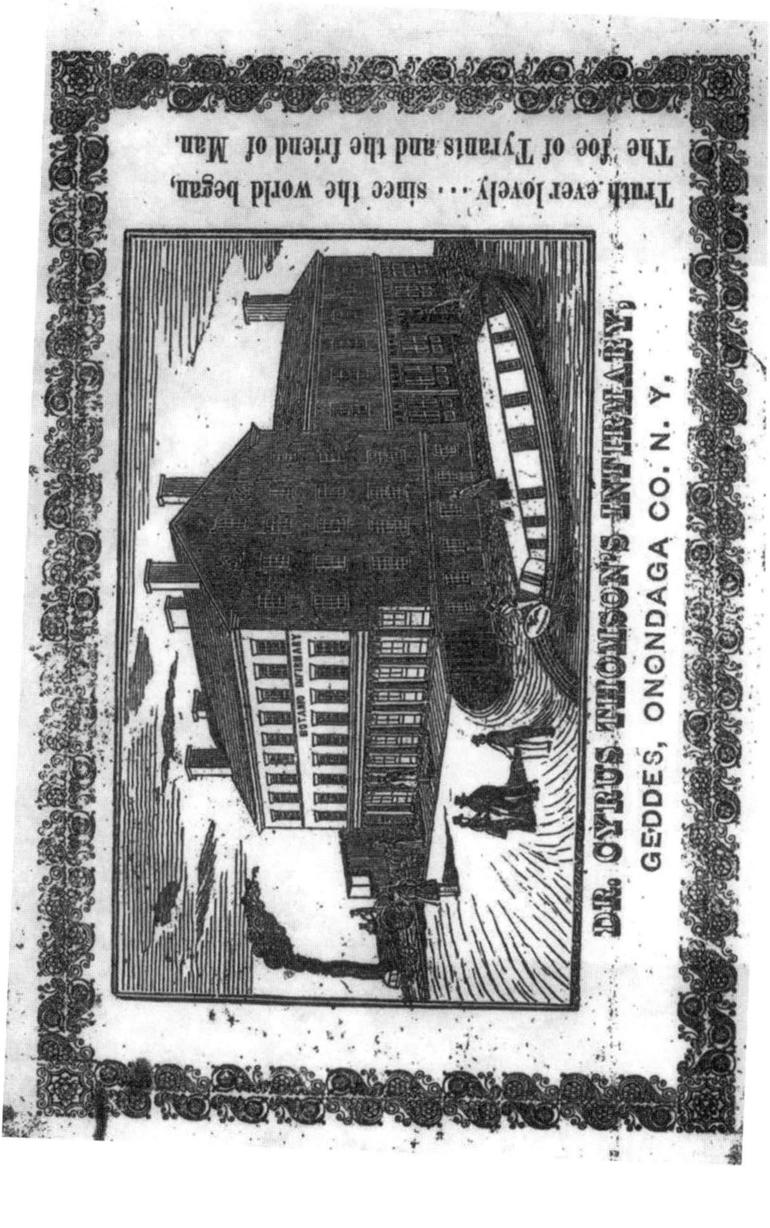
Truth ever lovely... since the world began,
The foe of Tyrants and the friend of Man.
BOTANIC INFIRMARY
DR. CYRUS THOMSON'S INFIRMARY,
GEDDES, ONONDAGA CO. N. Y.

Fig. 17. Advertisement for Dr. Cyrus Thomson's Infirmary in New York, 1843. Courtesy of John Ham Library, Brown University.

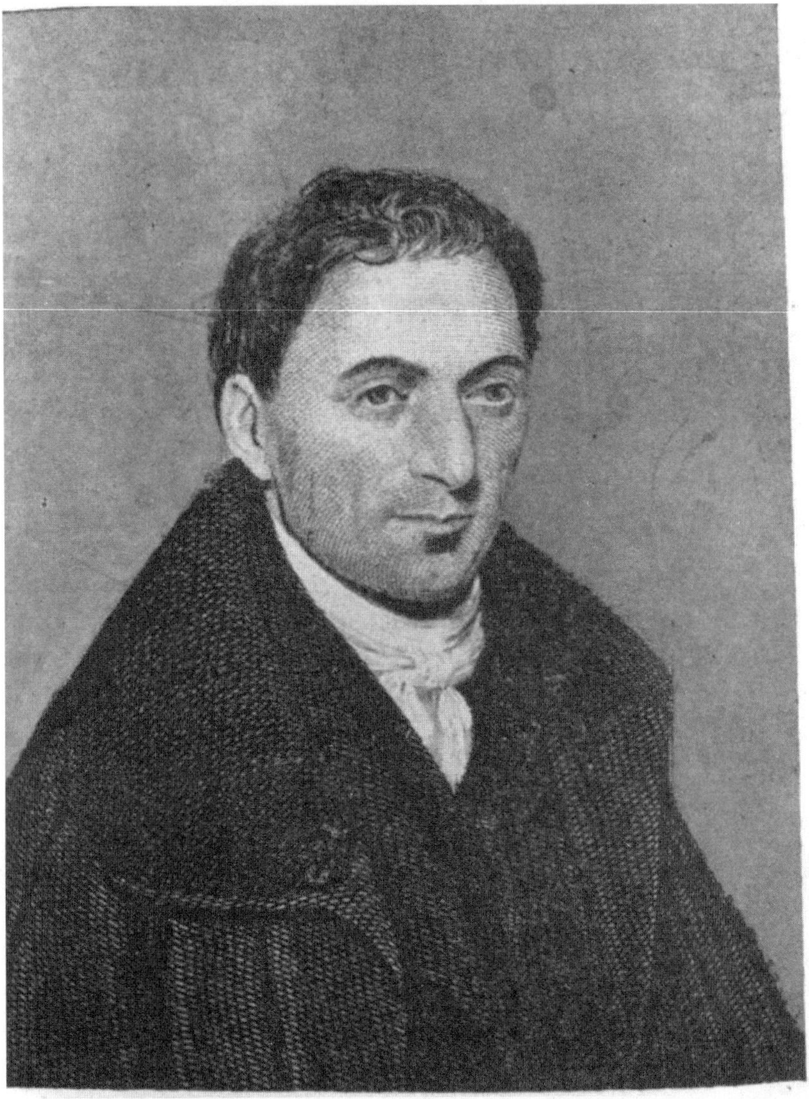

Fig. 18. Wooster Beach (1794–1868), founder of the Reformed Medical College of the City of New York. Courtesy of the Lloyd Library and Museum, Cincinnati.

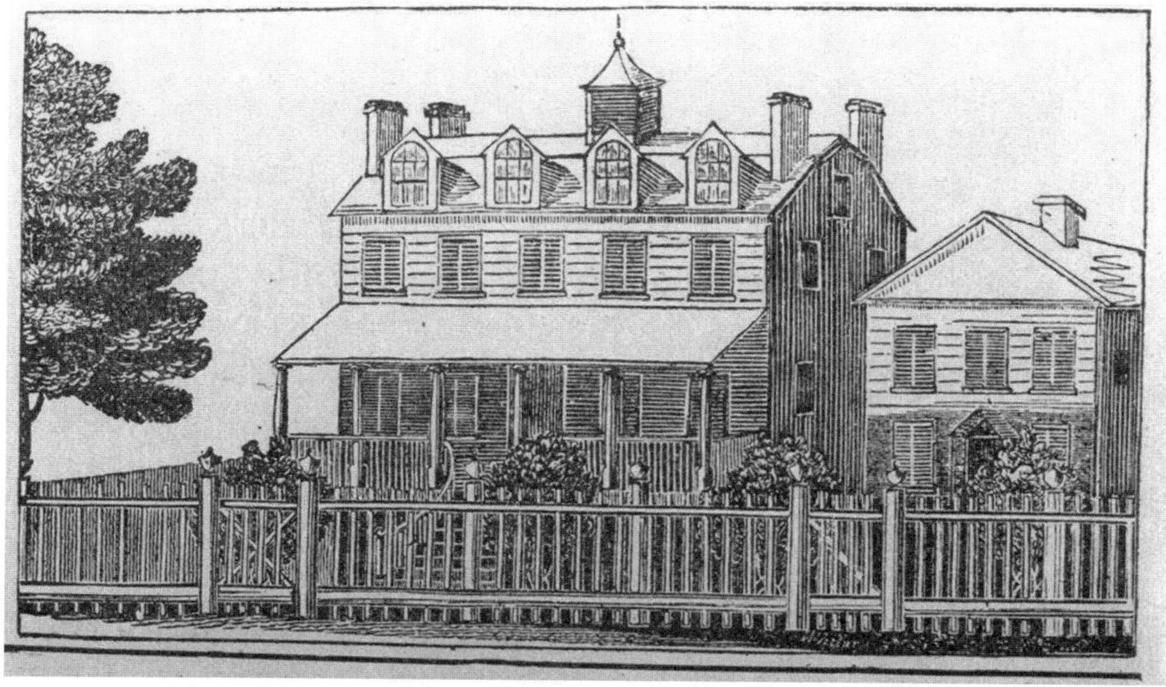

Fig. 19. Wooster Beach's Reformed Medical College of the City of New York, 1830. Courtesy of the Lloyd Library and Museum, Cincinnati.

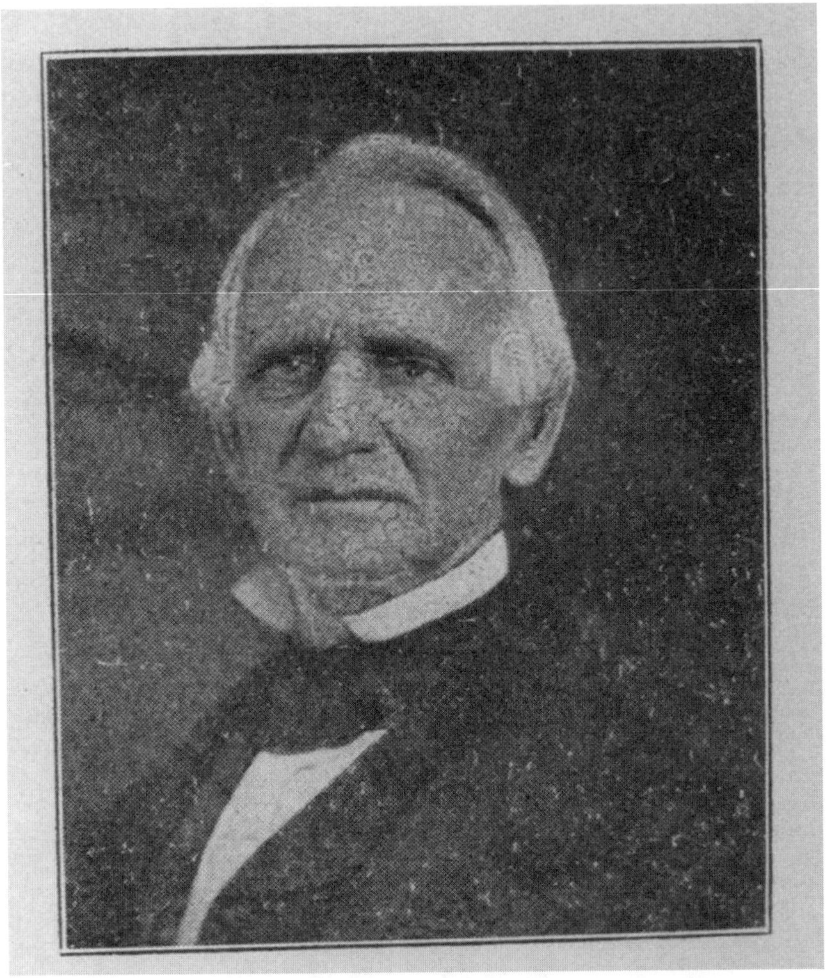

Fig. 20. Alva Curtis (1797–1881). Courtesy of the Lloyd Library and Museum, Cincinnati.

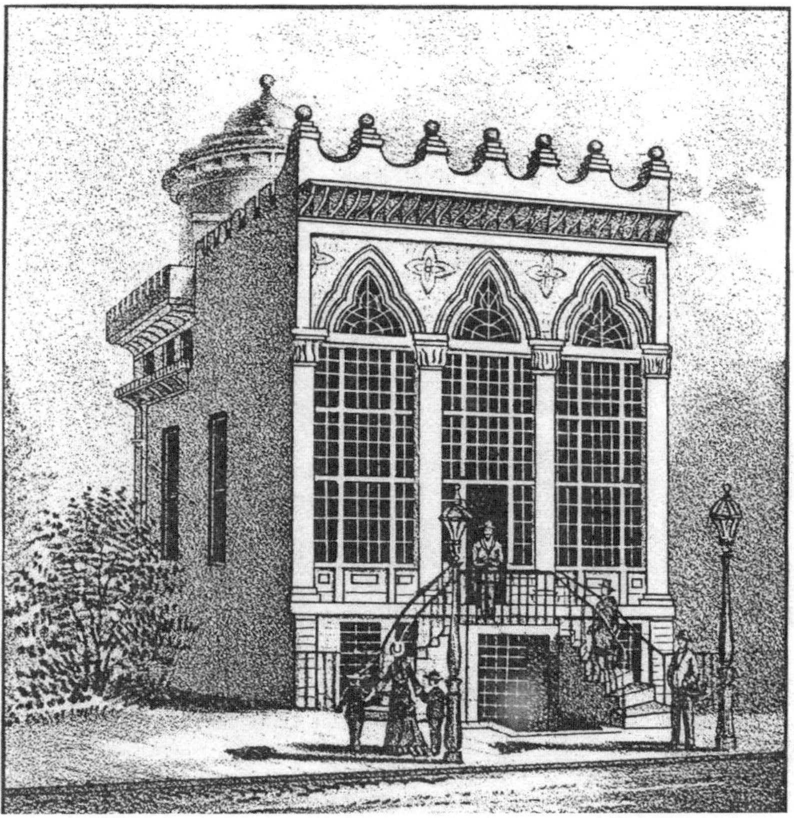

Fig. 21. Madame Trollope's Bazaar, home of Alva Curtis's American Medical Institute and Botanico-Medical College of Ohio, 1843. Courtesy of Lloyd Library and Museum, Cincinnati.

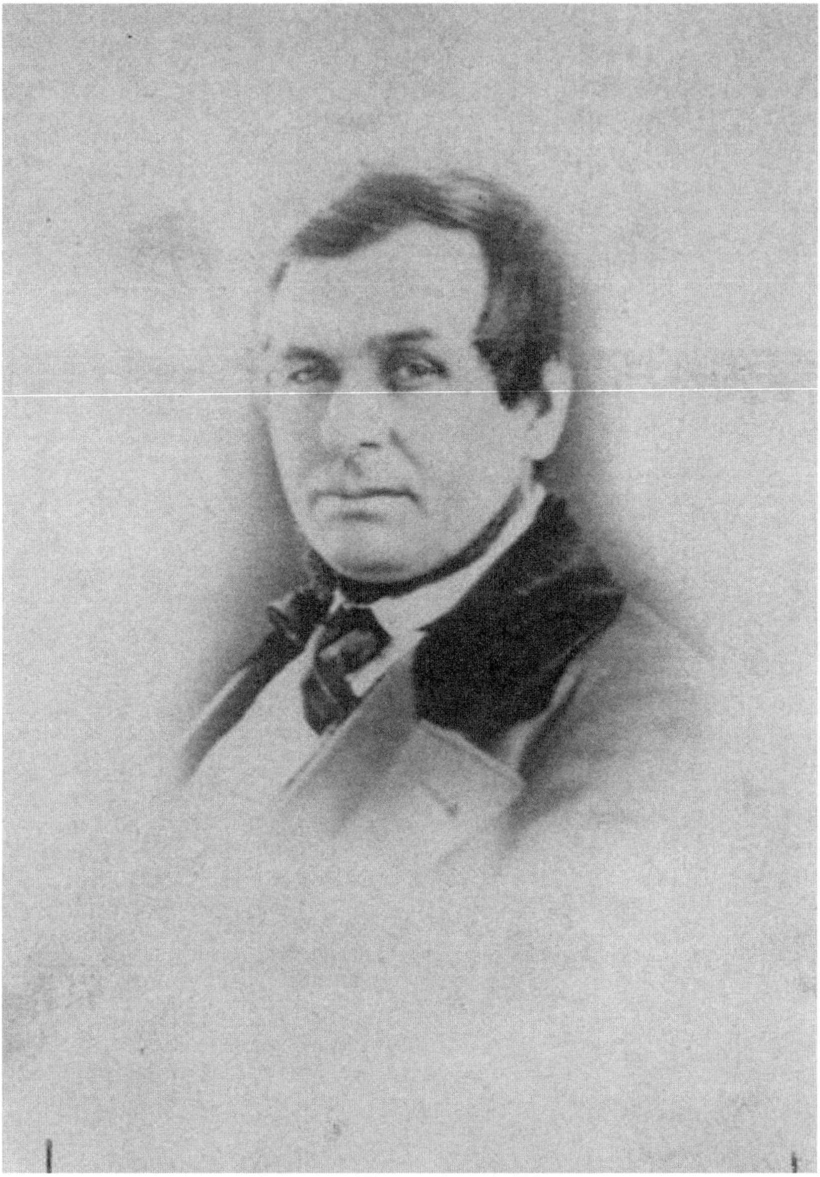

Fig. 22. Thomas Vaughan Morrow (1804–1850), founder of the Eclectic Medical Institute, Cincinnati. Courtesy of the Lloyd Library and Museum, Cincinnati.

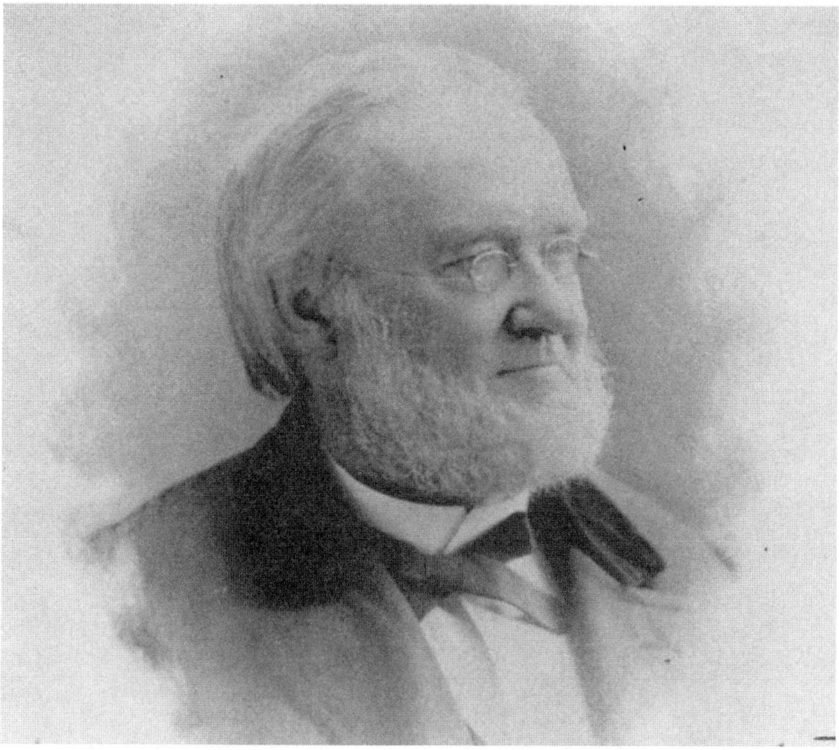

Fig. 23. Joseph Rodes Buchanan (1814–1899), dean of the Eclectic Medical Institute, Cincinnati Courtesy of the Lloyd Library and Museum, Cincinnati.

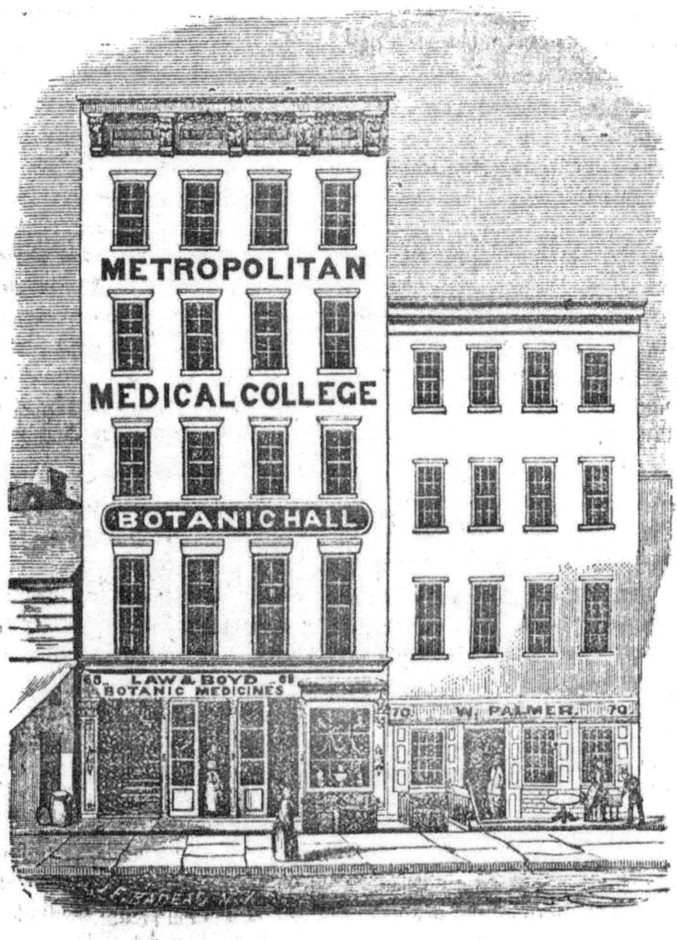

Fig. 24. Metropolitan Medical College at No. 68 East Broadway, New York City, 1852. Courtesy of the Lloyd Library and Museum, Cincinnati.

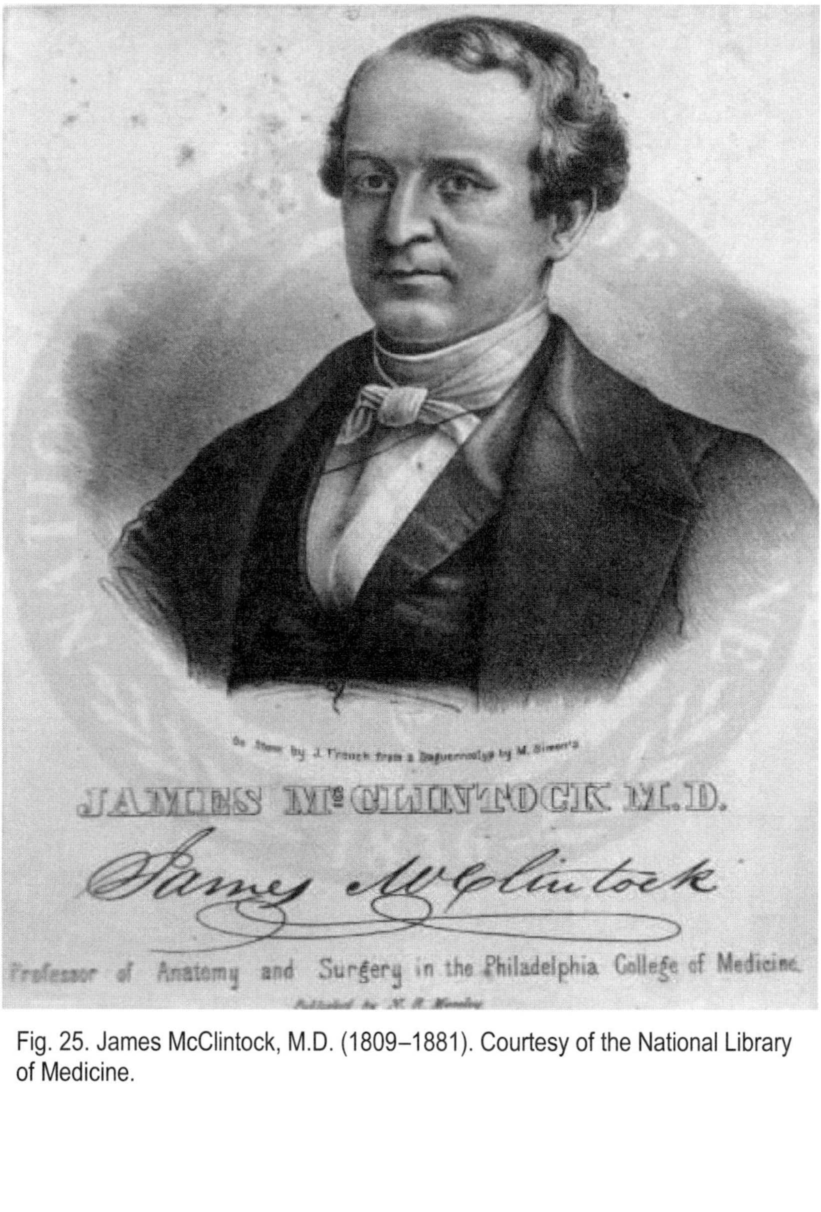
JAMES McCLINTOCK M.D.
Professor of Anatomy and Surgery in the Philadelphia College of Medicine

Fig. 25. James McClintock, M.D. (1809–1881). Courtesy of the National Library of Medicine.

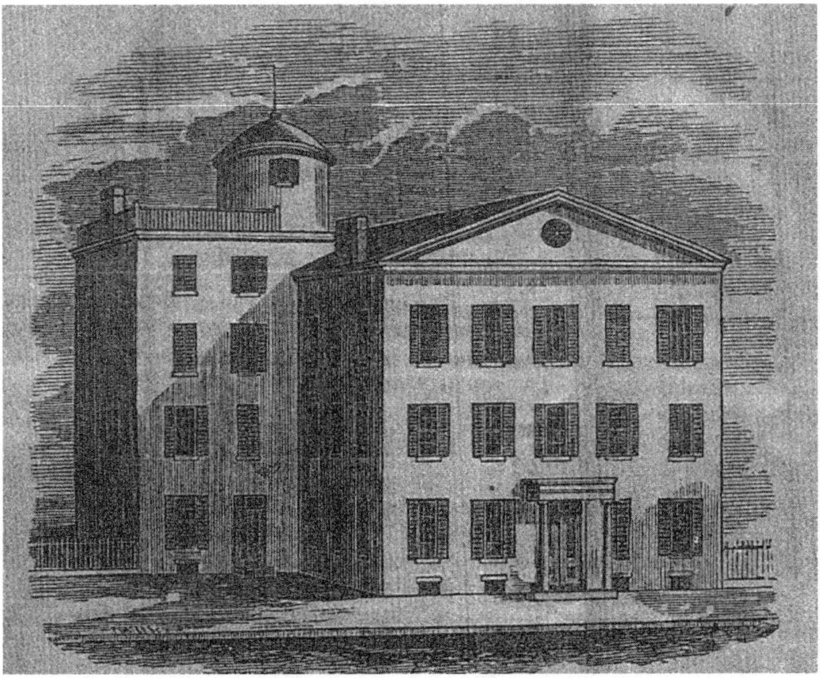

Fig. 26. The Eclectic Medical College of Philadelphia on Race Street below Fifth, 1860. Courtesy of the Lloyd Library and Museum, Cincinnati.

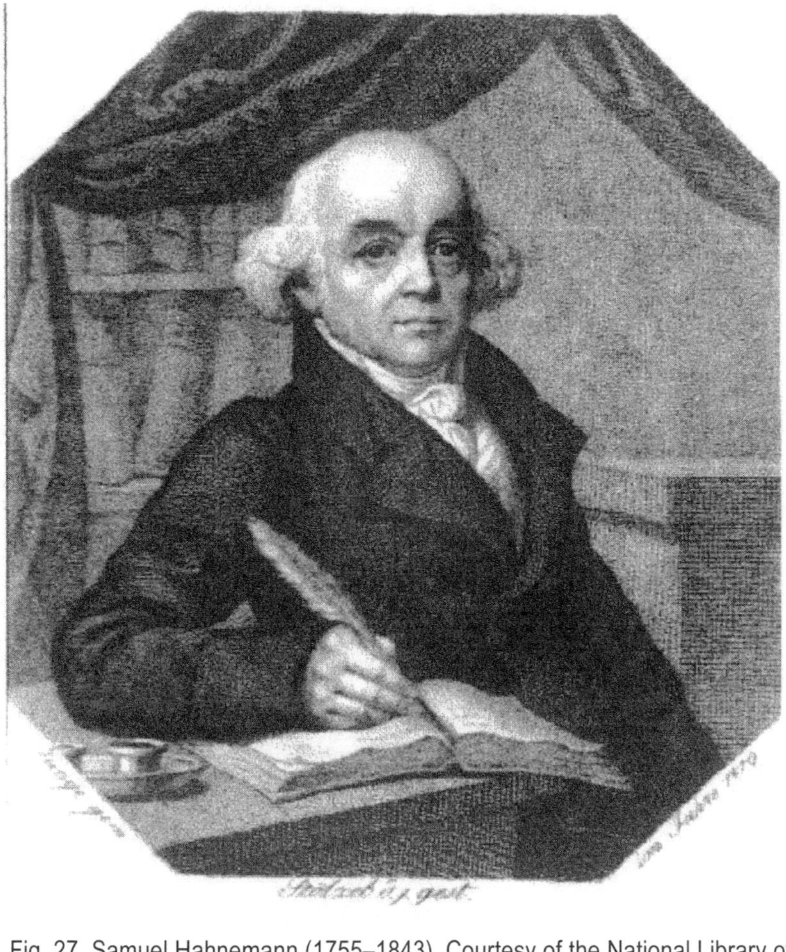

Fig. 27. Samuel Hahnemann (1755–1843). Courtesy of the National Library of Medicine.

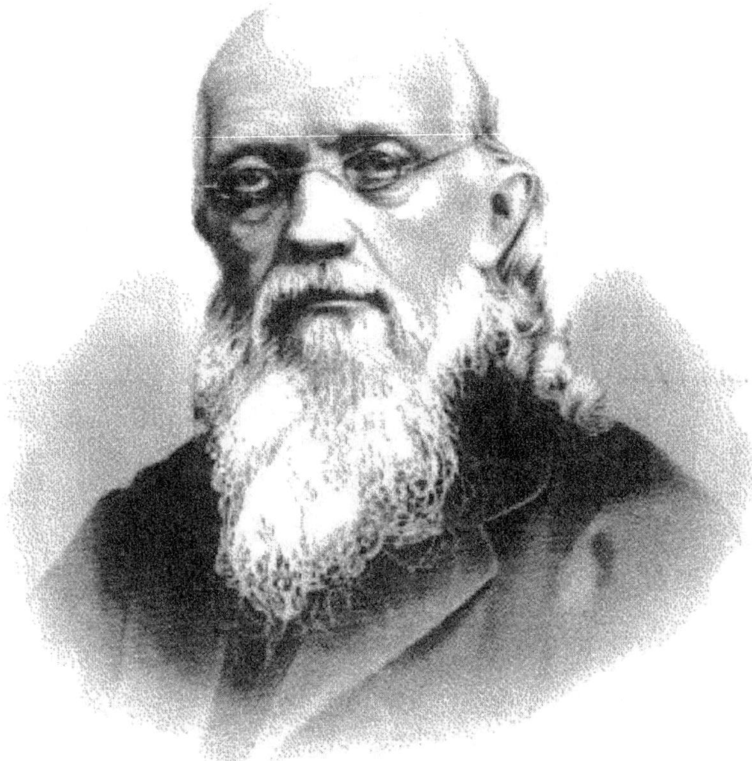

Fig. 28. Charles J. Hempel (1811–1879). Courtesy of the National Library of Medicine.

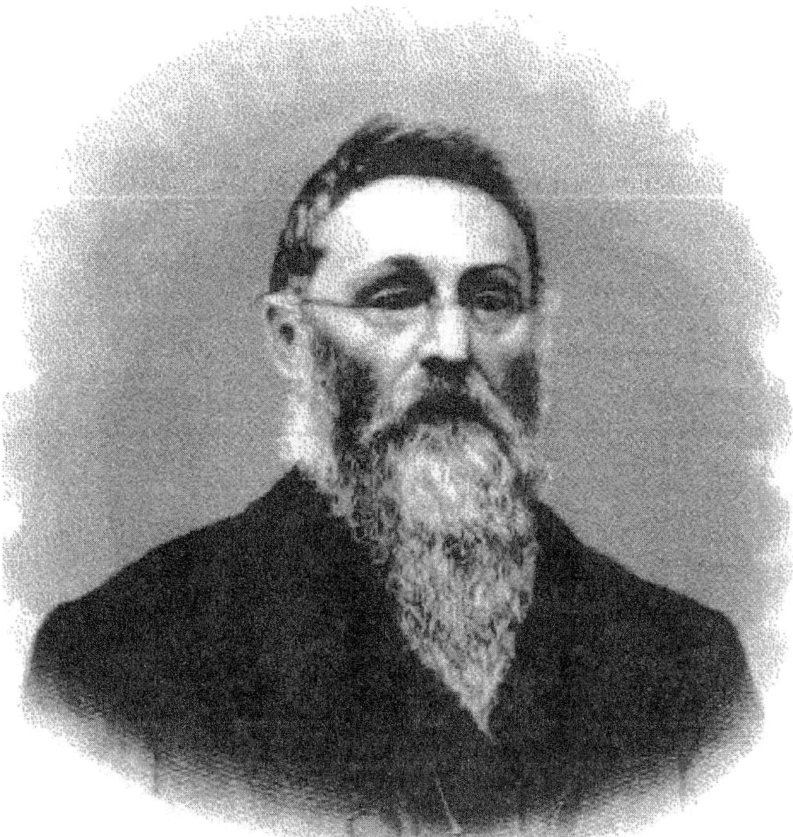

Fig. 29. Adolph Lippe (1812–1888). Courtesy of the National Library of Medicine.

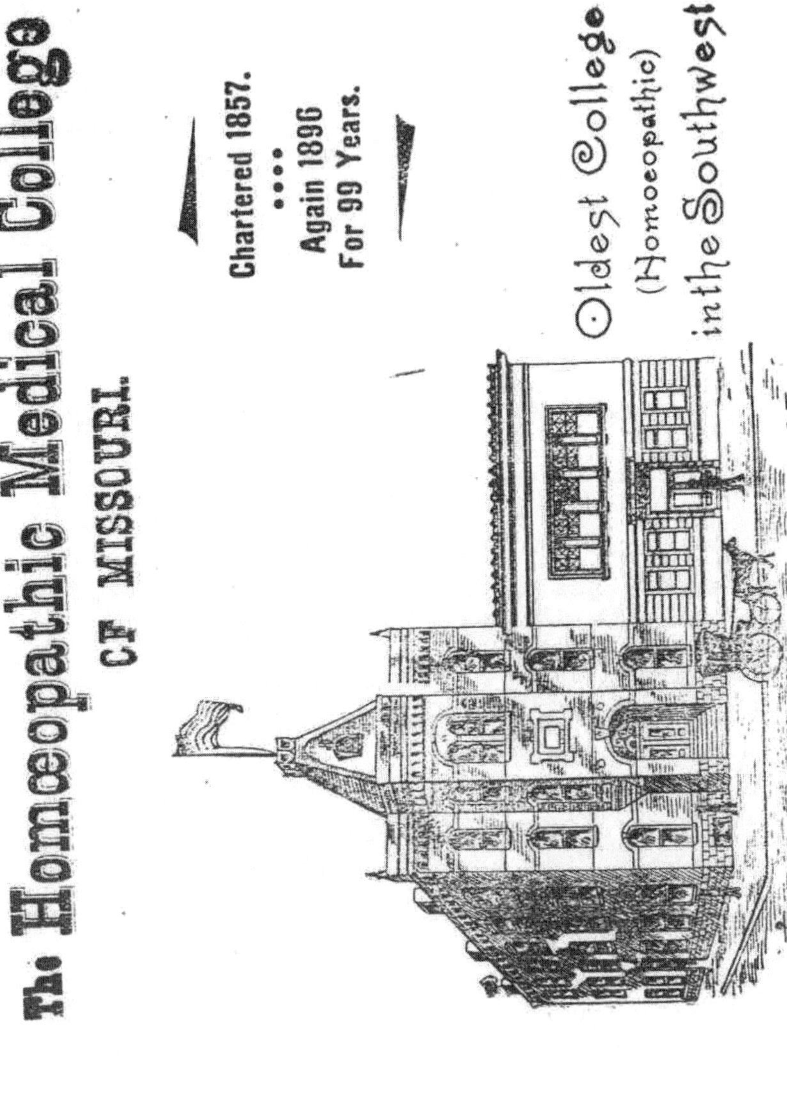
The Homoeopathic Medical College
OF MISSOURI.
Chartered 1857.
Again 1896
For 99 Years.
Oldest College
(Homoeopathic)
in the Southwest

Fig. 30. Homeopathic Medical College of Missouri. Courtesy of the Lloyd Library and Museum, Cincinnati.

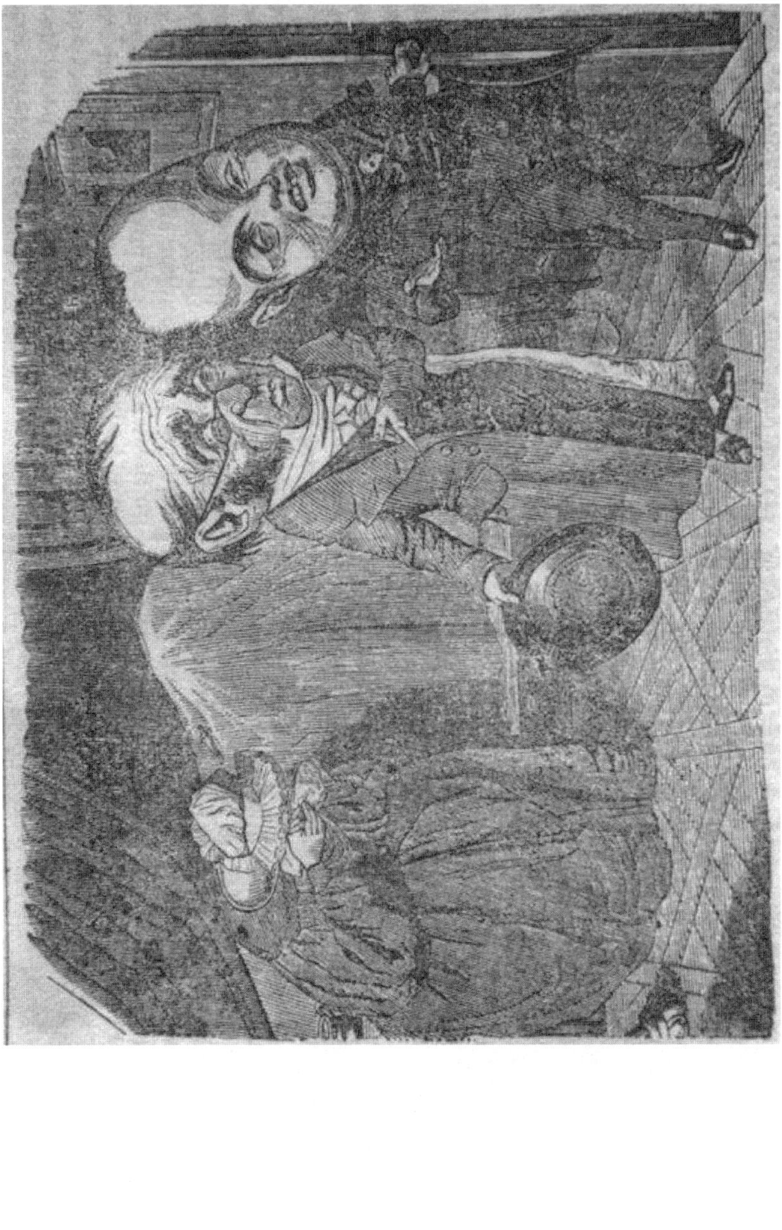

Fig. 31. Cartoon depicting "The Regulars in Consultation," 1841. Courtesy of the Lloyd Library and Museum, Cincinnati.

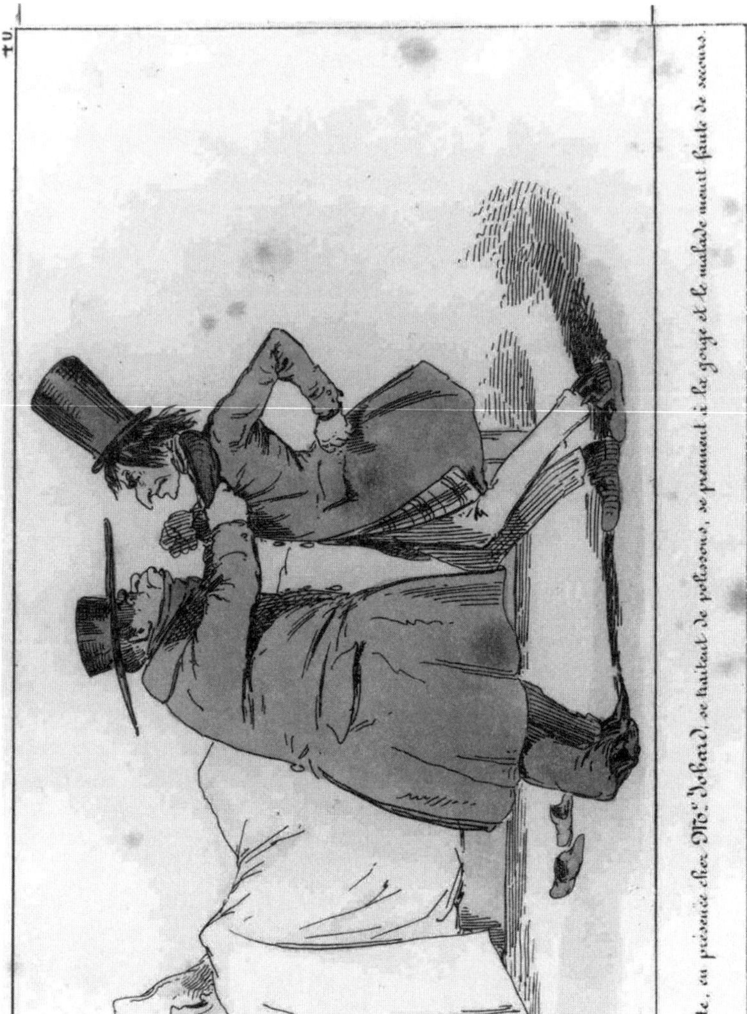
l'Homéopate et l'allopate, en présence chez Mr. Jobard, se traitent de polissons, se prennent à la gorge et le malade meurt faute de secours.

Fig. 32. Lithograph depiction of homeopath and allopath arguing the virtues of their medical systems over the bed of a patient (182?). By Henri Monnier (1805–1877). Courtesy of the National Library of Medicine.

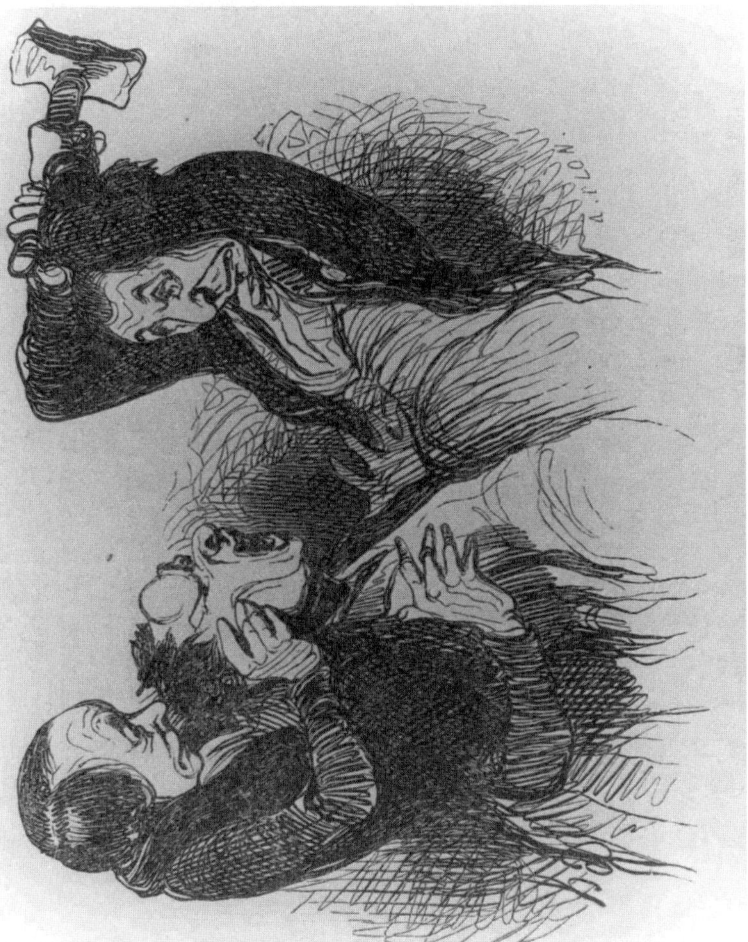

Fig. 33. Similia similibus curantur, or like cures like by Daumier from his illustrations for Fabre, 1841. Courtesy of the National Library of Medicine.

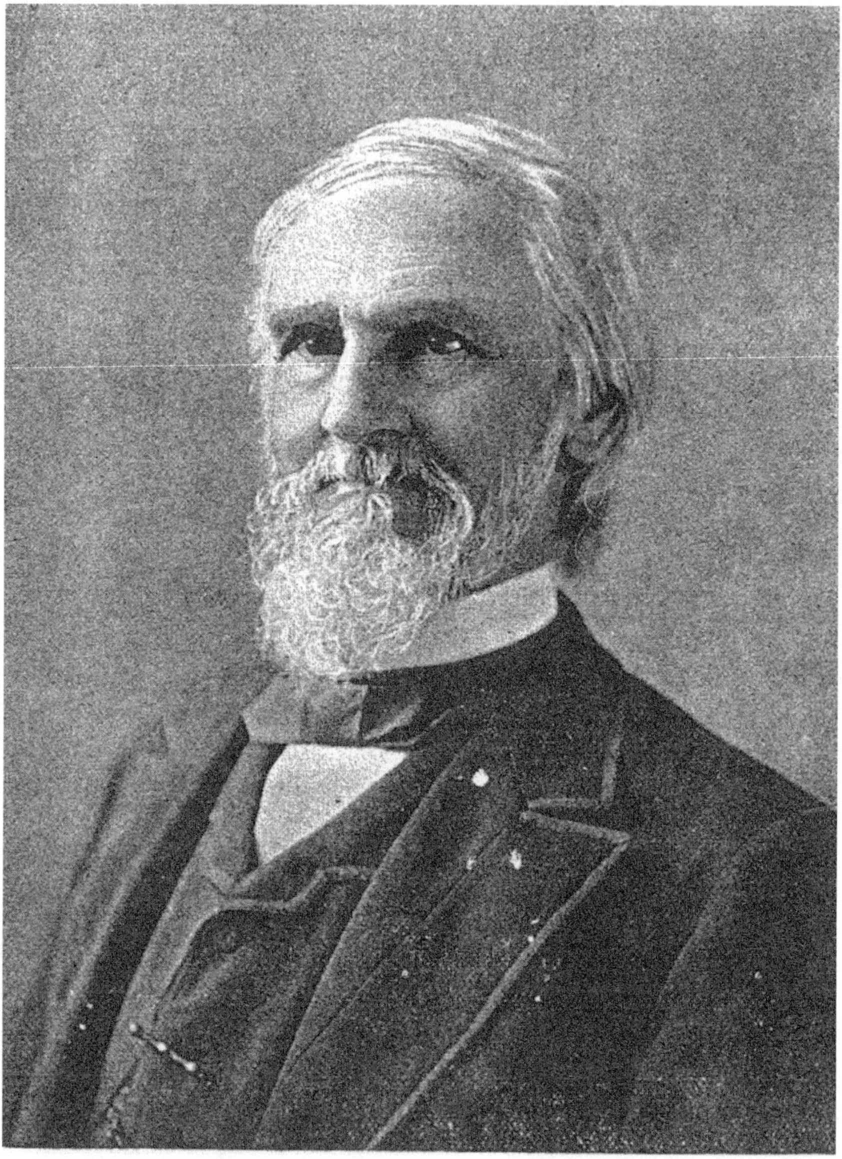

Fig. 34. Alexander Wilder (1823–1908), Secretary of the National Eclectic Medical Association. Courtesy of the Lloyd Library and Museum, Cincinnati.

APPENDIX A

Reform Medical Journals to 1909
(Botanic, Thomsonian, Physio-Medical, Homeopathic, and Eclectic)

	Title	Years	Location	Comments
1	*Alkaloidal Clinic*	1894–1905	Chicago	Monthly published by the Clinic Publishing Company. Succeeded by the *American Journal of Clinical Medicine.*
2	*Alumni News Letter*	1902	Chicago	Edited by T. E. Constain. Published three volumes.
3	*American Climates and Resorts*	1893–1895	Philadelphia	Monthly. Published by W. A. Chatterton. Intended for the laity.
4	*American Druggists' Circular and Chemical Gazette*	1857–1865	New York	Published nine volumes. Previously *Druggists' Circular and Chemical Gazette.*
5	*American Eclectic Medical Register*	1868	New York	Edited by Robert S. Newton
6	*American Eclectic Medical Review*	1866–1872	New York	Monthly. Edited by Robert S. Newton and E. Freeman. Published by J. F. Trow and Co. Later titled *New York Medical Review.*
7	*American Electro-Clinical Record*	1885	Chicago	Monthly journal of electricity. Published by W. A. Chatterton. A continuation of *The Medical Record.* Published but one year.
8	*American Health and Life*	1903	Chicago	Intended for laity.
9	*American Homeopath*	1879–1884	New York	Monthly. Published by A. L. Chatterton Pub. Co. and edited by E. C. Blumenthal. See *The American Homeopathist.*

	Title	Years	Location	Comments
10	*American Homeopathic Journal of Obstetrics and Gynaecology*	1885–1895	Ann Arbor; Chicago	Published by Advance Publishing Co. and edited by Phil Porter. Changed in 1895 to *Hahnemannian Advocate.*
11	*American Homeopathic Observer; a Monthly Journal Devoted to the Interests of Homeopathic Physicians*	1864–1885	Detroit	Monthly. Praised for bringing before the profession new provings, new remedies, and clinical cases illustrating the action of these medicines. Published by Edwin A. Lodge Homeopathic Pharmacy and edited by Edwin A. Lodge; Edwin M. Hale; Bushrod W. James; H. P. Gatchell; Thomas Nichol; L. Younghusband; E. W. Fish; Carl Muller; S. Lilienthal; Samuel A. Jones; and D. A. Colton. Younghusband's name was dropped in 1870 following disclosure of his fraudulent degrees. The prefix *American* was added in April 1864 to distinguish the journal from *The Homeopathic Observer* of England. Known as "Lodge's Journal." Discontinued after death of Lodge in 1885. Purchasers were also offered copies of *The Christian Unionist, The Christian at Work,* and *New Remedies.*
12	*American Homeopathic Record*	1867	New York	Published by J. T. S. Smith and Son and edited by H. M. Smith. Was to have been authorized by the American Institute of Homeopathy. Only one issue printed.
13	*American Homeopathic Review*	1858–1866	New York	Monthly. Published by J. T. S. Smith and Sons and edited by H. M. Smith; Roger G. Perkins; P. P. Wells; and C. Dunham. Discontinued after six volumes. Contained many studies of the materia medica and papers by Dr. Carroll Dunham. Opposed the *North American Journal of Homeopathy*. Tried to find a middle ground between the high and low dilutionists.
14	*American Homeopathist*	1864–1868	Cincinnati	Monthly. Published by Smith and Worthington and edited by Charles Cropper and James G. Hunt. Half professional and half lay journal. Adjunct to the Cleveland Homeopathic College. Miscellaneous monographs inserted in some volumes; included proceedings of Indiana Homeopathic Institute for 1867. Published for four years. Merged in 1868 with the *Ohio Medical and Surgical Reporter.*
15	*American Homeopathist*	1877	Chicago; New York	Monthly. Published by A. L. Chatterton and Co. and edited by J. P. Mills; C. E. Blumenthal et al. Changed name to *The American Homeopath* in 1879, and then back to *The American Homeopathist* in 1885, and then to *American Physician* in 1902.

	Title	Years	Location	Comments
16	*American Homeopathist*	1885–1902	New York	Monthly. Published by A. L. Chatterton and Co. Succeeded by *American Physician* in 1902.
17	*American Journal of Clinical Medicine*	1906–1924	Chicago	Monthly. Continuation of the *Alkaloidal Clinic.* Absorbed the *Chicago Medical Times* in 1911.
18	*American Journal of Electrology and Neurology*	1879–1880	New York	Quarterly. Published by Boericke and Tafel and edited by J. Butler. Continued in 1880 as *The Medico-Chirurgical Quarterly.*
19	*American Journal of Homeopathia*	1834–1835	New York	Bimonthly. Published by Moore and Payne and edited by John F. Gray; S. R. Kirby; and A. Gerald Hull. Ambitious and devoted to upholding strict homeopathy. Suspended publication in 1835 after four issues and resumed in 1840 as *Homeopathic Examiner.* First American homeopathic journal. Intended for the profession and intelligent laymen; not intended for dissemination to the public.
20	*American Journal of Homeopathic Materia Medica*	1867–1871	Philadelphia	Monthly. Published by King and Baird and edited by C. Hering and H. W. Martin. Organ of the Hahnemann Medical College of Philadelphia. Its object was to furnish the profession with a complete materia medica. Formerly called *The Journal of Homeopathic Clinics.* Published five volumes. Changed name in 1871 to *The American Journal of Materia Medica and Record of Medical Science.*
21	*American Journal of Homeopathic Materia Medica and Record of Medical Science*	1871–1876	Philadelphia	Published by J. M. Stoddart and edited by W. H. Bigler and A. R. Thomas. Organ of the Hahnemann Medical College of Philadelphia. Its object was to furnish the profession with a complete materia medica. Nine volumes published.
22	*American Journal of Homeopathy*	1838–1839	Philadelphia	Bimonthly. Published by W. L. J. Kiderlin and Company and edited by C. Hering; C. Lingen; C. Neidhard, et al. There was but one volume published. Reissued in 1839 as *Miscellanies on Homeopathy.*
23	*American Journal of Homeopathy*	1846–1854	New York	Semimonthly. Later became monthly. Published by C. G. Dean and edited by S. R. Kirby and R. A. Snow. On completion of second volume in April 1848, Snow resigned and Kirby continued alone as editor.
24	*American Journal of Indigenous Materia Medica and Repertory of Medical Science*	1860–1861	New York	Monthly. Founded by B. Keith

	Title	Years	Location	Comments
25	*American Journal of Materia Medica*	1860–1861	Chicago	Published by Halsey and King and edited by George E. Shipman. Only four numbers of the journal were published. Contained chiefly a record of provings.
26	*American Journal of Medical Reform, for the People and the Profession*	1851–1853	New York City	Monthly. Edited by J. D. Friend and H. M. Sweet. Continued as *Journal of Medical Reform for the People and the Profession.*
27	*American Journal of Medicine*	1852	Syracuse	Monthly. Published by S. H. Potter. Formerly the *American Medical and Surgical Journal.*
28	*American Journal of Medicine and Record of Innocent Medication*	1853	Philadelphia	Monthly. Edited by H. F. Johnson and assisted by the faculty of the American College of Medicine (eclectic).
29	*American Journal of Physiology*	1882–1884	Indianapolis	
30	*American Magazine Devoted to Homeopathy and Hydropathy*	1851–1854	Cleveland; Cincinnati	Monthly. Published and edited by J. H. Pulte and H. P. Gatchell; joined by C. D. Williams in 1854. Contained popular articles on anatomy, physiology, hygiene and dietetics. The second volume, published under the title of *The American Magazine of Homeopathy*. In 1854, it became a quarterly and was titled *Quarterly Homeopathic Magazine* and ceased to be a journal for popular reading.
31	*American Magazine of Homeopathy*	1852	Cleveland	Monthly. Published and edited by J. H. Pulte and H. P. Gatchell. Formerly *American Magazine Devoted to Homeopathy and Hydropathy.* Contained articles on water cure, movement cure, and health.
32	*American Medical and Surgical Journal*	1851–1852	Syracuse and Philadelphia	Monthly. Edited by S. H. Potter. In 1852 united with *New York Eclectic Medical and Surgical Journal* to form the *Union Journal of Medicine.*
33	*American Medical and Surgical Journal*	1855–1856	Cincinnati	Monthly. Conducted by S. H. Potter, E. H. Stockwell, and J. E. Kent. Formerly the *Syracuse Medical and Surgical Journal.* Continued in 1856 as the *American Medical Journal.*

	Title	Years	Location	Comments
34	*American Medical Journal*	1856–1857	Cincinnati	Monthly. Published by the faculty of the American Medical College. Edited by T. J. Wright. Continuation of the *American Medical and Surgical Journal*. Merged in 1857 with the *College Journal of Medical Science* of the Eclectic Medical Institute.
35	*American Medical Journal*	1873–1886	St. Louis	Monthly. Edited by S. H. Potter, J. W. Thrailkill, and G. H. Field. Supported eclectic medicine.
36	*American Medical Monthly*	1897–1904	Baltimore	Edited by E. C. Price. Previously titled *Southern Journal of Homeopathy.*
37	*American Medical Recorder*	1828–1829	Philadelphia	Founded by James Webster.
38	*American Physician*	1902–1908	Rahway, New York	Formerly *The American Homeopathist.*
39	*American Vegetarian and Health Journal*	1850–1854	Philadelphia	Monthly. Published by the American Vegetarian Society and edited by W. A. Alcott, T. L. Nichols, and Rev. William Metcafe.
40	*Amerikanische (Der) Deutsche*	1885	Chicago	Edited by K. Puscheck. Only a few volumes issued.
41	*Amerikanische (Der) Hausartz*	1894–1895	Essex, Iowa	Edited by Dr. Staads.
42	*Ann Arbor Alumnus*	1890	Ann Arbor	Quarterly. Edited by R. S. Copeland; V. D. Garwood; and W. H. Hodge. Devoted to the interests of the students and alumni of the Homeopathic Medical College of the University of Michigan. Three numbers issued.
43	*Ann Arbor Medical Advance*	1882–1884	Ann Arbor	Edited by J. P. Geppert, T. P. Wilson, and Henry Clay Allen. Formerly *Cincinnati Medical Advance.* In 1884 became *The Medical Advance.* In 1904 it merged with J. T. Kent's *Journal of Homeopathics* and became even more Hahnemannian in its approach to teaching pure homeopathy.

	Title	Years	Location	Comments
44	*Annual Journal of the Eclectic Medical Association of Michigan*	1871	Albion	Comprising the proceedings, constitution, bylaws, code of ethics, and annual address.
45	*Annual Journal of the Eclectic Medical Association of the State of Indiana*	1868–1869	Indianapolis	Annual.
46	*Annual Journal of the Illinois State Eclectic Medical Society*	1869–1875	Springfield	Annual. Published by the Illinois State Eclectic Medical Society.
47	*Annual Journal of the State Eclectic Medical Association of Michigan*	18??	Grand Rapids	Annual. Published by M. H. Clark and Co.
48	*Annual of Eclectic Medicine and Surgery*	1890–1897	Chicago	Founded by Finley Ellingwood and John V. Stevens. A yearly record of the observations, investigations and experiences of eclectic physicians.
49	*Annual of the Eclectic and Liberal Medical Association of Eastern Indiana*	1879	Lewisville	Annual. Edited by N. S. Smith
50	*Archives of American Medicine and Surgery*	1874	Macon	Published by the faculty of the College of American Medicine and Surgery.
51	*Argonaut*	1890–1892	Cleveland	Quarterly. Published and edited by K. B. Waite in the interest of the Cleveland Medical College.
52	*Argus*	1889	Cleveland	Published and edited by K. B. Waite. Formerly *The College Argus*. Represented the interests of the Cleveland Homeopathic Hospital College.
53	*Arkansas Eclectic Medical Journal*	1893–1895	Little Rock	Monthly. Edited by W. L. Leister. Name changed to *Southwestern Progressive Medical Journal.*
54	*Baltimore Family Health Journal*	1889–1891	Baltimore	Edited by Flora A. and Cora B. Brewster. Name changed in 1891 to *The Homeopathic Advocate and Health Journal* (1891–92). Intended for laity.

	Title	Years	Location	Comments
55	*Big Four*	1897	Kansas City	Bimonthly. Edited by C. W. Pyle.
56	*Boston Thomsonian Manual*	1844	Boston	Semimonthly. Edited by James S. Osgood. Title of volumes 7–8 of the *Thomsonian Manual.* The result of merging the *Thomsonian Manual* with the *Boston True Thomsonian.*
57	*Boston Thomsonian Manual and Lady's Companion*	1838–1840	Boston	Monthly. Published by Nathaniel S. Magoon and edited by Joseph P. Mendum. Title of volumes 5–6 of the *Thomsonian Manual.*
58	*Boston Thomsonian Medical and Physiological Journal*	1845–1846	Boston	Semimonthly. Edited by Benjamin Colby, Jr. and A. R. Porter. Editors arranged with Calvin Newton of Worcester to take over after 1846.
59	*Boston True Thomsonian*	1840–1843	Boston	Semimonthly. Published by Daniel L. Hale and edited by James Osgood. Published from the New England Thomsonian Depot. Merged with the *Thomsonian Manual* in 1844 to become the *Boston Thomsonian Manual.*
60	*Botanic Advertiser and Rhode Island Record of Modern Medical Reform: Commonly called the Thomsonian Practice*	1836–1840	Providence	Monthly. Published and edited by John A. Brown. Thomson accused Brown of being a mongrel.
61	*Botanic Advocate and Journal of Health*	1836–1839	Montpelier, Vt.	Monthly. Published by J. Wright and A. Holmes and edited by Wright. Dedicated to the use of barks, roots, and herbs; promised allegiance to Thomson's system and practice of medicine.
62	*Botanic Advocate and Thomsonian Family Physician*	1843–1844	New Haven	Monthly. Edited by Isaac J. Sperry and I. V. Wilson. Published on behalf of the Connecticut Botanical Society.
63	*Botanic Beacon*	1838	Tuscaloosa, Ala.	Published every six weeks.
64	*Botanic Investigator*	1835	Vicksburg, Miss.	Monthly. Edited and published by William W. Floyd. Did not exhibit any preference in its choice of botanic systems; believed the world had been damaged by system builders and so stood apart from Thomsonism.
65	*Botanic Journal, Devoted to the Interest of the Reformed Medial Practice*	1836–1837	Boston	Semimonthly. Published by E. G. House and edited by Samuel B. Emmons. Devoted to the interests of reformed medical practice.
66	*Botanic Ledger, and Family Journal of Health*	1839	Oxford, Oh.	Semimonthly, then monthly. Published and edited by Jesse Bennett and J. Lamborn.
67	*Botanic Luminary*	1836–1838	Saline; Adrian, Mich.	Monthly. Published and edited by Hiram Wright; after 1837 by S. W. King.

	Title	Years	Location	Comments
68	*Botanic Luminary*	1842	Hartford, Conn.	
69	*Botanic Medical Reformer and Home Physician*	1840–1842	Philadelphia	Monthly. Published by H. Hollembaek and Company; in May 1841 by Charles B. Barrett. Edited by Dr. Thomas Cooke. Steered an independent course; advanced the cause of botanic medicine through the union of the different sects.
70	*Botanic Register*	18??	Marion, Ala.	
71	*Botanic Sentinel*	183?	Philadelphia	Weekly. Published and edited by William Burton and Co.
72	*Botanic Sentinel and Literary Gazette. Devoted to the Only Rational and Scientific System of Medical Practice yet discovered, denominated the Thomsonian System*	1835–1837	Philadelphia	Weekly. Published by John Coates, Jr. and edited by William Henry Fonerden; after 1839 by Alexander C. Draper and Morris Mattson. Continued as the *Philadelphia Botanic Sentinel and Thomsonian Medical Revolutionist* (1837–39); and then the *Philadelphia Thomsonian Sentinel and Family Journal of Useful Knowledge* (1839–44).
73	*Botanico-Medical Investigator and Journal of Health*	1843	Springfield, Mass.	Published by Charles P. Kibbe and Paul W. Allen and devoted to medical reform and physical education.
74	*Botanico-Medical Recorder, or Impartial Advocate of Botanic Medicine, and the Principles Which Govern the Botanico-Medical Practice*	1837–1852	Columbus; Cincinnati	Fortnightly. Edited and published by Alva Curtis. Previously titled *Thomsonian Recorder* (1832–37). In 1851 became monthly. See also *Physiologico-Medical Recorder and Surgical Journal* (1849); *Physo-Medical Recorder and Surgical Journal* (1850); *Physo-Medical and Surgical Journal* (1851–52). Continued as *Physio-Medical Recorder* (1852–74).
75	*Botanico-Medical Reformer*	1844–1846	Mt. Vernon, Oh.	Monthly. Published and edited by John Kost.
76	*Botanic's Friend, and Herald of Truth*	1836	Philadelphia	
77	*British Journal of Homeopathy*	1851	New York	Quarterly. Published by William Radde and edited by J. J. Drysdale; J. R. Russell; and R. E. Dudgeon. American reprint.
78	*Brooklyn Homeopathic Hospital Bulletin*	1898	Brooklyn	

	Title	Years	Location	Comments
79	*Buchanan's Journal of Man*	1849–1856	Cincinnati	Monthly. Edited by Joseph Rodes Buchanan.
80	*Bulletin*	1878	St. Louis	Published by H. C. G. Luyties Homeopathic Pharmacy Company, with offices in St. Louis, Chicago, and New York.
81	*Bulletin*	1898	Cleveland	Published by the Cleveland Homeopathic College.
82	*Bulletin of Medical Instruction*	1894–1896	Boston	Edited by W. I. Talbot. Represented the Boston University School of Medicine.
83	*Bulletin of Medical Science*	1841–1846	Philadelphia	Quarterly. Formerly *Eclectic Journal of Medicine* (1836–40). Published by E. Barrington and G. D. Haswell. Edited by John Bell.
84	*California Eclectic Medical Journal*	1908–1921	Los Angeles	Monthly.
85	*California Homeopath*	1882–1893	San Francisco	Bimonthly. Published by Boericke and Schreck and edited by W. Boericke; W. A. Dewey; C. L. Tisdale; and H. R. Arndt, et al. Changed name in 1893 to *Pacific Coast Journal of Homeopathy*, and then to *Pacific Coast Homeopathic Bulletin*. The official organ of the state medical societies of California, Oregon, and Washington.
86	*California Medical Journal*	1880–1908	San Francisco	Monthly. Later titled *Los Angeles Journal of Eclectic Medicine;* and *California Eclectic Medical Journal.*
87	*California Medical Journal. A Monthly Devoted to the Advancement of Medicine, Surgery and the Collateral Sciences*	1880–1908	Oakland	Monthly. Edited by D. Maclean, J. H. Bundy and J. J. Kendrick.
88	*California Medical Times*	1877–1878	San Francisco	Quarterly. Edited by F. Hiller and S. Worth. First homeopathic periodical on the west coast. Four numbers issued.

	Title	Years	Location	Comments
89	*Carlisle Journal of Homeopathy*	1851	Carlisle, Pa.	Monthly. Published and edited by J. K. Smith. Intended as a popular journal bud did not survive past inaugural issue.
90	*Carnival Record*	1887	Philadelphia	A hospital fair paper for the Hahnemann Hospital Association of the Hahnemann Medical College of Philadelphia and the Lady Managers of the Children's Homeopathic Hospital of Philadelphia. Edited by C. F. McMichael; Miss L. Burling; and Miss A. Mason.
91	*Chicago Homeopath*	1854–1856	Chicago	Bimonthly. Published and edited by D. S. Smith; S. W. Graves; and R. Ludlam. Designed for the non-professional reader and was the best of its kind. Three volumes issued.
92	*Chicago Medical Review*	1880	Chicago	Bimonthly. Published by W. A. Chatterton and edited by Chandler and Engelhard. Only two issues published.
93	*Chicago Medical Times: A Monthly Journal Devoted to the Interests of Eclectic Medicine and Surgery*	1869–1888	Chicago	Edited by Robert A. Gunn; H. D. Garrison; W. H. Davis; A. L. Clark; Finley Ellingwood. Later titled *American Journal of Clinical Medicine.*
94	*Chironian*	1884–1905	New York	Semimonthly. Edited by E. H. Porter; P. W. Shedd; G. T. Hawley, et al. Published by the Homeopathic Medical College of New York.
95	*Cincinnati Eclectic and Edinburgh Medical Journal*	1859	Cincinnati	Monthly. Edited by Robert S. Newton and George W. L. Bickley. Published by E. Morgan and Sons. Title of volume 18 of the *Eclectic Medical Journal.*
96	*Cincinnati Journal of Homeopathy*	1851	Cincinnati	Monthly. Published by the Society of Homeopathic Physicians of Cincinnati and edited by B. Ehrmann; A. Miller; and G. W. Bigler. Published for one year. Contained editorial articles, extracts from other journals, reviews of books, proceedings of societies, and items of news.
97	*Cincinnati Medical Advance*	1873–1882	Cincinnati	Monthly. Published by J. P. Geppert and edited by T. P. Wilson; H. C. Allen, et al. Became *The Ann Arbor Medical Advance* (1882), the *Medical Advance* (1884); changed name in 1895 to *The Hahnemannian Advocate.*
98	*Cincinnati Medical Gazette*	1877–1879	Cincinnati	

	Title	Years	Location	Comments
99	*Cincinnati Medical Gazette and Recorder. A Journal of Medical Reform*	1880–1881	Cincinnati	Monthly. Edited by William H. Cook. Formed by consolidation of *Physio-Medical Recorder* with *Cincinnati Medical Gazette*. Suspended in 1881. Continued in 1883 as *Cincinnati Medical Recorder.*
100	*Cincinnati Medical Recorder. A Journal of Sanative Medicine*	1883–1884	Cincinnati	Semimonthly. Edited by William H. Cook. Title for 1880–81 was *Cincinnati Medical Gazette and Recorder.* Continued in 1884 as *Healthside.*
101	*Cleveland Homeopathic Reporter*	1900–1902	Cleveland	Published by J. R. Horner. Devoted to the interests of the Cleveland Homeopathic Medical College. Changed name to *Cleveland Medical and Surgical Reporter* in 1902.
102	*Cleveland Medical and Surgical Reporter*	1902–1912	Cleveland	Formerly the *Cleveland Homeopathic Reporter.*
103	*Clinic*	1875	Cleveland	Published by the faculty of the Cleveland Homeopathic College. Only a few numbers published.
104	*Clinical Record*	1889	Chicago	Monthly. Published and edited by W. A. Chatterton. Record of clinical medicine, surgery, and materia medica. Published only a few issues.
105	*Clinical Reporter*	1888–1911	St. Louis	Monthly. Published by Schultz Pub. Co. and later Foulon and Co. Edited by I. D. Foulon; J. M. Kershaw; and D. M. Gibson. Product of the faculty of the Homeopathic Medical College of Missouri. United with *The St. Louis Journal of Homeopathy* in 1895 and then the *St. Louis Journal of Homeopathy and Clinical Reporter* (1895–97). Then became *The Clinical Reporter* (1897–1911).
106	*Clinical Review*	1885–1887	Cleveland	Monthly journal of medicine and surgery. Edited by C. L. Cleveland.
107	*Clinique: A Monthly Abstract of the Clinics and of the Proceedings of the Clinical Society of the Hahnemann Hospital of Chicago*	1880–1927	Chicago	Monthly. Published by the Hospital Board and edited by R. Ludlam; Clifford Mitchell; H. V. Halbert; T. Bacmeister; C. A. Weirick; and Rhoda Pike Barstow. The official organ of the Hahnemann Medical College in Chicago and later amalgamated with Chicago Homeopathic Medical College. Consolidated with *Medical Era* in 1904. Passed into the control of the Illinois Homeopathic Medical Association in 1918 with T. Bacmeister as editor.

	Title	Years	Location	Comments
108	*College Argus*	1889	Cleveland	Quarterly. Published by F. W. Roberts and edited by K. B. Waite and F. Kraft. Publication of the Cleveland Homeopathic Hospital College. Became *The Argus* after two volumes.
109	*College Journal*	1860	St. Louis	Bimonthly. Published by the St. Louis Homeopathic College. Only two numbers published.
110	*College Journal of Medical Science*	1856–1859	Cincinnati	Monthly. Established by the faculty of the Eclectic Medical Institute. Edited by J. R. Buchanan; John King; John W. Hoyt; William Sherwood; C. H. Cleaveland; and I. G. Jones. In 1857, both the *Worcester Journal of Medicine* and the *American Medical Journal* merged with it. Succeeded by the *Journal of Rational Medicine*.
111	*Compass*	1890–1895	Detroit	Monthly. Published by Wilton and Wetherbee and edited by S. H. Knight. Became the *Grace Hospital Gazette* in 1895.
112	*Correspondenzblatt der homoopathischen Aertze, herausgegeben durch die Nord Amerikanische Akademie der Homeopathischen Heilkunst zu Allentown an der Lecha*	1835–1837	Allentown	Published by the North American Academy of Homeopathia and edited by C. Hering. Fourteen numbers only appeared.
113	*Cresset*	1887	New York	Published for the New York Homeopathic Medical College and Hospital for Women.
114	*Critic and Medical Inquirer*	1853	Cincinnati	Monthly. Published by J. Kost, A. B. Wright, and Z. P. Glass.
115	*Critique*	1897–1909	Denver	Edited by S. S. Kehr and J. W. Mastin. Formerly the *Denver Journal of Homeopathy*. Claimed the largest circulation of a medical journal in the West. Ended with the Denver Homeopathic Medical College closed its doors.
116	*Curopathist*	1873–1874	Indianapolis	Monthly. Edited by J. T. Boyd. Intended for the laity and devoted to the interest of reformers in medicine.

	Title	Years	Location	Comments
117	*Dayton Herald of Health*	1851	Dayton	Edited by H. Wigand and intended for the laity.
118	*Denver Journal of Homeopathy*	1894–1897	Denver	Edited by S. S. Smythe; S. S. Kehr; and J. W. Mastin. Changed name to *The Critique* (1897) at the end of the third volume.
119	*Deutsche (Der) Amerikanische Homeopathische Zeitschrift*	1885		Edited by K. Puscheck.
120	*Doctor (The)*	1876	Baltimore	Published during fair to support the Baltimore Homeopathic Free Dispensary. Only a few numbers issued.
121	*Donation (The)*	1891	Philadelphia	Edited by B. W. James and issued in aid of fair held for benefit of the Children's Homeopathic Hospital of Philadelphia. One number issued.
122	*Dr. Ryan's Monthly Homeopathic Review*	18??		
123	*Drugs and Medicines of North America*	1884–1887	Cincinnati	Quarterly. A publication devoted to the historical and scientific discussion of the botany, pharmacy, chemistry, and therapeutics of the medicinal plants of North America, their constituents, products, and sophistications. Published by J. U. and C. G. Lloyd.
124	*Duncan Brothers' Homeopathic Pharmacy Bulletin*	1881	Chicago	Issued irregularly as an adjunct to Duncan Brothers' Pharmacy.
125	*Eastern Medical Journal*	1883–1887	Worcester, Mass.	Monthly. Eclectic journal edited by A. J. Marston.
126	*Echo (The)*	1875	New York	Edited by H. Sedley. Published in thirteen numbers during the New York Homeopathic Hospital Fair.
127	*Eclectic (The). A Monthly Magazine of Useful Knowledge*	1870	Cincinnati	Monthly. Published by John M. Scudder.

	Title	Years	Location	Comments
128	*Eclectic and American Journal of Medicine*	1852	Rochester	Formerly *Eclectic Journal of Medicine.* Also titled the *New York Eclectic Medical and Surgical Journal.* Later titled *Union Journal of Medicine.*
129	*Eclectic and Medical Botanist*	1832–1833	Columbus	Semimonthly. Published by Scott and Wright. Edited by Harvey D. Little and William Hance.
130	*Eclectic and Medical Botanist, Devoted Principally to Improvements in the Botanic Practice of Medicine*	1832–1833	Columbus	Semimonthly. Edited and published by Harvey D. Little and William Hance. Supported Horton Howard's "improved" botanical system; fought battle against *Thomsonian Recorder*; continued as the *Eclectic Journal of Science.*
131	*Eclectic and University Journal of Philadelphia*	1865	Philadelphia	Founded by William Paine. Formed by the consolidation of the *Eclectic Medical Journal of Philadelphia* with the *University Medical and Surgical Journal of Philadelphia.*
132	*Eclectic and University Medical and Surgical Journal of Philadelphia*	1865	Philadelphia	Monthly. Edited by W. Paine. Title of volume 8 of the *Eclectic Medical Journal of Philadelphia.*
133	*Eclectic Health Journal*	1892	Salt Lake City	Published by Richard A. Hasbrouck.
134	*Eclectic Journal and Family Adviser*	1894	Carthage, Missouri	Founded and edited by W. W. Johnston and W. H. Price.
135	*Eclectic Journal of Medicine*	1836–1840	Philadelphia	Monthly. Edited by John Bell. Published by Barrington and Haswell. Later titled *Bulletin of Medical Science.*
136	*Eclectic Journal of Medicine*	1851–1852	Rochester	Edited by Levi Reuben and L. C. Dolley. Formerly *Eclectic Medical and Surgical Journal*. Later titled *Eclectic and American Journal of Medicine.*
137	*Eclectic Journal of Medicine: Designed for Popular and Professional Reading*	1852	Rochester	Monthly. Published by A. Strong and Co.
138	*Eclectic Journal of Science; a Weekly Publication, Devoted to Improvements in Botanic Medicine, and the Diffusion of Useful Scientific Knowledge*	1834–1835	Columbus, Ohio	Weekly. Edited by William Hance. Title of 1832–33 volume was the *Eclectic and Medical Botanist*. Devoted to improvements in botanic medicine.

	Title	Years	Location	Comments
139	*Eclectic Medical Advocate; a Monthly Journal of Medicine, Surgery, and the Kindred Sciences*	1884–1885	New York	Monthly. Edited by Joseph A. House; A. Wilder. Published by the Eclectic Publishing Company. Formerly titled the *Medical Tribune; Journal Devoted to Medicine, Surgery, and the Collateral Sciences.* Continued in 1885 as the *Medical Advocate. A Monthly Journal of Medicine, Surgery, and the Kindred Sciences.*
140	*Eclectic Medical and College Journal*	1860	Cincinnati	Title of volume 19 of the *Eclectic Medical Journal.*
141	*Eclectic Medical and Surgical Journal*	1849–1851	Rochester	Formerly the *New York Eclectic Medical and Surgical Journal.* Later titled *Eclectic Journal of Medicine.*
142	*Eclectic Medical and Surgical Journal*	1884–1886	Des Moines	Monthly. Edited and published by O. H. P. Shoemaker.
143	*Eclectic Medical Gleaner*	1894–1912	Cincinnati	Bimonthly. Edited by W. E. Bloyer.
144	*Eclectic Medical Journal*	1849–1888	Cincinnati	Monthly. Edited by Joseph R. Buchanan; T. V. Morrow; R. S. Newton; and J. K. Scudder. Formerly titled the *Western Medical Reformer,* the *Cincinnati Eclectic and Edinburgh Medical Journal,* and the *Eclectic Medical and College Journal.*
145	*Eclectic Medical Journal*	1883	Indianapolis, Ind.	Monthly. Edited by A. J. Smith and Mrs. Joyce F. Hobson. Continued as the *Indiana Eclectic Medical Journal.*
146	*Eclectic Medical Journal and Organ of the Georgia Eclectic Medical College*	1879–1880	Georgia	
147	*Eclectic Medical Journal of Pennsylvania*	1863–1880	Philadelphia	Bimonthly. Edited by the faculty of the Eclectic Medical College of Pennsylvania. A continuation of the *Quarterly Eclectic Medical Journal of Pennsylvania.* In 1864 John Buchanan became editor. Some numbers titled the *Journal of Progressive Medicine.*

	Title	Years	Location	Comments
148	*Eclectic Medical Journal of Philadelphia*	1858–1871	Philadelphia	Monthly. Edited by William Paine. A continuation the *Middle States Medical Reformer and Journal of Health*. Merged in 1865 with the *University Medical and Surgical Journal of Philadelphia* and became the *Eclectic and University Medical and Surgical Journal of Philadelphia*. Later titled the *Philadelphia University Journal of Medicine and Surgery*.
149	*Eclectic Medical Record and Herald of Health; a Quarterly Journal Devoted to the Eclectic Practice of Medicine, Surgery, and the Laws of Life*	1870	New York	Quarterly. Edited by Luke D. Broughton.
150	*Eclectic Medical Record and Psychological Review*	1869	Indianapolis	Founded by J. C. Lewis.
151	*Eclectic Medical Review*	1847–1848	Pittsburgh, Pa.	Monthly. Edited by A. W. Ewing and J. W. Whitaker.
152	*Eclectic Repertory and Analytical Review, Medical and Philosophical*	1811–1821	Philadelphia	Quarterly. Edited by A. Finley. Later titled *Journal of Foreign Medical Science and Literature*.
153	*Eclectic Review*	1890–1915	New York	Monthly. G. W. Boskowitz
154	*Eclectic Scalpel; a Journal of Health and Reform, Adapted to Popular and Professional Reading and the Exposure of Quackery in Medicine*	1868	Brookville, Ohio	Monthly. Edited by Alpheus Dove.
155	*Eclectic Star. Devoted to Health, Literature, and Medical Science*	1883–1886	Atlanta	Monthly. Published and edited by S. F. Salter.
156	*Electro-Clinical Record*	1885	Chicago	Published and edited by W. A. Chatterton.
157	*Faith's Record*	1871	Chicago	Monthly. Published and edited by G. E. Shipman. Served the Chicago Foundlings' Home.

	Title	Years	Location	Comments
158	*Fall River and Middleboro' Medical Inquirer*	1846	Mass.	
159	*Family Journal of Health*	1860–1860	Cincinnati	Monthly. Published by Johnson, Stephens and Morgan and edited by J. M. Scudder.
160	*Family Journal of Homeopathy*	1854	St. Louis	Monthly. Published by the Association of Physicians and edited by D. White and J. T. Temple. Published for one year and intended for the laity.
161	*Family Medical Investigator*	1871	Kansas City	Edited by J. Field and intended for the laity.
162	*Fitchburg Homeopathic Hospital News*	1896	Fitchburg, Mass.	
163	*Fonerden's Botanic Journal*	1841	Forsyth, Ga.	Title of volume 3 of the *Southern Botanic Journal.*
164	*Gentry's Record of Homeopathic Materia Medica*	1895	Chicago	
165	*Georgia and Tennessee Eclectic Medical Journal*	1882	Atlanta	Monthly. Title of volume 4 of *Georgia Eclectic Medical Journal.*
166	*Georgia Botanic Journal and College Sentinel; Devoted to the Cause of Medical Reform*	1847–1848	Macon	Monthly. Edited by J. T. Coxe and M. S. Bellenger. Continued as the *Southern Botanico-Medical Reformer.*
167	*Georgia Eclectic Medical Journal; Devoted to Liberal Medicine, Hygiene, and Sanitary Science*	1879–1889	Atlanta	Monthly. Edited by J. R. Borland et al. Formerly the *Georgia and Tennessee Eclectic Medical Journal*. Later titled *Modern Eclecticism.*
168	*Globule (The)*	1869	Philadelphia	Published by "Young Folks." In aid of the Homeopathic Hospital Fair. Three numbers issued.

	Title	Years	Location	Comments
169	*Grace Hospital Gazette*	1895	Detroit	Published by Grace Hospital. Formerly titled *The Compass.*
170	*Graham Journal of Health and Longevity*	1837–1839	Boston	Weekly. Edited by David Campbell. Designed to illustrate and sustain the principles and science of human life as taught by Sylvester Graham.
171	*Granite State Medical Revolutionist and Hygienic Advertiser*	1850	Manchester	Edited by J. M. Hawkes
172	*Guilder (The)*	1900	New York City	Organ of the New York Medical College and Hospital for Women.
173	*H.H.H. Record*	1883	Pittsburgh	Issued daily in aid of fair held by the Ladies' Association of the Pittsburgh Homeopathic Hospital.
174	*Hahnemann Advocate*	1889	Rochester	Monthly. Published by Committee of Hospital. Organ of Hahnemann Homeopathic Hospital of Rochester.
175	*Hahnemann Monthly*	1866	Cleveland	Published by the Hahnemann Life Insurance Company. Circulated gratuitously as an advertising medium of the Hahnemann Life Insurance Company. Only a few issues ever published.
176	*Hahnemann Publishing House Circular*	1883	Philadelphia	Edited by F. E. Boericke and published irregularly as an advertiser of new books.
177	*Hahnemannian (The) Advocate*	1895–1902	Chicago	Edited by H. W. Pierson. Represented Hering Medical College and high potency homeopathy. Formerly *The Medical Advance.*
178	*Hahnemannian (The) Institute*	1850–1852	Philadelphia	Published by the Hahnemann Medical College of Philadelphia and edited by students. Formerly *The Institute.*

	Title	Years	Location	Comments
179	*Hahnemannian (The) Monthly*	1865–1949	Philadelphia	Published by King and Baird; Boericke and A. J. Tafel. Edited by J. H. P. Frost; Adolph Lippe; Robert J. McClatchey; W. H. Winslow; E. A. Farington; Pemberton Dudley; Clarence Bartlett; and W. W. Van Baun. Intended to communicate the views of the faculty of the Homeopathic Medical College of Pennsylvania.
180	*Hahnemannian (The) Periscope*	1901	San Francisco	Published by the Hahnemann Medical College of the Pacific.
181	*Hahnemannian Pulse*	1892	Chicago	Student's paper issued by the Hahnemannian Medical College of Chicago.
182	*Health (The) Homeopathy*	1900	Chicago	Edited by H. M. Pierson
183	*Health (The) Record*	1885–1892	Corning, N.Y.	Quarterly. Edited by M. S. Purdy. Intended for laity. First movement-cure journal published in America.
184	*Health and Life*	1880–1882	Philadelphia	Quarterly. Edited by Starkey and Palen. Emphasized the compound oxygen treatment process. Intended for the laity.
185	*Healthside. A Monthly Journal Devoted to the Interests of Sound Bodies and Long Life*	1884	Cincinnati	Published and edited by William Wesley Cook. Prior title was the *Cincinnati Medical Recorder.*
186	*Herald (The) of Health and Homeopathy*	1890	San Francisco	Monthly. Published by Boericke and Runyon and edited by W. Boericke. Intended for laity.
187	*Herald of Progressive Medicine. The Eclectic or American System of Medical Practice*	1873	Atlanta	Published and edited by W. T. Park.
188	*Home Papers*	1866	Chicago	Monthly. Published and edited by C. S. Halsey. Intended for laity. Published for only one year.

	Title	Years	Location	Comments
189	*Homeopath (Der) und Diaetische Hausfreund*	1853–1854	Buffalo	Monthly. Published by Lewis and Baar and edited by Dioclesian Lewis. Intended for circulation among the German laity. Only a few numbers published.
190	*Homeopath (The)*	1858	New York	Semimonthly. Published by Charles T. Hurlburt and edited by Charles E. Blumenthal. Intended to popularize the system. Published one year.
191	*Homeopath (The)*	1858	Philadelphia	Published by Boericke and Tafel and edited by C. Hering and A. Lippe. Devoted to pointing out the mistakes in the symptomen-codex. Generated controversy with the *Philadelphia Journal of Homeopathy*.
192	*Homeopathic (The) Advocate and Guide to Health*	1851	Keen, N.H.	Monthly. Published and edited by D. White. Intended for popular reading. Continued for a year.
193	*Homeopathic (The) Courier*	1881	St. Louis	Monthly. Published by H. L. Verdier and edited by J. T. Boyd; J. T. Kent; W. C. Richardson; and J. W. Thrasher. Two volumes issued.
194	*Homeopathic (The) Expositor*	1866	Milwaukee	Monthly. Published and edited by J. S. Douglas and Perrine. Intended for the laity. Only published for a few months.
195	*Homeopathic (The) Expositor*	1879–1882	Ithaca	Quarterly. Published by E. J. Morgan, Jr. and edited by Morgan and A. M. Baldwin. Intended for the laity.
196	*Homeopathic (The) Guide*	1895	Louisville	Intended for the laity.
197	*Homeopathic (The) Leader*	1883	New York	Edited by W. Y. Cowl and only two numbers issued.
198	*Homeopathic (The) Student*	1895	Chicago	Published by the Chicago Homeopathic Medical College and edited by C. W. Weirick. Succeeded by *The Chicago Homeopathic Medical College Bulletin* in 1904. Ceased publication with the consolidation of Chicago Homeopathic College and Hahnemann Medical College in 1904.

	Title	Years	Location	Comments
199	*Homeopathic (The) Sun*	1868	New York City	Monthly. Published by William Radde and edited by F. W. Hunt. Devoted to popular homeopathic information, particularly life insurance. Published for just a few months.
200	*Homeopathic Advocate and Health Journal*	1891–1892	Baltimore	Monthly. Published by Advocate Pub. Company and edited by Flora A. and Cora B. Brewster; E. C. Price et al. Intended for laity. Formerly the *Baltimore Family Health Journal.* Published in the interest of the Maryland Homeopathic Hospital.
201	*Homeopathic Envoy*	1890–1918	Philadelphia; Lancaster	Monthly. Published and edited by E. P. Anshutz. Popular journal.
202	*Homeopathic Examiner*	1840–1847	New York	Monthly. Published by Ludwig Felt and Co.; W. Dean; and Radde. Edited by A. Gerald Hull; J. F. Gray; and C. J. Hempel. Discontinued from December 1843 to August 1845 when a new series was commenced by Drs. John F. Gray and Charles J. Hempel. Formerly *The American Journal of Homeopathy.*
203	*Homeopathic Eye, Ear and Throat Journal*	1895–1911	Lancaster	Monthly. Edited by A. B. Norton; J. L. Moffat; and A. W. Palmer. Official organ of the Ophthalmological, Otological and Laryngological Society (1911–1919). In 1911 became *Journal of Ophthalmology, Otology and Laryngology.*
204	*Homeopathic Hospital Envoy*	1896–1902	Denver	Supported by the ladies auxiliary of the Denver Homeopathic Hospital on Champa Street.
205	*Homeopathic Hospital Reporter*	1868	Cleveland	Published by the Cleveland Homeopathic Hospital.
206	*Homeopathic Independent*	1868–1869	St. Louis	Published by J. Conzelman and edited by Conzelman; J. T. Temple; T. G. Comstock et al. Lasted for one year.
207	*Homeopathic Journal of Materia Medica, Chemistry and Pharmacology*	1867	Chicago	Monthly. Published by Williams and Dwight Homeopathic Pharmacists of Chicago. Lasted less than a year.
208	*Homeopathic Journal of Obstetrics and Diseases of Women and Children*	1879–1885	New York City	Quarterly. Published by A. L. Chatterton and edited by H. Minton; L. L. Danforth; P. Porter; G. W. Winterburn; B. F. Underwood; and G. F. Honan. Name changed in 1886 to *Homeopathic Journal of Obstetrics, Gynaecology, and Paedology.*

	Title	Years	Location	Comments
209	*Homeopathic Journal of Obstetrics, Gynaecology and Paedology*	1886–1904	New York City	Published by A. L. Chatterton and edited by Phil Porter; G. W. Winterburn; B. F. Underwood; and G. F. Honan. Formerly *The Journal of Obstetrics and Diseases of Women and Children.* Became *The Journal of Surgery, Gynecology and Obstetrics* in 1905.
210	*Homeopathic Journal of Surgery and Gynecology*	1898	New York	Published by the Medical Century Company and became part of *The Medical Century* magazine.
211	*Homeopathic Medical News Letter*	1851–1852	St. Louis	Monthly. Published and edited by J. Granger; T. J. Vastine; and T. G. Comstock. Intended for the patients of the editors. Published for one year.
212	*Homeopathic News*	1854–1856	Philadelphia	Published by Boericke and Tafel and edited by Adolphus Lippe and Constantine Hering. Published in eight pages and purported to be an independent advertising sheet. Published the errors of *Jahr's New Manual.*
213	*Homeopathic News*	1871–1879	St. Louis	Monthly. Published by H. C. G. Luytties and Company and edited by C. H. Goodman; R. G. A. Meier; W. T. Helmuth et al. Name changed to *Monthly Homeopathic News* in 1879. Continued as trade journal until 1890 and then pirated other publications without credit.
214	*Homeopathic News*	1876	Kansas City	Monthly. Published by Feld and Riley and edited by J. Feld. Trade journal for the Kansas City Homeopathic Pharmacy.
215	*Homeopathic Physician*	1881–1893	Philadelphia	Monthly. Published by Bedell and Brothers and edited by E. L. Lee and Walter James. Devoted to high potency homeopathy. Designed to disseminate the popular views of homeopathic science.
216	*Homeopathic Pioneer*	1845–1846	Syracuse	Monthly. Published and edited by H. Hull Cator and L. M. Tracy. Provided extracts from other journals, reviews of books and case records. Published for one year.
217	*Homeopathic Quarterly*	1869	Buffalo	Published and edited by R. Gregg. Devoted to the elucidation of Gregg's theory of phthisis pulmonalis. Two volumes published.
218	*Homeopathic Record*	1878	Chicago	Published and edited by W. F. Morrison.

	Title	Years	Location	Comments
219	*Homeopathic Recorder*	1885–1959	Philadelphia	Bimonthly then became a monthly. Published by Boericke and Tafel and edited by J. T. O'Connor; C. F. Millspaugh; E. P. Anshutz et al. Official organ of publishers. Merged with *Journal of the American Institute of Homeopathy* and in 1928 Boericke and Tafel passed control over by the American Institute of Homeopathy. High class trade journal. Intent of new editor was to be "Simon-pure" in homeopathy.
220	*Homeopathic Semi-Monthly Magazine*	1869	St. Louis	Edited by J. Conzelman.
221	*Homeopathic Times*	1875–1881	New York City	Monthly. Published and edited by E. Guernsey; A. K. Hills; and J. B. Gilbert. Consolidation of *Medical Union* and *The New York Journal of Homeopathy*. Name changed to *The New York Medical Times* in 1881 and continued until 1882.
222	*Homeopathischer (Der) Hausfreud*	1857	Hermann, Mo.	Edited by J. Conzelman and published for only a short time.
223	*Homeopathist (The)*	1850–1852	Buffalo	Semimonthly and then monthly. Published and edited by D. Lewis. Lasted about two years and intended to spread the knowledge of homeopathy among the people. Lewis sold homeopathic medicines in Buffalo.
224	*Homeopathist (The)*	1859	Vermont, Il.	Edited by J. M. Blaisdell. Intended to diffuse knowledge of homeopathy among the people. Lasted only a short time.
225	*Homeopathist (The)*	1859	Springfield, Mass.	Monthly. Published by J. M. Buzzell and edited by Buzzell and D. White. Intended to be a popular sheet. Only three or four numbers issued. Used to advertise Dr. Buzzell's private hospital in Springfield.
226	*Homeopathist (The)*	1870–1874	New York	Published by the Homeopathic Mutual Life Insurance Company of New York and edited by E. B. Holmes.
227	*Homoeopatische (Der) Bote*	1886–1892	St. Louis	Edited by W. F. Bockstruck and published irregularly.

	Title	Years	Location	Comments
228	*Homoeopatische (Der) Zeitschrift*	1883	Newark, N.J.	
229	*Hospital (The) Visitant*	1894–1896	Portland	
230	*Hospital Bazaar*	1874	Chicago	Edited by Miss Kate N. Daggett. Published in aid of the Hahnemann Hospital Charity Fair. Seven numbers issued.
231	*Hospital Leaflet*	1889	Rochester	Monthly. Published by Lady Supervisors of the Hospital. Published in interest of the Rochester Homeopathic Hospital.
232	*Hospital Leaflet*	1895	Buffalo	Monthly. Published by the Board of Association Managers and devoted to the interests of the Buffalo Homeopathic Hospital.
233	*Hospital Messenger*	1887	Philadelphia	Published by the Executive Board of the Women's Homeopathic Association of Pennsylvania during the fair at St. George's Hall. Edited by Mrs. Charles Reese.
234	*Hospital News*	1888	Minneapolis	One issue published under the auspices of the Homeopathic Hospital.
235	*Hospital Tidings*	1895–1945	Philadelphia	Name changed in 1946 to *Hahnemann Hospital Tidings.*
236	*Humphrey's Journal of Specific Homeopathy*	1855–1863	Auburn, N.Y.	Monthly. Published and edited by F. Humphreys. Intended for the laity.
237	*Independent Botanic Advocate*	1839–1841	Hartford	Monthly. Published by the Connecticut Botanic Medical Society and edited by Doctors Wilson and Isaac J. Sperry. Later became *Botanic Advocate and Thomsonian Family Physician.*
238	*Independent Botanic Register*	1835–1836	Columbus	Monthly. Published and edited by Thomas Hersey. *Jewett's Advertiser* was a companion to this journal.

	Title	Years	Location	Comments
239	*Independent Medical Investigator*	1879	Greenfield, Ind.	Founded by S. S. Boots and J. L. Marsh.
240	*Indiana Eclectic Medical Journal*	1884–1888	Indianapolis	Monthly. Edited by G. W. Pickerill and Joyce F. Hobson. Formerly titled *Eclectic Medical Journal.* In 1884 the *Independent Medical Investigator* merged with it.
241	*Indiana Medical Journal*	1881–1882	Indianapolis	Monthly. Edited by Daniel Lesh and Samuel S. Boots. Published by the trustees of the Indiana Eclectic Medical College. In 1881 the *Independent Medical Investigator* merged in this journal.
242	*Indianapolis Polyclinic*	1898–1901	Indianapolis	Succeeded by *Physio-Medical Record.*
243	*Indicator (The)*	1893	Cleveland	Edited by B. B. Viets. Organ of Cleveland Homeopathic Medical Hospital.
244	*Investigator (The)*	1879	Richmond, Va.	Intended for the laity.
245	*Iowa Eclectic Medical Journal*	1884	Des Moines	Founded by O. H. P. Shoemaker.
246	*Iowa Homeopathic Journal*	1907–1920	Des Moines	Monthly. Edited by J. G. Huntoon. Journal of the Hahnemann Medical Association of Iowa.
247	*Iowa Medical Journal*	1884	Des Moines	Founded by J. G. Hill and edited by Hill and H. O. Conoway.
248	*Jewett's Advertiser*	1835–1836	Columbus	Quarterly. Published by Col. Moses Jewett and edited by Thomas Hersey. Companion to the *Independent Botanic Register.* Advertised medicines employed in the iatroleptic practice, or curing diseases principally by external application and friction.

	Title	Years	Location	Comments
249	*Journal (The) of Electro-Therapeutics*	1890–1892	New York	Monthly. Published by A. L. Chatterton and Company and edited by W. H. King.
250	*Journal of American Medicine and Surgery. A Monthly Journal Devoted to Medicine and Surgery*	1882	Atlanta	Monthly. Eclectic magazine edited by S. F. Salter. A continuation of *The Reformer.*
251	*Journal of Eclectic Medicine*	1891	Morristown, Tenn.	
252	*Journal of Education and of Physiological and Medical Reform*	1866	Cincinnati	Published by A. Moore and edited by Alva Curtis. See *Journal of Education and of Physiological and Medical Reform.*
253	*Journal of Education and of Physiological and Medical Reform*	1866	Cincinnati	Monthly. Edited by Alva Curtis.
254	*Journal of Foreign Medical Science and Literature*	1821–1824	Philadelphia	Quarterly. Edited by William Price, Dr. Emlen, and John D. Godman. Previously titled *Eclectic Repertory and Analytical Review, Medical and Philosophical.* In 1825 merged with the *American Medical Recorder.*
255	*Journal of Health of the Metropolitan Medical College*	1859–1860	New York City	Monthly. Edited by H. M. Sweet, George Newby, and H. P. Herdman.
256	*Journal of Homeopathic Clinics*	1867–1871	Philadelphia	Edited by C. Hering and H. N. Martin. Ceased after nine volumes. Title change in 1871 to *American Journal of Homeopathic Materia Medica and Record of Medical Sciences.*
257	*Journal of Homeopathics*	1889–1890	New York	Monthly. Published and edited by H. Hitchcock. Discontinued after two volumes. Devoted to the philosophy of homeopathy.
258	*Journal of Homeopathics*	1897–1903	Philadelphia	Edited by J. T. Kent. Merged with *Medical Advance* in 1903. Devoted to high potency homeopathy.
259	*Journal of Medical Reform for the People and the Profession*	1854–1857	New York City	Monthly. Edited by William H. Cook. In 1854 Isaac M. Comings became editor, followed by Joseph D. Friend and H. M. Sweet. Formerly the *American Journal of Medical Reform, for the People and the Profession.*

	Title	Years	Location	Comments
260	*Journal of Ophthalmology, Otology, and Laryngology*	1889–1929	New York City; Lancaster	Quarterly. Published by A. L. Chatterton and edited by G. S. Norton; C. Deady; J. L. Moffat; M. Leal et al. Official organ of the Ophthalmological, Otological and Laryngological Society (1911–1929). Merged in 1911 with *Homeopathic eye, Ear and Throat Journal*. In 1918 the journal merged with the *Journal of the American Institute of Homeopathy*.
261	*Journal of Orificial Surgery*	1892–1901	Chicago	Monthly. Published by Pratt and Holbrook and edited by E. H. Pratt. Published nine volumes.
262	*Journal of Pediatrics*	1902–1903	Buffalo	Edited by J. C. Chadwick.
263	*Journal of Progressive Medicine*	1872	Philadelphia	Bimonthly. Edited by John Buchanan. Also titled *Eclectic Medical Journal of Pennsylvania*.
264	*Journal of Rational Medicine*	1860–1862	Cincinnati	Monthly. Edited by C. H. Cleaveland. A continuation of the *College Journal of Medical Science*.
265	*Journal of Surgery, Gynecology and Obstetrics*	1905–1910	New York City	Bimonthly. Published by A. L. Chatterton. Formerly *Homeopathic Journal of Obstetrics, Gynaecology and Paedology*.
266	*Journal of the American Institute of Homeopathy*	1909–present	Cleveland	Monthly. Later became a quarterly. Superceded the *Medical Century*. Published by the Board of Trustees of the American Institute of Homeopathy. Merged with *The Homeopathic Recorder* (1927). Journal included bureaus of clinical medicine, homeopathy, materia medica, pedology, and sanitary science. Each article was followed by full discussion.
267	*Kansas Medical Journal*	1883	Topeka; La Cygne	Monthly. Edited and published by J. Milton Welch.
268	*Keystone (The)*	1889–1905	Buffalo	Monthly. Published by Keystone Pub. Company and edited by J. T. Cooke; L. B. Lee; E. Hilliard; and Jessie Shepard. Under the auspices of the Women's Aid Society of the Buffalo Homeopathic Hospital.

	Title	Years	Location	Comments
269	*Keystone Medical Journal*	1881–1884	Tunkhannock and Tyrone, Pa.	Founded by H. P. Piper; A. B. Woodware.
270	*L'Homoion*	1859–1860	New Orleans	Monthly. Edited by Dr. Taxil. Published thorough December 1860.
271	*L'Homoion*	1861	New Orleans	Monthly. Edited by L. Caboche. Official journal of the Societe Hahnemannienne de la Nouvelle Orleans.
272	*Library of Homeopathic Classics*	1907	New York	Edited by Shedd. Supplement to the *New York Journal of Homeopathy.*
273	*Lobelia Advocate and Thomsonian Medical Recorder; A Medical Family Journal Devoted to the Advocacy of Thomsonian Rights and Medical Principles*	1838–1839	Carroll County; Baltimore (1838)	Monthly. Published and edited by John Rose. Dedicated to reporting the activities of the Senate and House of Delegates regarding all medical matters, obtaining a Thomsonian emancipation from Maryland lawmakers, supporting botanic physicians, and documenting the errors of regular medicine.
274	*Lobelian and Rhode Island Medical Review*	1838–1839	Newport	Monthly. Charles Gardener, proprietor; C. B. Peckham, editor.
275	*Los Angeles Journal of Eclectic Medicine*	1904–1908	Los Angeles	Became *California Medical Journal;* and later *California Eclectic Medical Journal.*
276	*Louisville Journal of Medicine and Surgery*	1838	Louisville	Merged with *Western Journal of Medical and Physical Sciences* (Cincinnati).
277	*Madison Homeopathist*	1854	Madison	Monthly. Published and edited by Drs. Bowen and Giles. Lasted for only a few months. Intended for the laity.
278	*Maine Medical Journal. Devoted to Eclecticism*	1882	Lewistown	Monthly. Edited by W. Wadworth and A. J. Marston. Continued as *Eastern Medical Journal.*
279	*Maine Thomsonian Recorder and Family Journal of Health*	1838–1840	Portland	Semimonthly. Published and edited by Benjamin Colby, Jr. Merged with the *Thomsonian Medical Advertiser.*

	Title	Years	Location	Comments
280	*Massachusetts Eclectic Medical Journal. Devoted to Medicine and General Science*	1881–1885	Boston	Monthly. Edited by H. G. Barrows; G. H. Merkel; and Robert A. Reid. Continued as *Massachusetts Medical Journal.*
281	*Massachusetts Medical Journal*	1886–1888	Boston	Monthly. Edited by Robert A. Reid. Formerly the *Massachusetts Eclectic Medical Journal.*
282	*Materia Medica Journal*	1896	Chicago	Edited by H. C. Allen. Homeopathic in context.
283	*Medical Advance*	1884–1898	Ann Arbor	Semimonthly. Was for years printed in the basement of Pulte Medical College by Prof. T. P. Wilson. When he removed to the University of Michigan the magazine went with him to Ann Arbor. Formerly the *Ann Arbor Medical Advance.* Became *Hahnemannian Advocate* in 1898. Merged with *Journal of Homeopathics* to develop true homeopathy into a science. Represented the traditions of Hering, Dunham, and Lippe.
284	*Medical Advocate. A Monthly Journal of Medicine, Surgery, and the Kindred Sciences*	1885–1887	New York	Edited by Joseph A. House and Alexander Wilder. Formerly the *Eclectic Medical Advocate; A Monthly Journal of Medicine, Surgery, and the Kindred Sciences.*
285	*Medical Advocate; Devoted to the Cause of Advocating the Thomsonian System of the Practice of Medicine on Botanical Principles*	1827–1828	Boston	Monthly. Published and edited by Eleazer G. House.
286	*Medical and Scientific News*	1896–1898	Elkhart, Ind	Formerly *The National Medical Exchange Monthly Bulletin.*
287	*Medical and Surgical Record*	1889–1892	Omaha	Edited by D. A. Foote and E. F. Allen. Continuation of *The Surgical Record* (1888–1889).
288	*Medical Arena*	1892–1903	Kansas City	Edited by S. C. Delap. Was first titled *The Medical Standard* and one issue published under this name. Then became *The Keynote of Homeopathy.* It then became *Medical Arena.* Championed the Kansas City Homeopathic Medical College. Abandoned homeopathy in 1903 and became eclectic.

	Title	Years	Location	Comments
289	*Medical Argus*	1890–1891	Kansas City, Mo.	Monthly. Edited by F. F. Casseday. Eight volumes issued. Devoted to homeopathy and the collateral sciences.
290	*Medical Aurora, A Family Journal of Health*	184?	Columbus	Monthly. Published and edited by Zimri Hussey. Founded to advocate and defend the theory and practice of medicine as taught in the Literary and Botanico-Medical College at Columbus. Hussey owned and managed the school's infirmary and was one of the original trustees. He was committed to sustaining the Thomsonian system provided it was also scientific.
291	*Medical Call*	1881–1888	Quincy, Il.	Quarterly. Published by O. H. Crandall and edited by Crandall and W. D. Foster. Continued through three or four volumes.
292	*Medical Century*	1893–1915	Chicago; New York	Published by Medical Century Company and edited by C. E. Fisher and W. A. Dewey. It first absorbed *The New Remedies*, and then the *Northwestern Journal of Homeopathy.* In 1893 it acquired *Medical Era* and later combined with *The Homeopathic Journal of Surgery and Gynecology.*
293	*Medical Counselor*	1879–1886	Chicago	Monthly. Published by W. A. Chatterton and edited by H. R. Arndt; N. B. Delamater; and J. B. Mills. Changed with volume eleven to *Medical Counselor and Michigan Journal of Homeopathy* and moved to Grand Rapids, Michigan. In 1889 it became *The Medical Era,* and in 1893, it became *The Medical Century.*
294	*Medical Counselor and Michigan Journal of Homeopathy*	1886–1889	Grand Rapids	Semimonthly. Edited by H. R. Arndt and D. A. MacLachlan. See *Medical Counselor*. Merged with *Medical Era.*
295	*Medical Current*	1886–1896	Chicago	Monthly. Published by W. A. Chatterton and edited by H. Sherry; W. E. Reed; E. F. Storke; and W. A. Smith. A continuation of *The American Electro-Clinical Record.*
296	*Medical Debates*	1899	New York	
297	*Medical Eclectic. Devoted to Reformed Medicine, General Science and Literature*	1873–1882–	New York	Semimonthly. Published by the Eclectic Medical College of the City of New York. Edited by Alexander Wilder; R. S. Newton.

	Title	Years	Location	Comments
298	*Medical Era*	1883–1903	Chicago	Published by Gross and Delbridge and edited by C. Gatchell; C. E. Fisher; R. N. Tooker; J. E. Gross; and T. D. Williams. Became *Medical Century* in 1893, and then returned back to *Medical Era*. Became the official organ of the Illinois Homeopathic State Medical Association. Became *The Clinique* in 1902.
299	*Medical Era*	1896–1902	Detroit	Merged with *Medical Counselor and Michigan Journal of Homeopathy.*
300	*Medical Forum*	1904–1907	Kansas City	Monthly. Edited by W. E. Cramer and C. Ott.
301	*Medical Free Press*	1892–1895	Indianapolis	Founded by G. W. Pickerill
302	*Medical Freedom*	1871	Manchester, N.H.	Published by J. Heygood.
303	*Medical Gleaner*	1889–1893	Cleves, Oh.	Monthly. Published by W. C. Cooper; W. E. Bloyer. Became *Eclectic Medical Gleaner.*
304	*Medical Herald*	1881	St. Louis	Monthly. Edited by C. H. Goodman and C. W. Taylor. One copy issued.
305	*Medical Independent. Devoted to Domestic Medicine, Physiology, Hygiene, Science, Arts, and Information for the People*	1870–1872	Philadelphia	Weekly. Edited by William Paine. Continued as the *National Independent.*
306	*Medical Institute of Philadelphia*	1886–1905	Philadelphia	Monthly. Published by the Hahnemann Institute and edited by J. W. LeSeur; W. S. Morris et al. Changed name in 1889 to *The Medical Institute of the Hahnemann Medical College of Philadelphia.*. In 1893 it became *The Institute*, and then T*he Hahnemannian Institute*. The student publication of the Hahnemann College.
307	*Medical Investigator*	1847	Bloomington, Ind.	Monthly. Printed at the Christian Record Office and devoted to botanic medicine.

	Title	Years	Location	Comments
308	*Medical Investigator*	1856	St. Louis	Edited by D. White. Intended as a weekly homeopathic newspaper. Published for only a few months.
309	*Medical Investigator*	1861–1874	Chicago	Bimonthly. Published by C. S. Halsey and edited by T. C. Dunhcan; E. M. Hale; R. Ludlam; and G. E. Shipman. Intended as newspaper for the profession and advertising sheet for the publishers: Eleven volumes issued. Changed name to *The Medical Investigator and Business Advertiser*. In 1875 it became *The United States Medical Investigator.*
310	*Medical Investigator and Business Advertizer*	1863	Chicago	Published by C. F. Halsey. Formerly *Medical Investigator.*
311	*Medical Journal of Reform*	1852–1854	New York City	Monthly. Edited by Joseph D. Friend. Official journal of the Metropolitan Medical College.
312	*Medical Liberator. The Official Organ of the Iowa Medical Liberty League*	1886–1888	Des Moines	Weekly. Edited by J. Winfield Scott. Formerly the *Weekly Magnet.* In 1888 continued as *National Liberator,* Boston.
313	*Medical Library*	1886–1888	New York City	Bimonthly. An eclectic review of medical literature.
314	*Medical Magazine*	1901–1903	Milwaukee	Edited by H. B. Dale
315	*Medical Mirror; A Monthly Journal Devoted to the Interests of Liberal Medicine*	1874	New York City	Monthly. Edited by Robert A. Gunn and Benjamin J. Stow. Continuation of the *Monthly Mirror.*
316	*Medical Mission Herald*	1895	Chicago	Intended for the laity.
317	*Medical News*	1889	Orrville, Oh.; Elkhart, Ind.	Quarterly. Edited by H. A. Mumaw. Became the *Medical News and Bulletin.*

	Title	Years	Location	Comments
318	*Medical News and Bulletin*	1888–1889	Orrville, Oh.	Formerly *The Medical News*. Became *The Semi-Monthly Bulletin of the Western Exchange Bureau.*
319	*Medical News-Paper; Or, the Doctor and Physician*	1822–1825	Boston	Edited by Elias Smith. One of the earliest journals to support Thomson's practice of medicine.
320	*Medical Recorder*	1852–1853	Memphis	Title of volume 1 of the *Memphis Medical Recorder.*
321	*Medical Reformer*	1837	Washington, Ga.	Semimonthly. Published by M. J. Kappell and edited by James W. Price.
322	*Medical Reformer*	1851	Memphis	Monthly. Published and edited by Samuel R. Jones. Devoted to the advancement of the medicine taught at the Botanico Medical College of Memphis.
323	*Medical Reformer*	1864	Philadelphia	Monthly. Eclectic magazine edited by M. N. Miller.
324	*Medical Reformer and Progressionist*	1870–1871	Macon	Monthly. Published by the reform medical profession and edited by J. T. Coxe.
325	*Medical Reformer and Progressionist*	1871	Macon, Ga.	
326	*Medical Reformer and Temperance Advocate*	1853	New York City	Founded and edited by I. M. Comings.
327	*Medical Reformer. By a Physician*	1823	New York City	Monthly. Advocated botanic approach to medicine.
328	*Medical Review*	1873–1876	Indianapolis	Monthly. Edited by J. A. Brown and W. C. Cooper. Dedicated to the advancement of "liberal medicine."
329	*Medical Student*	1888–1905	Boston	Monthly. Undergraduate publication of Boston University. Editor chosen by students.

	Title	Years	Location	Comments
330	*Medical Topics*	1890	Chicago	Quarterly. Published by W. A. Chatterton. Two numbers published.
331	*Medical Tribune; Journal Devoted to Medicine, Surgery, and the Collateral Sciences*	1878–1884	New York	Monthly. Edited by Robert A. Gunn and Alexander Wilder. Merged into the *Eclectic Medical Advocate*. Advocate of "free medicine."
332	*Medical Truth. Devoted to Reformed Medicine and General Science*	1883–1884	New York	Monthly. Published and edited by H. W. Duszowski.
333	*Medical Truth-Teller*	1846	Rochester	Founded by J. Gates.
334	*Medical Union*	1873–1875	New York	Published by C. T. Hurlburt and edited by E. Guernsey; J. C. Minor; C. E. Blumenthal et al. Merged with *New York Journal of Homeopathy* to become *The Homeopathic Times* in 1875. Two volumes published.
335	*Medical Visitor*	1885–1905	Chicago	Monthly. Published by T. S. Hoyne and edited by W. A. Smith and H. B. Dale. Directory of homeopathy physicians and published in place of *Dr. Hoyne's Annual Directory*. Passed into the hands of Halsey Brothers, homeopathic pharmacists of Chicago.
336	*Medical World*	1881		Edited by C. H. Goodman and C. W. Taylor.
337	*Medico-Chirurgical Quarterly*	1880	New York.	Edited by J. Butler and G. M. Dillow. Published single volume. Formerly *The American Journal of Electrology and Neurology.*
338	*Memphis Journal of Medicine; Devoted to the Advancement of Reformed Medicine*	1853–1857	Memphis, Tenn.; Holly Springs, Miss.	Monthly. Edited by T. C. Gayle, R. H. Harrison, and Jerome Cochrane.
339	*Memphis Medical Journal of the Progressive Medical and Physical Sciences*	1851–1852	Memphis	Monthly. Edited by H. J. Hulce.
340	*Memphis Medical Recorder*	1852–1858	Memphis	Bimonthly. Also titled *Medical Recorder.*

	Title	Years	Location	Comments
341	*Michigan Journal of Homeopathy*	1848–1854	Detroit	Monthly. Published by G. W. Pattison and edited by John Ellis and E. H. Drake. Published irregularly; contained articles addressed more to the laity than the profession. Two volumes issued.
342	*Michigan Journal of Homeopathy*	1872	Detroit	Quarterly. Published and edited by E. R. Ellis. The second rendition was the product of the faculty of the Detroit Homeopathic College. Contained the announcement of the Detroit College, and matters of interest to the medical profession. Four issues published.
343	*Middle States Medical Reformer and Advocate of Innocuous Medication*	1854–1857	Milford, Del. (1854–55); Millville, Pa. (1855–57); Bloomsburg, Pa. (1857)	Monthly. Published and edited by Palemon John and John S. Prettyman. Formerly the *Middle States Medical Reformer and Journal of Health.* In 1858 continued as the *Eclectic Medical Journal of Philadelphia.*
344	*Middle States Medical Reformer and Journal of Health*	1855	Millville, Pa.	Monthly. Published and edited by Palemon John and John S. Prettyman. Volume 3–4 of the *Middle States Medical Reformer and Advocate of Innocuous Medication.*
345	*Milwaukee Homeopathic Medical Reporter*	1848	Milwaukee	Monthly. Published and edited by L. M. Tracy and J. Douglas. Criticized for advertising the journal's two editors.
346	*Minneapolis Homeopathic Magazine*	1892–1903	Minneapolis	Monthly. Published by the Minneapolis Pharmacy Company and edited by H. C. Aldrich. Published ten volumes.
347	*Minnesota Homeopath*	1854	St. Paul	Bimonthly. Edited by G. Hatfield. Published only a few numbers.
348	*Minnesota Medical and Surgical Journal*	1866–1887	Minneapolis	
349	*Minnesota Medical Mirror*	1881–1885	Cambridge City	Monthly. Edited by N. M. Cook. Devoted to the progress made in eclectic medicine, surgery, and pharmacy.

	Title	Years	Location	Comments
350	*Minnesota Medical Monthly*	1886–1888	Minneapolis	Published by T. Gardiner and edited by W. E. Leonard; P. M. Hall; R. D. Matchan et al. Published two volumes.
351	*Miscellanies on Homeopathy*	1838–1839	Philadelphia	Published by L. J. Kiderlin and Company. Edited by C. Hering; C. Loingen; C. Neidhard et al. Thought to be one of the best books for physicians and laymen on homeopathy. Formerly *The American Journal of Homeopathy.*
352	*Mistletoe*	1891–1892	Philadelphia	Edited by R. S. Pencer, Mr. G. A. Barrows et al. Published for the benefit of the Hahnemann Hospital of Philadelphia.
353	*Modern Eclecticism*	1889	Atlanta	Formerly *Georgia Eclectic Medical Journal; Devoted to Liberal Medicine, Hygiene, and Sanitary Science.*
354	*Monthly Homeopathic News*	1871–1903	St. Louis	Monthly. Published by H. C. G. Luyties and R. G. A. Meier. Edited by H. C. G. Luyties; W. T. Helmuth; and C. H. Goodman. Formerly *The Homeopathic News.*
355	*Monthly Mirror. Devoted to Free Thought in Medicine, Science, and General Literature*	1873–1874	New York	Monthly. Edited by Robert A. Gunn.
356	*Monthly Record*	1857–1909	New York	Published by Five Points House and in connection with the Five Points House of Industry that was under homeopathic control.
357	*Munson's Homeopathic Bulletin*	1872–1892	St. Louis	Monthly. Published by Munson Homeopathic Pharmacy and edited by J. W. Munson. A gratuitous advertising journal.
358	*National (The) Medical News*	1891	Orrville, Oh.	Formerly *The Semi-Monthly Bulletin of the Western Exchange Bureau.* Later became *The National Medical Exchange Monthly Bulletin* (1891).
359	*National Independent*	1872	Philadelphia	Weekly. Edited by William Y. Leader and Dr. William Paine. Formerly the *Medical Independent.*
360	*National Liberator*	1888	Boston	Formerly *Medical Liberator.* The official organ of the Iowa Medical Liberty League.

	Title	Years	Location	Comments
361	*National Medical Exchange Monthly Bulletin*	1888–1900	Elkhart, Ind.	Formerly *The National Medical News.* Later became *The Medical and Scientific News.*
362	*Nature's Arcana. Devoted to Medical Reform, Science, Art, Literature, and General Intelligence*	1872–1873	Boston	Bimonthly.
363	*Nebraska Medical Journal. An Eclectic Monthly*	1884	Lincoln	Monthly. Edited by W. S. Latta, E. B. Guild, and J. M. Keys.
364	*New England Botanic, Medical and Surgical Journal*	1847–1851	Worcester	Semimonthly. Published and edited by Calvin Newton. Formerly titled *New England Medical Eclectic and Guide to Health.* Continued as *Worcester Journal of Medicine.*
365	*New England Eclectic Medical Journal. Devoted to the Interests of Progressive Medicine*	1873	Enfield Center, N.H.	Monthly. Proprietor and editor Eli G. Jones.
366	*New England Eclectic Medical Journal; A Monthly Journal Devoted to the Interests of Progressive Medicine*	1872	Auburn, Me.	Monthly. Edited by Eli G. Jones of Union Village, Vermont.
367	*New England Medical Eclectic*	1859	Worcester	Monthly. Editor W. C. George.
368	*New England Medical Eclectic and Guide to Health*	1846–1847	Worcester	Semimonthly. Founded and edited by Calvin Newton. Name changed in 1847 to *New England Botanic, Medical and Surgical Journal.*
369	*New England Medical Gazette. A Monthly Journal of Homeopathic Medicine, Surgery, and the Collateral Sciences*	1866–1905	Boston	Monthly. Published by S. Whitney and Otis Clapp and Sons. Edited by H. C. Angell; I. T. Talbot; H. C. Clapp; C. F. Nichols; W. Wesselhoeft; C. A. Chase; J. L. Coffin et al. Devoted to the progress of homeopathy in New England. Considered "progressive" in character and viewed high and low attenuations as "open questions" to be treated fairly. Represented the interests of the Boston University School of Medicine.
370	*New Jersey Eclectic Medical and Surgical Journal*	1874–1876	Newark	Devoted to liberal medicine, general science, and literature. Edited by Edward Fishblatt.

	Title	Years	Location	Comments
371	*New Remedies*	1889–1892	Chicago	Bimonthly. Published by Gross and Delbridge and edited by J. E. Gross; M. E. Hale et al. Merged in 1892 with *The Medical Century.*
372	*New York Amusement Gazette*	1888	New York City	Daily bulletin of the fair for the benefit of the Homeopathic Free Hospital.
373	*New York and Chicago Medical and Surgical Journal*	1881	Philadelphia	Monthly. Founded by E. N. Fishblatt. Formerly *New York Medical and Surgical Journal.*
374	*New York Eclectic Medical and Surgical Journal*	1877–1880	New York	Bimonthly. Edited by Edward N. Fishblatt. Formerly *New Jersey Eclectic Medical and Surgical Journal.* In 1880 continued as the *New York Medical and Surgical Journal.*
375	*New York Eclectic Medical and Surgical Journal. Adapted to Popular and Professional Reading*	1849–1852	Syracuse; Rochester	Monthly. Edited by William W. Hadley; S. H. Potter; R. Reuben; and L. C. Dolley. United with *American Medical and Surgical Journal,* forming the *Union Journal of Medicine.*
376	*New York Eclectic Medical Journal*	1876	New York	Title of volume 3 of *The Medical Eclectic.*
377	*New York Eclectic Medical Review. A Monthly Record of Medicine and the Collateral Sciences*	1866–1866	New York	Monthly. Edited by R. S. Newton; Edwin Freeman; P. Albert Morrow. Later called *American Eclectic Medical Review.*
378	*New York Journal of Homeopathy*	1846–1854	New York City	Biweekly and then monthly after 1848. Published and edited by S. R. Kirby and R. A. Snow. Discontinued after 1854.
379	*New York Journal of Homeopathy*	1873–1875	New York City	Monthly. Published by Carle and Grener and edited by W. T. Helmuth; T. F. Allen; S. A. Jones et al. Merged with *The Medical Union* to become *The Homeopathic Times* in 1875. Two volumes published. Prepared under auspices of the New York Homeopathic Medical College. Became *The New York Medical Times.*
380	*New York Medical and Pathological Journal*	1858–1859	New York	Monthly. Edited by W. W. Hadley.

	Title	Years	Location	Comments
381	*New York Medical and Surgical Journal*	1880–1881	New York	Monthly. Edited by Edward N. Fishblatt. Formerly the *New York Eclectic Medical and Surgical Journal.* Continued in 1881 as *New York and Chicago Medical and Surgical Journal.*
382	*New York Medical Eclectic*	1878–1882	New York	Edited by R. S. Newton. Volumes 5–9 of the *Medical Eclectic.*
383	*New York Medical Intelligencer, or Eclectic Gazette*	1845	New York	Published every alternate Wednesday. Edited by D. S . Meikleham.
384	*New York Medical Review*	1873	New York	Monthly. Formerly the *American Eclectic Medical Review.* Edited by E. S. McClellan.
385	*New York Medical Times*	1881–1896	New York	Monthly. Published by E. P. Coby and Company. Formerly *The Homeopathic Times*. Went over to allopathy.
386	*New York Thomsonian; A Botanico-Medical Journal*	1847–1848	Stillwater, N.Y.	Biweekly. Published and edited by Addison Bassett. Continuation of the *Poughkeepsie Thomsonian, a Semi-Monthly Family Journal of Health.*
387	*North American Homeopathic Journal*	1851–1855	New York City	Quarterly. Published by William Radde and edited by Constantine Hering; E. E. Marcy; and J. W. Metcalf. Suspended operations in November 1853 following the resignation of Hering and the poor health of Metcalf. Resumed in August 1856 as *The North American Journal of Homeopathy.* Prominent feature was report of provings and clinical cases.

	Title	Years	Location	Comments
388	*North American Journal of Homeopathy, a Quarterly Magazine of Medicine and the Auxiliary Sciences*	1856–1923	New York City	Quarterly. Published by William Radde and edited by John C. Peters (N.Y.); E. E. Marcy (N.Y.); William H. Holcombe (Natchez, Miss.); Henry C. Preston (Providence, R.I.). In 1860, the editorial board changed; and again in 1861, bringing in a broader range of regional editors. Took public issue with the editorial policies of *The Philadelphia Journal of Homeopathy.* Was accused of being in league with eclecticism and "other empirical schools" and with contributing "to render our house fearfully divided against itself." John C. Peters of New York was the chief editor until 1861 when F. G. Snelling took over. With the tenth volume, the journal dropped the words, "A Quarterly Magazine of Medicine and the Auxiliary Sciences" from its title. In 1870, the journal began a new series under editors F. W. Hunt and Samuel Lilienthal. Quarterly changed to monthly in 1885. Editorship changed in 1885 to G. M. Dillow and in 1892 to Eugene H. Porter. Formerly *The North American Homeopathic Journal.*
389	*North Western Journal of Homeopathy*	1858	Chicago	Quarterly. Published by the Association of Homeopathic Physicians and edited by Cowell and Halsey. Claimed to be a new series of the journal conducted by G. E. Shipman. Purported to be a magazine of medicine and the auxiliary sciences and edited by an association of homeopathic physicians. Lasted only one issue.
390	*North Western Sanitarian*	1894	Kenosh, Wisc.	Intended for the laity.
391	*Northern Ohio Medical and Scientific Examiner*	1848–1849	Cleveland; Columbus	Published by Oliver and Gilmen. Edited by A. W. Oliver; J. Wheeler; C. D. Williams; J. Gilman; and W. B. Waterman. Named changed to *Ohio Medical Examiner* after four issues.
392	*Northwestern Annalist*	1876–1877	Dubuque, Ia.	Quarterly. Edited by E. A. Guilbert. Dedicated to introducing homeopathy into the University of Iowa. Only four numbers issued.
393	*North-Western Journal of Homeopathia*	1848–1852	Chicago	Monthly. Published and edited by George E. Shipman. Continued for four years. Contributions from the best writers on homeopathy. Included extracts and reports from foreign periodicals.
394	*Northwestern Journal of Homeopathy*	1889–1891	Cedar Rapids, Ia.	Monthly. Published by Medical Pub. Company and edited by A. C. Cowperthwaite. Merged in 1893 with *Medical Century.*

	Title	Years	Location	Comments
395	*Occidental*	1869	St. Louis	Monthly. Published by J. V. Hogan and edited by G. S. Walker and T. G. Comstock. Organ of the Homeopathic Mutual Life Insurance Company. Published less than a year.
396	*Ohio Medical and Surgical Reporter*	1867–1877	Cleveland	Bimonthly. Published by Beckwith and Company; Witte and Company (1868). Edited by T. P. Wilson and G. W. Barnes; H. H. Baxter (1870) et al. Organ of the Cleveland Homeopathic Hospital College and the profession of Ohio. Formerly *The American Homeopathist.*
397	*Oregon Physio-Medical Journal*	1866–1868	Salem	Bimonthly. Published and edited by J. C. Sheldon. Continued as the *Pacific Physio-Medical and Surgical Journal.*
398	*Pacific Coast Journal of Homeopathy*	1893–1940	San Francisco	Quarterly. Published by the Journal Pub. Company and edited by William Boericke.
399	*Pacific Physio-Medical and Surgical Journal*	1868	Salem	Formerly *Oregon Physio-Medical Journal.*
400	*Paine's Journal of Domestic Medicine*	1873–1874	Philadelphia	Monthly. Edited by William Paine.
401	*Pellet (The)*	1872	Boston	Edited by J. B. Aldrich and J. M. Bugbee. A record of the Massachusetts Homeopathic Hospital Fair.
402	*Pellet (The)*	1876	Brooklyn	Published in the interest of the Brooklyn Homeopathic Hospital Fair. One number was issued yearly.
403	*Pellet (The)*	1884	Cincinnati	Edited by Mrs. W. Owens; Miss F. E. Worthington; and Stella Hunt. Published during the fair held in aid of the Ohio Hospital for Women and Children.
404	*Pellet (The)*	1886	Chelsa, Mass.	Edited by Mrs. C. A. Richardson and Mrs. H. Sawyer. Published by the Chelsea Massachusetts Hospital Aid Association.

	Title	Years	Location	Comments
405	*People's Health Journal of Chicago*	1885–1892	Chicago	Monthly. Published by the People's Health Journal Company and edited by L. D. Rogers and S. Ida Wright Rogers. Intended for the laity. Devoted to health, hygiene and preventive medicine.
406	*People's Medical Monthly*	1886	Chicago	Monthly. Published and edited by Edwin F. Rush.
407	*Periscope*	1878	Dubuque, Ia.	Bimonthly. Published by the Remedial Instrument Company and edited by R. S. Gee. Organ of the Remedial Instrument Company and devoted to physical, mental, and moral culture.
408	*Pharmacy Bulletin*	1881	Chicago	Published by Duncan Brothers.
409	*Phi Alpha Gamma Quarterly*	1901		Quarterly. National fraternity magazine.
410	*Phials*	1900–1905	Ann Arbor	Annual. Published by Parker and Snyder.
411	*Philadelphia Botanic Sentinel and Thomsonian Revolutionist; Devoted to the Thomsonian System of Medical Practice*	1837–1839	Philadelphia	Fortnightly. Edited by Morris Mattson. Originally titled the *Botanic Sentinel and Literary Gazette* (1835–37); continued as the *Philadelphia Thomsonian Sentinel and Family Journal of Useful Knowledge* (1939–44).
412	*Philadelphia Homeopathic Journal*	1838	Philadelphia	Published by the Association of Homeopathic Physicians and edited by Constantine Hering, Lingen, and Neidhard. Six numbers of thirty-six pages each issued. Subsequently published under title of *Miscellanies on Homeopathy*.
413	*Philadelphia Journal of Homeopathy*	1852–1856	Philadelphia	Monthly. Published by Rademacher and Jacob F. Sheek. Edited by William A. Gardiner; Alvan E. Small (1854); John Geary (1855). Originally intended to uphold strict Hahnemannian view of homeopathy. Contained clinical records, monographs on special diseases, studies of the materia medica, provings of remedies, editorial articles, etc. Considered strong reference source.
414	*Philadelphia Thomsonian Medical Journal*	1853–1854	Philadelphia	Monthly. Edited by John W. Comfort.

	Title	Years	Location	Comments
415	*Philadelphia Thomsonian Sentinel and Family Journal of Useful Knowledge: Devoted to the Thomsonian System of Medical Practice*	1839–1844	Philadelphia	Semimonthly. Published by John Coates, Jr. Originally the *Botanic Sentinel and Literary Gazette* (1835–37), then the *Philadelphia Botanic Sentinel and Thomsonian Revolutionist* (1837–39).
416	*Philadelphia University Journal of Medicine and Surgery*	1871	Philadelphia	Founded by Joseph Longshore; E. D. Buckman. Title of vols. 9–14 of the *Eclectic Medical Journal of Philadelphia.*
417	*Physician's and Surgeon's Investigator*	1880–1889	Buffalo	Monthly. Published by the Physicians and Surgeons Association. Edited by S. W. Wetmore; A. A. Hubbell; S. N. Brayton; A. S. Couch; F. P. Lewis; G. W. Lewis; L. A. Bull; and J. M. Lee. Issued ten volumes. Edited by the faculty of the College of Physicians and Surgeons of Buffalo.
418	*Physiologico-Medical Recorder and Surgical Journal*	1849–1852	Cincinnati	Monthly. Published and edited by Joseph Brown and E. H. Stockwell. Originally the *Botanico-Medical Recorder* (1837–52); also the *Physo-Medical Recorder and Surgical Journal* (1850).
419	*Physio-Medical Journal*	1877–1888	Indianapolis	Monthly. Published and edited by the Physio-Medical Journal Publishing Company. Formerly the *Physio-Medical Journal and Reform Advocate.* Edited by George Hasty.
420	*Physio-Medical Journal and Reform Advocate*	1875–1876	Indianapolis	Monthly. Edited and published by the journal committee appointed by the Indiana State Physio-Medical Convention. Became the *Physio-Medical Journal.*
421	*Physio-Medical Record*	1902–1907	Indianapolis	Official organ of the American Association of Physio-Medical Physicians and Surgeons. Formerly *Indianapolis Polyclinic.*
422	*Physio-Medical Recorder; Or, Impartial Advocate of Sanative Medicine and the Principles Which Govern the Physio-Medical Practice*	1852–1874	Cincinnati	Monthly. Published and edited by Alva Curtis; purchased in 1855 by William H. Cook. Originally titled the *Botanico-Medical Recorder* (1837–52); suspended from Jan. 1861 to Feb. 1862; united with the *Cincinnati Medical Gazette* in 1880, forming the *Cincinnati Medical Gazette and Recorder.*
423	*Physo-Medical and Surgical Journal*	1851–1852	Cincinnati	Monthly. Published and edited by E. H. Stockwell. Originally the *Physo-Medical Recorder and Surgical Journal.*
424	*Physo-Medical Era*	1849	Mount Vernon, Oh.	Monthly. Edited by M. K. Hard and D. W. Bloom. Dedicated to the pure and sanative system of medication.

	Title	Years	Location	Comments
425	*Physo-Medical Recorder and Surgical Journal*	1850	Cincinnati	Monthly. Published and edited by E. H. Stockwell. Originally the *Physiologico-Medical Recorder and Surgical Journal* (1849); renamed the *Physo-Medical and Surgical Journal* (1851–52).
426	*Popular Homeopathic Journal*	1866	Elgin, Il.	Monthly. Published by Smith and Lee and edited by C. A. Jaeger. Devoted to promote the cause of homeopathy and to enlighten the public on its theories and its superiority in practice over other systems of medicine. Six numbers issued.
427	*Popular Medical Examiner*	1885	New York	Monthly. Published by the New York Medical Examiner Company and edited by W. M. Cate. Intended for the laity.
428	*Post Graduate Bulletin*	1897	Chicago	
429	*Poughkeepsie Thomsonian, A Semi-Monthly Family Journal of Health*	1838–1847	Poughkeepsie, N.Y.	Semimonthly. Founded by A. H. Platt and Thomas Lapham; in 1845, Abial Gardener. Edited by George L. LeRow; replaced in 1839 by A. H. Platt; in 1845, by Abial Gardener. Continued as the *New York Thomsonian; A Botanico Medical Journal.*
430	*Practicien (le) Homeopathique*	1857–1858	New Orleans	Monthly. Published and edited by L. Caboche. Continued a little more than a year.
431	*Proceedings and Papers of the Michigan Eclectic Medical Association*	1897	Michigan	Annual
432	*Proceedings of the Annual Meeting of the Minnesota State Eclectic Medical Society*	1870	Owatonna	Annual
433	*Proceedings of the Eclectic Physicians of Cincinnati and Covington*	1853	Cincinnati	Annual
434	*Proceedings of the Illinois State Eclectic Medical Society*	1869–1875	Springfield	Annual

	Title	Years	Location	Comments
435	*Proceedings of the Indiana Eclectic Medical Association for Indianapolis*	189?	Indianapolis	Annual
436	*Proceedings of the Ohio State Eclectic Medical Association*	1865–1872	Ohio	Annual
437	*Proceedings of the Southern and Western States Reform Medical Association*	1869	Griffin	Annual. Included the proceedings of the Georgia State Association, and prospectus of the *Medical Progressionist.*
438	*Proceedings of the Texas Eclectic Medical Association*	1893	Texas	Annual
439	*Progress (The)*	1903–1909	Denver	Edited by D. A. Strickler. Resulted from split among Colorado homeopaths in 1903. Claimed to represent the interests of the Denver Homeopathic Medical College.
440	*Publishers (The) Record*	1883	Chicago	Monthly. Published by W. A. Chatterton and edited by C. H. Evans. Journal of information concerning books and periodicals on medical and related subjects.
441	*Pulte (The) Quarterly*	1890–1893	Cincinnati	Quarterly. Published by Pulte Medical College and edited by T. M. Stewart et al. Published in the interests of the Pulte Medical College, its alumni and the profession.
442	*Quarterly Bulletin*	1904	Philadelphia	Organ of Hahnemann of Philadelphia
443	*Quarterly Bulletin of Homeopathic Literature*	1871–1885	Philadelphia; New York	Quarterly. Published by Boericke and Tafel. Succeeded by *The Homeopathic Recorder*
444	*Quarterly Eclectic Medical Journal of Pennsylvania*	1862	Philadelphia	Quarterly. Edited by Henry Hollembaek. Continued as *Eclectic Medical Journal of Pennsylvania.*

	Title	Years	Location	Comments
445	*Quarterly Homeopathic Journal*	1849–1854	Boston	Published by Otis Clapp and edited by A. C. Becker; J. E. Birnstill; B. De Gersdoff; and J. A. Tarbell. Mainly devoted to the translation and republication of homeopathic news gathered from Germany, France, and England. Recognized two groups of homeopaths: those who accepted the theories of psora and infinitesimals, and those who did not.
446	*Quarterly Homeopathic Magazine*	1854	Cleveland	Edited by J. H. Pulte; H. P. Gatchel; and C. D. Williams. The editors made frequent use of European homeopathic literature. Formerly *The American Magazine Devoted to Homeopathy and Hydropathy*. One volume issued.
447	*Quarterly Journal of Eclectic Medicine and Surgery*	1909	Cincinnati	Quarterly. Published by the National Eclectic Medical Association.
448	*Record (The)*	1873	Boston	Published by Otis Clapp and Son. Issued irregularly by the Homeopathic Association of Boston University.
449	*Reformed Medical Journal*	1832	New York	Edited by W. Beach and H. D. Sheppard.
450	*Reformer (The)*	1881	Atlanta	Later titled *Journal of American Medicine and Surgery. A Monthly Journal Devoted to Medicine and Surgery.*
451	*Regular (The) Physician*	1884	Havanna, N.Y.	Quarterly. Edited by A. P. Hollett. Organ of the Southern Tier Homeopathic Medical Society.
452	*Rhode Island Medical Reformer; A Family Journal for the Promotion of Health and Longevity*	1843	Providence	Semimonthly. Founded and edited by by B. Franklin Clark.
453	*Rochester Medical Truth Teller: And Monthly Journal of Health*	1844–1846	Rochester	Monthly. Published by E. Shepard and edited by Justin Gates. Known as a Thomsonian botanical publication.
454	*Saint Louis Clinical Review*	1878–1884	St. Louis	Monthly. Published by Maynard and Company and edited by P. G. Valentine; W. B. Edmonds; S. B. Parsons; F. Kraft; and J. M. Kershaw. United with *The St. Louis Periscope and Homeopathic Medicine and Surgery* to form *The St. Louis Periscope and Clinical Review.*

	Title	Years	Location	Comments
455	*Saint Louis Eclectic Medical Journal*	1874–1883	Saint Louis	Monthly. Edited by George H. Field. Continued as *Saint Louis Medical Journal.*
456	*Saint Louis Journal of Homeopathy*	1895	St. Louis	Published by Schultz Publishing Company. Joined with *Clinical Reporter.* Became *Saint Louis Journal of Homeopathy and Clinical Reporter* (1895).
457	*Saint Louis Journal of Homeopathy and Clinical Reporter*	1895–1897	St. Louis	Published by Schultz Publishing Company. Formerly *Saint Louis Journal of Homeopathy.* Became *The Clinical Reporter* in 1897.
458	*Saint Louis Medical Journal*	1884–1888	Saint Louis	Monthly. Edited by George H. Field. Formerly *Saint Louis Eclectic Medical Journal.*
459	*Saint Louis Periscope and Clinical Review*	1884–1886	St. Louis	Published by F. W. Nixon and edited by W. B. Edmonds; S. B. Parsons; F. Kraft et al. Formed by the merger of *The Saint Louis Periscope of Homeopathic Medicine* and *The Saint Louis Clinical Review.*
460	*Saint Louis Periscope of Homeopathic Medicine and Surgery*	1884	St. Louis	Monthly. Edited by E. C. Franklin. United with *The Saint Louis Clinical Review* to become *The Saint Louis Periscope and Clinical Review.*
461	*Sanitary Gleanings*	1884–1885	Philadelphia	Published by Shermon and Company and edited by B. W. James. Intended for laity. Only twelve numbers published.
462	*Semi-Monthly Bulletin of the Western Exchange*	1889	Orrville, Oh.	Formerly *The Medical News and Bulletin.* Later became *The National Medical News.*
463	*Similibus (The)*	1872	New York	Edited by Mrs. Carroll Dunham; and Mrs. Henry D. Paine. Published for the benefit of the Homeopathic Surgical Hospital. Complete in ten numbers.
464	*Social Reformer and Herald of Universal Health*	1844	Boston	Semimonthly. Published and edited by John Allen and Joseph A. Whitmarsh. Favored botanic medicines.
465	*Southern (The) Journal of Health*	1885	Atlanta; Ashville, N.C.	Edited by H. P. Gatchell and intended for the laity.

	Title	Years	Location	Comments
466	*Southern Botanic Journal*	1837–1841	Augusta; Forsyth, Ga.	Biweekly. Published by Harvey and Carlisle and edited by D. F. Nardin; 1838, J. L. Wood and William H. Fonerden. Dedicated to the friends of the Thomsonian system.
467	*Southern Botanic Journal*	1846	Forsyth, Ga.	Semimonthly. Edited by William H. Fonerden.
468	*Southern Botanico-Medical College Journal*	1842–1843	Forsyth, Ga.	Monthly. Edited by L. Bankston; Hugh Quin; I. M. Comings; and J. H. Hand.
469	*Southern Botanico-Medical Journal. Devoted to the Principles and Practice of Medicine, as Originated by Dr. Samuel Thomson*	1841–1842	Forsyth, Ga.	Semimonthly. Edited by H. Lee. Journal later removed with college to Macon.
470	*Southern Botanico-Medical Reformer*	1849–1851	Macon, Ga.	Quarterly. Edited by M. S. Thomson. A continuation of the *Georgia Botanic Journal and College Sentinel.*
471	*Southern Homeopathic Pellet*	1884–1885	Austin, Tx.	Renamed *Southern Journal of Homeopathy.*
472	*Southern Journal of Homeopathy*	1885–1897	Austin, Tx.; New Orleans	Monthly. Published and edited by C. E. Fisher. Formerly *Southern Homeopathic Pellet*. In 1897 it became *The American Medical Monthly.*
473	*Southern Medical Reformer*	1845	Forsyth, Ga.	Monthly. Founded by S. F. Salter and edited by Henry M. Price. Published for the Southern Botanico-Medical College at Macon and Forsyth; the most intellectual of the periodicals; founded on the belief that, for Thomsonian practice to succeed, it must have its foundation in schools dedicated to practicing medicine.
474	*Southern Medical Reformer*	1847–1848	Petersburg, Va.	Monthly. Published by the Scientific and Eclectic Medical Institute and edited by Henry M. Price.
475	*Southern Medical Reformer*	1881	Atlanta	Founded by S. F. Salter.
476	*Southern Medical Reformer and Review*	1852–1860	Macon, Ga.	Monthly. Edited by J. T. Coxe; L. Bankston; and J. Kost.

	Title	Years	Location	Comments
477	*South-Western (The) Homeopathic Journal and Review*	1847–1850	St. Louis	Monthly. Edited by John T. Temple and Thomas Houghton. Extended through three volumes. First homeopathic periodical published in the West.
478	*Southwestern Eclectic Medical Journal*	1895	Hillsboro, Tx.	Bimonthly. Founded by W. L. Fowler.
479	*Southwestern Medical Advocate*	1847	Memphis	Monthly. Published by the Botanico Medical College of Memphis and edited by James Conquest Cross and William Byrd Powell.
480	*Southwestern Progressive Medical Journal*	1898–1901	Rogers, Ark.	Edited by W. L. Leister
481	*Student Newsletter and Hospital Tidings*	18??	Chicago	Published by the Chicago Homeopathic Medical College.
482	*Sugar Pills*	1874	Cincinnati	In aid of the Homeopathic Free Dispensary at Seventh and Mound Streets. Six numbers issued.
483	*Surgical (The) Record*	1889	Omaha	Bimonthly. Published by A. L. Stonecypher and edited by E. F. Allen and D. A. Foote. Name changed to *The Medical and Surgical Record* in 1889.
484	*Syracuse Clinic*	1898–1900	Syracuse	Published by the Clinic Publishing Company and edited by E. E. Keeler. Name changed to *Good Health Clinic.*
485	*Syracuse Homeopathic Hospital Record*	1899	Syracuse	
486	*Syracuse Medical and Surgical Journal*	1854–1855	Syracuse	Monthly. Edited by S. H. Potter. Formerly *American Medical and Surgical Journal.* Continued as the *Union Journal of Medicine.*
487	*Texas (The) Homeopathic Pellet*	1883–1884	Austin, Tx.	Monthly. Published and edited by C. E. Fisher. Medical journal devoted to the missionary interests of homeopathy. In 1884 changed name to *The Southern Homeopathic Pellet*, then to *Southern Journal of Homeopathy* in 1885. In 1897, it became the *American Medical Monthly.*

	Title	Years	Location	Comments
488	*Thomsonian*	1838	Poughkeepsie	Semimonthly. Published by A. H. Platt and Thomas Lapham and edited by George LeRow. Continued as the *Poughkeepsie Thomsonian, A Semi-Monthly Family Journal of Health* (1838–47). A family journal of health devoted exclusively to support the dissemination of the Thomsonian system of medical practice.
489	*Thomsonian Advertiser*	1844–1845	Boston	Founded and edited by James Osgood and A. B. Porter.
490	*Thomsonian Advocate or an Appeal to the Citizens of Connecticut*	1836	New Haven	Published by the New Haven County Botanic Society and edited by Bennett W. Sperry.
491	*Thomsonian Botanic Watchman*	1834–1835	Albany	Monthly. Published and edited by John Thomson.
492	*Thomsonian Defender*	1835–1836	Maryville, Tenn.	Monthly. Founded and edited by William Spillman. Spillman reported that fifty-three of Thomson's vegetable medicines grew in eastern Tennessee.
493	*Thomsonian Manual; Or, Advocate of the Principles Which Govern the Thomsonian System of Medical Practice*	1835–1844	Boston	Bimonthly. Founded by James Howarth and Co.; followed by Samuel Thomson and George A. Chapman; Natianiel S. Magoon. Edited by Nathaniel S. Magoon; 1837, Jeremiah P. Chapman; Morris Mattson; Joseph P. Mendum and E. L. Gray. Recognized as the official organ of Samuel Thomson. Editors faced constant meddling by Samuel Thomson. Title changed in 1838 to the *Boston Thomsonian Manual and Lady's Companion*; in 1844 it merged with the *Boston True Thomsonian to become the Boston Thomsonian Manual.*
494	*Thomsonian Medical and Physiological Journal*	18??	Boston	Merged in 1846 into the *New England Medical Eclectic.*
495	*Thomsonian Medical Independent*	1845	Boston	
496	*Thomsonian Messenger*	1841–1843	Norwich	Monthly. Founded by O. B. Lyman.
497	*Thomsonian Physician*	18??	New Ipswich	Published by S. W. King. Political and medical journal.
498	*Thomsonian Recorder*	1837	Louisville	Published and edited by M. L. Lewis. When Alva Curtis dropped *Thomsonian* from the *Recorder's* title, Lewis took the title, promising to adhere to the strict principles of Thomsonism.

	Title	Years	Location	Comments
499	*Thomsonian Recorder; Or, Impartial Advocate of Botanic Medicine, and the Thomsonian Practice*	1832–1837	Columbus, Oh.	Biweekly. Founded by Jarvis Pike and Company; in 1836, Alva Curtis. Edited by Thomas Hersey; 1835, Alva Curtis. First botanic medicine periodical devoted to Thomsonism and published in the West. Later became *Botanico-Medical Recorder* in 1837; also the *Physiologico-Medical Recorder and Surgical Journal* (1849); also the *Physo-Medical Recorder and Surgical Journal* (1850); also the *Physo-Medical and Surgical Journal* (1851–52); in 1852, name changed to *Physio-Medical Recorder.* It continued until 1880 when, after Curtis's death, the journal consolidated with another magazine, then reappeared as the *Cincinnati Medical Gazette and Recorder* from 1880 to 1885 when it became extinct.
500	*Thomsonian Scout*	1841–1842	Burlington	Monthly. Founded and edited by William S. Johnson and Pierce Standish.
501	*Thomsonian Sentinel*	1841	Philadelphia	See the *Philadelphia Thomsonian Sentinel and Family Journal of Useful Knowledge.*
502	*Thomsonian Spy*	1838	Manchester, Vt.	Monthly. Published and edited by Ezra Edson and Silas Wilcox.
503	*Thomsonian Trumpet*	1839	Shippensburg, Pa.	Monthly. Published and edited by John F. Weishampel. Intended as family journal with focus toward women; discontinued after several printings. Discouraged with his prospects, Weishampel sold his equipment and headed West.
504	*Thomsonian Vindicator*	1837	New York City	Semimonthly. Published by the Friendly Botanic Society and edited by S. W. Frisby.
505	*Transactions of the American Institute of Homeopathy*	1867–1909	Boston	Annual. Published by the American Institute of homeopathy. Some sessions were held in conjunction with international congresses.
506	*Transactions of the Annual Convention of the Wisconsin State Eclectic Medical Society*	187?	Milwaukee	Annual
507	*Transactions of the Connecticut Eclectic Medical Association*	1887	Bridgeport	Annual
508	*Transactions of the Eclectic Medical Association of the State of Indiana*	1865–1900	Indianapolis	Annual.

	Title	Years	Location	Comments
509	*Transactions of the Eclectic Medical Association of the State of Pennsylvania*	1878–1879	Johnstown	
510	*Transactions of the Eclectic Medical Society of the State of California*	1874–1896	Oakland	Annual
511	*Transactions of the Eclectic Medical Society of the State of New York*	1863–1900	Albany	Annual
512	*Transactions of the Eclectic Medical Society of the State of New Jersey*	1875–18??	Newark	Annual
513	*Transactions of the Illinois State Eclectic Medical Society*	1884–1885	Chicago	Annual
514	*Transactions of the Iowa State Eclectic Medical Society*	1868–1881	St. Louis	Annual
515	*Transactions of the Massachusetts Eclectic Medical Society*	1901	Boston	Annual
516	*Transactions of the Michigan Eclectic Society*	1900–1902	Paw Paw-	Annual
517	*Transactions of the Michigan State Society of Rational Medicine*	1881	Detroit	Annual
518	*Transactions of the National Eclectic Medical Association*	1852;1870–1889	Rochester	Annual
519	*Transactions of the New York State Eclectic Medical Society*	1850–1852	Syracuse	Annual

	Title	Years	Location	Comments
520	*Transactions of the North Western Ohio Eclectic Medical Association*	1882–1914	Ohio	Annual
521	*Transactions of the Ohio State Eclectic Medical Association*	18??	Ohio	Annual
522	*Transactions of the Physico-Medical Association of Ohio*	1870	Cincinnati	Annual
523	*Transactions of the Physico-Medical Society of the State of New York*	18??	New York	Annual
524	*Transactions of the Physio-Medical Association of Indiana*	1874–18??	Spiceland, Ind.	Annual. Published 12 volumes
525	*Transactions of the Physio-Medical Society of Indiana*	1868–1871	Indiana	Annual
526	*Transactions of the State Eclectic Medical and Surgical Society of Michigan*	1876–1889	Kalamazoo	Annual.
527	*True Thomsonian*	1843	Boston	Supported the cause of Dr. Morris Mattson against Samuel Thomson
528	*Union Journal of Medicine*	1853	Syracuse	Monthly. Edited by Levi Reuben and S. H. Potter. Formerly the *New York Eclectic Medical and Surgical Journal.* Formed by consolidation of *New York Eclectic Medical and Surgical Journal,* and *American Journal of Medicine*. Continued as the *Syracuse Medical and Surgical Journal.*
529	*United States Journal of Homeopathy*	1860–1863	New York	Quarterly. Published by C. T. Hurlburt and edited by E. E. Marcy and Henry C. Preston et al. Marcy and Preston withdrew from the *North American Journal of Homeopathy* and associated with fifty-two other homeopathic physicians to publish this journal. It continued for two years and then merged into the *North American Journal of Homeopathy* in 1863. The editors recognized only one therapeutic law, that of *similia similibus curantur,* and under no circumstances would admit that it was one of several laws of cure. Such admissions were for the eclectic and ultra-allopathist, but not the homeopath.

	Title	Years	Location	Comments
530	*United States Medical and Surgical Journal; A Quarterly Magazine of the homeopathic Practice of Medicine and Medical Science in General*	1865–1875	Chicago	Quarterly. Published by C. S. Halsey and edited by George E. Shipman; A. E. Small et al. First published under the auspices of the Western Institute of Homeopathy. Later issued by A. E. Small, R. Ludlam, W. Danforth, and R. N. Foster, all of the Hahnemann Medical College of Chicago. Merged in 1875 into *The United States Medical Investigator.*
531	*United States Medical Investigator*	1875–1892	Chicago	Semimonthly. Founded by Duncan Brothers; W. E. Reed; and W. A. Chatterton. Edited by C. H. Evans and T. C. Duncan. See *Medical Investigator.*
532	*University (The) Homeopathic Observer*	1903–1905	Michigan	Organ of the medical department of the University of Michigan, Ann Arbor.
533	*University Journal of Medicine and Surgery*	1866–1868	Philadelphia	Monthly. Edited by W. Paine. Formerly *Eclectic and University Medical and Surgical Journal of Philadelphia.* Later named *Philadelphia University Journal of Medicine and Surgery.*
534	*University Medical and Surgical Journal of Philadelphia*	1864	Philadelphia	Monthly. Published by Joseph S. Longshore; I. Loukens; and Charles Murphy. Organ of the Penn Medical University of Philadelphia. Consolidated with the *Eclectic Medical Journal of Philadelphia* forming the *Eclectic and University Medical and Surgical Journal of Philadelphia.* Continued as *Eclectic Medical Journal of Philadelphia.*
535	*Wayside (The)*	1888	Nappanee, Il.	Quarterly. Edited by H. W. Mumaw. Intended for the laity and devoted to physical and social culture. Four numbers issued.
536	*Weekly Magnet*	1886	Des Moines, Iowa	Weekly. Became *Medical Liberator: the Official Organ of the Iowa Medical Liberty League.*
537	*West-American Review*	1853	Cincinnati	Founded by G. W. L. Bickley.
538	*Western (The) Homeopathic Observer*	1863–1871	St. Louis	Monthly. Published by H. G. C. Luyties. Edited by William Tod Helmuth; G. S. Walker; and E. C. Franklin. Contained short and interesting articles for the profession. Discontinued at the close of the seventh volume.

	Title	Years	Location	Comments
539	*Western (The) Journal of Homeopathy*	1859	St. Louis	Monthly. Published by Strong and Company and edited by E. C. Franklin. Intended for the homeopathic profession in the Mississippi Valley as a means of communication among them.
540	*Western and Southern Medical Recorder*	1841–1843	Lexington	Monthly. Edited by James Conquest Cross. Merged in 1843 with *Western Lancet.*
541	*Western Botanic Recorder*	1835–1836	Louisville	Published by E. H. Clapp and edited by M. L. Lewis.
542	*Western Journal of the Medical and Physical Sciences*	1828–1838		Formerly titled *Western Medical and Physical Journal, Original and Eclectic.* Later titled *Louisville Journal of Medicine and Surgery*, and *Western Journal of Medicine and Surgery.*
543	*Western Lancet*	1842–1850	Cincinnati	Monthly. Published by Robinson and Jones.
544	*Western Medical and Physical Journal, Original and Eclectic*	1827–1828	Cincinnati	Monthly. Founded by Hatch and Nichols. Later titled *Western Journal of the Medical and Physical Sciences.*
545	*Western Medical Reformer*	1836–1848	Worthington	Monthly. Thomas Vaughan Morrow; I. G. Jones. Later titled *Eclectic Medical Journal.*
546	*Western Medical Reformer and Eclectic Journal*	1847–1848	Cincinnati	Volume 7 of *Western Medical Reformer.*
547	*Western Medical Reformer. A Monthly Journal of Medical and Chirurgical Science*	1836–1848	Worthington; Cincinnati	Monthly. Edited and published by the medical professors of Worthington College. Also called *Western Medical Reformer and Eclectic Journal.* Continued as the *Eclectic Medical Journal.*
548	*Western Medical Truth-Teller and Physiological Journal*	1846	Hillsborough, Il.	
549	*Western New York Journal of Homeopathy*	1846–1854	New York	Published and edited by S. R. Kirby and R. A. Snow. Only one number was published and this was reprinted under the title of *The American Journal of Homeopathy.*
550	*Western Quarterly Journal of Practical Medicine*	1837	Cincinnati	Edited by John Eberle, assisted by A. G. Smith; J. Moorhead; J. Locke; I. Cobb; and J. T. Shotwell.
551	*Wisconsin (The) Medical Record*	1885	Wisconsin	Edited by E. F. Storke. Issued only one number. Represented interests of Wisconsin Homeopathic Medical Society.

	Title	Years	Location	Comments
552	*Woonsocket Sentinel and Thomsonian Advocate*	1842–1843	Woonsocket, R.I.	Weekly. Edited by Willing Vose and George W. Davis. Devoted to reformed practice, health, temperance, news, and miscellany.
553	*Worcester Journal of Medicine*	1852–1856	Worcester	Monthly. Published by Calvin Newton and edited by Newton, H. G. Newton, F. H. Kelly, R. O. Williams, and A. J. Howe. Formerly the *New England Botanic, Medical and Surgical Journal* (1847–51).

[Sources include National Library of Medicine, *Index-Catalogue of the Library of the Surgeon-General's Office, United States Army, Series III* (10 volumes; Washington D.C.: Government Printing Office, 1918–1952); Thomas Lindsley Bradford, *Homeopathic Bibliography of the United States, From the Year 1825 to the Year 1891, Inclusive* (Philadelphia: Boericke and Tafel, 1892); "American Homeopathic Periodicals," *The American Observer*, IX (1872), 576–89; W. A. Dewey, "History of the Periodical Literature of the Homeopathic School," in William Harvey King, *History of Homeopathy and Its Institutions in America: Their Founders, Benefactors, Faculties, Officers, Hospitals, Alumni, etc., With a Record of Achievement of Its Representatives in the World of Medicine* (4 volumes; New York: Lewis Publishing Company, 1905); Jay Yasgur, "Homeopathic Journals of the United States," *Pharmacy in History*, XL (1998), 39–54; *First Search Database; Google Search Engine.*]

APPENDIX B

Reform Medical Colleges to 1915
(Botanic, Thomsonian, Physio-Medical, Homeopathic, and Eclectic)

	Name of School	Years	Location	Comments
1	Reformed Medical College of the City of New York	1826–1840	New York City	Eclectic. Opened on Eldridge Street by Wooster Beach (1794–1868) under title of U.S. Infirmary. Name changed in 1829 to Reformed Medical Academy and in 1830 to Reformed Medical College of the City of New York. First sectarian medical college in the United States. Graduates received elaborate certificate in lieu of a diploma. Not recognized by the New York Board of Regents. Unchartered.
2	Reformed Medical College of Ohio	1830–1840	Worthington	Eclectic. Better known as the Medical Department of Worthington College or simply as Worthington Medical College. First chartered sectarian medical college in the United States. Staffed by faculty of the Reformed Medical College of the City of New York led by John J. Steele and later by Thomas Vaughan Morrow. Distinguished itself from Thomsonism. Official organ was *Western Medical Reformer*. Closed as a result of resurrection riot in 1839 and lost charter in 1840. Morrow continued to instruct students at Worthington until 1842.
3	North American Academy of the Homeopathic Healing Art	1835–1841	Allentown, Pa.	Homeopathic. Founded in 1835 and incorporated in 1836. Teaching was entirely in German. Extinct around 1841. Last meeting of the directors was in 1842.
4	Botanico-Medical College and Infirmary	1836–1839	Columbus	Independent Thomsonian. Founded by Alva Curtis and operated without a state charter. Was organized contrary to Samuel Thomson's bias against the establishment of medical schools. Became intellectual center for the Independent Thomsonians. Later known in eastern states as physiopathists and in the Middle West as physio-medicals. Incorporated in 1839 as the Literary and Botanico-Medical Institute of Ohio.

	Name of School	Years	Location	Comments
5	College of Medicine, Botanic	1836–1846	New York City	Botanic. Founded by Isaac S. Smith, whose father, Elisha Smith, was author of *The Botanic Physician* (1830) and founder of the New York Association of Botanic Physicians. When Elisha died, his efforts were taken up by Isaac who organized reform physicians around a medical college. School affected by dissension among faculty. Not recognized by the New York Board of Regents. Extinct about 1846.
6	Literary and Botanico-Medical Institute of Ohio	1839–1869	Columbus; Cincinnati (1841)	Independent Thomsonian. Formerly Botanico-Medical College and Infirmary of Alva Curtis. First chartered Thomsonian medical college and the first with the word "botanic" in its official name. Chartered as the Literary and Botanico-Medical Institute of Ohio. Moved from Columbus to Cincinnati in 1841. By 1845, the college was advertising itself as the University of the Literary and Botanico-Medical College of the State of Ohio at Cincinnati. In 1847, school divided into a Literary and Scientific Department under Alva Curtis and a Medical Department under Joseph Brown, E. M. Parritt, E. H. Stockwell, J. A. Powers, and R. C. Carter. The Medical Department became known as the Physopathic Medical College of Ohio. When Curtis broke with Brown and Stockwell, he amended the charter to form the Physio-Medical Department of the Literary and Scientific Institute in 1851. The *Botanico-Medical Recorder* was his official organ. In 1854, Curtis brought William H. Cook to Cincinnati to be dean of college. Official organ became the *Physio-Medical Recorder*. Cook became displeased with Curtis's handling of diplomas and left to establish his own Physio-Medical Institute in 1859. Curtis's college declined and school's charter expired in 1869.
7	American Medical College of Ohio	1839–1857	Cincinnati	Eclectic. Founded by L. E. Jones and friends of T. V. Morrow. Intended to rival the Eclectic Medical Institute. Ended for lack of funds and students. Merged into the Eclectic Medical Institute in 1857. Jones reinstated on faculty of the Eclectic Medical Institute.

	Name of School	Years	Location	Comments
8	Southern Botanico-Medical College	1839–1884	Forsyth, Ga.; Macon, Ga.	Independent Thomsonian. Founded by Lanier Bankston and soon became battleground between Independent Thomsonians and eclectics. Moved to state capital at Macon in 1845. Changed name in 1854 to the Reform Medical College of Georgia thereby reflecting the dominant influence of eclectic thinking within the faculty. Closed in 1861 due to Civil War and revived in 1874 at Macon as the College of American Medicine and Surgery (eclectic). Moved to Atlanta in 1881 where it united in 1884 with another institution and adopted the name Georgia College of Eclectic Medicine and Surgery. It was the first sectarian medical college in the South.
9	Reformed Medical School of Cincinnati	1842–1845	Cincinnati	Eclectic. Organized by Thomas Vaughan Morrow following repeal of charter for Worthington Medical College. Provided course of lectures at the Hay Scales House at Sixth and Vine Streets. Unchartered. Immediate predecessor of the Eclectic Medical Institute which was incorporated March 10, 1845.
10	Eclectic Medical Institute	1845–1910	Cincinnati	Eclectic. Successor to Worthington Medical College which removed to Cincinnati in 1843 and reopened as the Reformed Medical School of Cincinnati. In 1845 it was chartered as the Eclectic Medical Institute. First use of the word "eclectic" in the name of a medical college. Also first medical school in America to accept women for study and graduation in medicine. Offered a medical degree in homeopathy for one year. Absorbed the American Medical College in 1857 and the Eclectic College of Medicine and Surgery in 1859. Name changed to Eclectic Medical College in 1910. Coeducational since 1871. School dissolved in 1939 and charter surrendered in 1942. Last class graduated in 1939. Official organ was the *Eclectic Medical Journal.* The first and the last eclectic medical school in the United States.
11	Alabama Medical Institute	1845–1846	Wetumpka	Independent Thomsonian. Chartered by secessionist faculty who left the Southern Botanic-Medical College. Gave one session from November 1845 to February 1846 and then closed. Too many of Alabama's botanical advocates preferred to receive their education in the North.

	Name of School	Years	Location	Comments
12	Worcester Medical School	1846–1859	Worcester	Independent Thomsonian before becoming eclectic. Opened in 1846 by Calvin Newton as a physio-medical branch institution under the degree authority of the Southern Botanico-Medical College in Macon, Georgia. School changed its name to Worcester Botanico-Medical College in 1847. Newton's *New England Medical Eclectic and Guide to Health* was the official organ of college. Arrangement abrogated and made with the Scientific and Eclectic Medical Institute of Virginia in Petersburg. Reorganized as New England Botanico-Medical College in 1849 and then as the Worcester Medical College in 1851 when it secured its own charter. Gained affiliation with Syracuse Medical College in 1852. Conferred first degree of M.D. upon a woman (Dr. Lucinda Hall) in New England. The school went on hard times and suspended its classes after moving to Chapman Hall in Boston in 1856. Closed doors in 1859.
13	Memphis Institute	1847–1851	Memphis	Eclectic. Charter granted to William Byrd Powell who, disappointed with the direction taken at the Botanico-Medical College of Memphis, organized a college to include teaching in arts, science, law, and medicine. Powell occupied the chair of cerebral physiology. Faculty consisted of Powell, R. S. Newton, Z. Freeman, and J. Milton Sanders. Suspended in 1851.
14	Botanico-Medical College of Memphis	1847–1861	Memphis	Independent Thomsonian. Incorporated as the Memphis Institute by Michael Gabbert and James Seaver. Its official organ was the *Southwestern Medical Advocate* edited by William Byrd Powell. Originally Thomsonian but came under influence of eclectics. Took name of Eclectic Medical Institute of Memphis in 1859 and closed in 1861, a victim of the resinoid craze and the financial consequences stemming from the Civil War.
15	Scientific and Eclectic Medical Institute of Virginia	1847–1851	Petersburg	Independent Thomsonian. Short lived due to strenuous disagreements between Thomsonian and eclectic factions within the faculty. Moved increasingly to eclectic philosophy. Unable to maintain enrollments. Closed in 1851.
16	Medical School of Fredonia	1847–1848	Fredonia	Eclectic. Organized by Stephen H. Potter and Orin Davis. Moved in 1848 to Rochester, taking the name of Eclectic Medical Institute of New York. Unchartered.

	Name of School	Years	Location	Comments
17	Physopathic Medical College of Ohio	1847–1880	Cincinnati	Physio-medical. Organized by faculty of the Literary and Botan co-Medical College of Ohio in 1847 when school separated its Literary and Scientific Institute from its department of medicine. Medical department included Joseph Brown, E. M. Parritt, E. H. Stockwell, J. A. Powers, and R. C. Carter. Represented themselves as the heirs of the Medical Department of the Literary and Botanico-Medical College of Ohio. In 1851 it repudiated the principles of Thomson, condemned the practice of steam and puke, and severed all ties with Alva Curtis. The *Physio-Medical Recorder and Surgical Journal* was the school's official organ.
18	Eclectic Medical Institute of New York	1848–1849	Rochester	Eclectic. Formerly the Medical School of Fredonia in New York. In 1848 it moved to Rochester, taking the name Eclectic Medical Institute of New York. In 1849 it merged with the Randolph Eclectic Medical Institute and moved to Syracuse, becoming the Central Medical College of New York that in 1850 became the Rochester Eclectic Medical College. Not recognized by the New York Board of Regents. Unchartered. Espoused eclectic medical philosophy.
19	Eclectic Medical College	1848	Louisville	Eclectic. Chartered by Legislature in 1848. Extinct.
20	Randolph Eclectic Medical Institute	1848–1849	Rochester	Eclectic. Organized in 1848. A year later it merged with the Eclectic Medical Institute of New York and moved to Syracuse, becoming the Central Medical College of New York. In 1850 it became the Rochester Eclectic Medical College. Not recognized by the New York Board of Regents.
21	Homeopathic Medical College of Pennsylvania	1848–1869	Philadelphia	Homeopathic. Incorporated in 1848 and lectures commenced same year. First class graduated in 1849. In 1869 it united with Hahnemann Medical College of Philadelphia and took the latter title. Became Hahnemann Medical College and Hospital of Philadelphia in 1885.
22	Boston Female Medical College	1848–1874	Boston	Eclectic. Founded by Samuel Gregory. Chartered in 1850 as New England Female Medical College. Original faculty was eclectic and then homeopathic faculty became dominant in the 1860s. Merged in 1874 into the Medical Department of Boston University.
23	American Reform Medical Institute	1849–1850	Louisville	Eclectic. Initiated by Dr. A. H. Baldridge who left the Eclectic Medical Institute of Cincinnati in protest when it established a chair of homeopathy. Faculty included both eclectic and botanic physicians. Closed after two sessions.

	Name of School	Years	Location	Comments
24	Worcester Medical College	1849	Worcester	Independent Thomsonian before becoming eclectic. Organized in 1849 as New England Botanico-Medical College; reorganized in 1852 as Worcester Medical College, Eclectic. Moved to Boston in 1857 and to Worcester in 1858. Extinct in 1859. Revived in 1914 as Middlesex College of Medicine and Surgery.
25	Rochester Eclectic Medical College	1849–1852	Rochester	Eclectic. Organized at Syracuse in 1849 as the Central Medical College of New York by the union of the Eclectic Medical Institute of New York with the Randolph Eclectic Medical Institute. In 1850 it moved to Rochester and became the Rochester Eclectic Medical College. Not recognized by the New York Board of Regents. Extinct by 1852.
26	Central Medical College	1849–1850	Syracuse; Rochester	Eclectic. Chartered and formed as a result of merger of Randolph Eclectic Medical Institute and the Eclectic Medical Institute of New York. Adopted policy of coeducation in 1849. Graduated second woman (Dr. Lydia Folger Fowler) in U.S. with degree of M.D. Serious dissension among faculty caused trustees to dismiss many. In 1850 it became Rochester Eclectic Medical College. Not recognized by the New York Board of Regents.
27	Western College of Homeopathic Medicine	1849–1857	Cleveland	Homeopathic. Incorporated in 1849 and lectures commenced in 1850. First class graduated in 1850. Named changed in 1857 to Western Homeopathic College; in 1870 to Homeopathic Hospital-College and absorbed the Homeopathic Medical College for Women. In 1894 it became the Cleveland University of Medicine and Surgery. In 1898 it joined Cleveland Medical College (Homeopathic) to form Cleveland Homeopathic Medical College.
28	Thomsonian College	1850–185?	Barbourville, Ga.	Independent Thomsonian. Unchartered. Extinct.
29	Syracuse Medical College	1850–1855	Syracuse	Eclectic. Organized in 1850 by dismissed professors of Central Medical College. Absorbed Central Medical College in 1852. Not recognized by the New York Board of Regents. Extinct by 1855.
30	Female Medical College of Pennsylvania	1850–1852	Philadelphia	Eclectic. Difficulty in securing faculty for a women's college led do several irregulars (eclectics) appointed among the first professors. Name changed in 1867 to Woman's Medical College of Pennsylvania. Eclectic influence did not remain long. Eclectic faculty moved to the New England Female Medical College of Samuel Gregory.

	Name of School	Years	Location	Comments
31	New England Female Medical College	1850–1874	Boston	Eclectic. Formerly Boston Female Medical College founded by Samuel Gregory. Original faculty was eclectic and then homeopathic faculty became dominant in the 1860s. Merged in 1874 into the Medical Department of Boston University.
32	Physio-Medical Department	1851–1869	Cincinnati	Physio-medical. When Curtis broke with Brown and Stockwell, he formed the Physio-Medical Department of the Literary and Scientific Institute in 1851. The *Botanico-Medical Recorder* was his official organ. In 1854, Curtis brought William H. Cook to Cincinnati to be dean of college. Official organ became *Physio-Medical Recorder.* Displeased with Curtis's handling of diplomas, Cook left and established his own Physio-Medical Institute in 1859. Curtis's college declined and school's charter expired in 1869.
33	Eclectic Medical College of Philadelphia	1850–1864	Philadelphia	Eclectic. Organized by doctors Thomas Cooke, James McClintock, Joseph Sites, Henry Hollemback, and P. F. Sweet. First term held in spring of 1851. Its official organ was the *American Medical and Surgical Journal.* Merged with Penn Medical College to become Philadelphia University of Medicine and Surgery, thus dropping the term "eclectic" from title.
34	Metropolitan Medical College of the City of New York	1852–1862	New York City	Mixed. Organized in 1852 at 68 East Broadway. So constituted that both eclectics and physiopaths served as trustees and faculty. Principal leader of college was Isaac Miller Comings. Credibility of college undermined when faculty agreed to give diplomas to first-term matriculants as well as to some individuals who were not students at all. William H. Cook resigned in protest. Ultimately dominated by the more liberal eclectics. Charter revoked in 1862. Diplomas not recognized by the New York Board of Regents.
35	American Medical College of Ohio	1852–1857	Cincinnati	Eclectic. Founded by Dr. L. E. Jones and A. H. Baldridge in opposition to the Eclectic Medical Institute. Also included S. H. Potter and E. H. Stockwell from the Syracuse Medical College. Continued until 1857 when it merged with Eclectic College of Medicine and Surgery (1856–1859).

	Name of School	Years	Location	Comments
36	Penn Medical College	1853–1881	Philadelphia	Mixed. Incorporated in 1853 and lectures commenced same year. Established by Dr. Joseph S. Longshore and his associates and named for William Penn. Founded on principles of eclecticism, homeopathy, and the chrono-thermal system of Samuel Dickson of London. Nearly one third of graduates were women. Adopted a "progressive education" curriculum that was graded. Merged with the Eclectic Medical College of Philadelphia in 1864. Name changed to Philadelphia University of Medicine and Surgery. Suspended from 1867 to 1874. Extinct 1881.
37	American College of Medicine	1853–1880	Philadelphia	Eclectic. Founded by Mr. Joseph S. Fisher as rival to the Eclectic Medical College of Pennsylvania. Held but a single term of lectures and then suspended for lack of financial support. Reorganized in 1858 to become two associate institutions: Eclectic Medical College of Pennsylvania (diploma mill) under Dr. John Buchanan; and American College of Medicine under William Paine. American College of Medicine sold in 1865 to become Philadelphia University of Medicine and Surgery. Engaged in selling diplomas.
38	Independent Medical School of Philadelphia	1854	Philadelphia	Homeopathic. Chartered in 1854 and prospectus provided by Constantine Hering and Adolph Lippe. Never organized.
39	Homeopathic College of Vermont	1854	Vermont	Homeopathic. Never recognized by the Vermont State Society.
40	Reform Medical College of Georgia	1854–1874	Macon	Eclectic. Formerly Southern Botanico–Medical College. Eclectic in philosophy. Closed in 1861 and revived in 1874 at Macon as College of American Medicine and Surgery.
41	Hahnemann Medical College and Hospital	1855–1922	Chicago	Homeopathic. First Class graduated in 1860. In 1904 college absorbed Chicago Homeopathic Medical College.
42	Eclectic College of Medicine and Surgery	1856–1859	Cincinnati	Eclectic. Created from schism in the Eclectic Medical Institute and became a serious competitor. Incorporators included Joseph R. Buchanan, William Sherwood, James C. C. Holenshade, John King, C. H. Cleaveland, and others. Its official organ was the *College Journal.* In 1859 it merged with the Eclectic Medical Institute.
43	Eclectic Medical College of Pennsylvania	1856–1880	Philadelphia	Eclectic. Diploma mill owned by John Buchanan

	Name of School	Years	Location	Comments
44	Botanic Medical College	1857–1861	Memphis	Independent Thomsonian. In 1859 reorganized as the Eclectic Medical Institute and became extinct in 1861.
45	Western Homeopathic Medical College	1857–1864	St. Louis	Homeopathic. Incorporated in 1857 and lectures commenced in 1859. First class graduated in 1860. No sessions held between 1861 and 1864. Reopened in 1864 as Homeopathic Medical College of Missouri.
46	Western Homeopathic College	1857–1870	Cleveland	Homeopathic. Formerly Western College of Homeopathic Medicine. Became the Homeopathic Hospital-College in 1870.
47	American College of Medical Science	1858	New York	No information available.
48	Eclectic Medical Institute	1859–1861	Memphis	Eclectic. Formerly the Botanico-Medical College of Memphis whose faculty were invited to join the Eclectic Medical Institute of Cincinnati. All but James Conquest Cross and William Byrd Powell left. Following loss of the founding faculty to Cincinnati, the Memphis Institute took name of Eclectic Medical Institute of Memphis. Closed in 1861. Extinct.
49	Physio-Medical Institute	1859–1885	Cincinnati	Physio-medical. Organized by William H. Cook, editor of the *Physio-Medical Recorder,* and formerly of the Syracuse and Metropolitan Medical Colleges in New York. Competed with the Physio-Medical College of Alva Curtis who, in his later years, became involved with selling diplomas. Stopped classes in 1862 because of Civil War and resumed in 1863. College closed in 1885 and Cook moved to Chicago with several of the faculty where he opened the Chicago Physio-Medical Institute.
50	Homeopathic Medical College of the State of New York	1860–1869	New York City	Homeopathic Incorporated in 1860 and lectures commenced same year. First class graduated in 1861. Assumed title of New York Homeopathic Medical College in 1869; New York Homeopathic Medical College and Hospital in 1887; New York Homeopathic Medical College and Flower Hospital in 1909; and New York Medical College and Flower Hospital in 1936.
51	Brooklyn Academy of Medicine	1861–1888	Brooklyn, N.Y.	Eclectic. Charter revoked.
52	Michigan School of Homeopathy and Surgery	1863	Detroit	Homeopathic. Extinct.
53	New York Medical College for Women	1863–1866	New York City	Homeopathic. Incorporated in 1863. First class graduated in 1864. Assumed title of New York Medical College and Hospital for Women in 1866. Became extinct in 1918.

	Name of School	Years	Location	Comments
54	Homeopathic Medical College of Missouri	1864–1909	St. Louis	Homeopathic. Reorganized in 1882 and absorbed Hering Medical College and St. Louis College of Homeopathic Physicians and Surgeons. Became extinct in 1909.
55	Philadelphia University of Medicine and Surgery	1865–1880	Philadelphia	Eclectic. Incorporated in 1853 as the American College of Medicine in Pennsylvania and the Eclectic Medical College of Philadelphia. In 1856 became the Eclectic Medical College of Pennsylvania. Title changed in 1865 to Philadelphia University of Medicine and Surgery. Extinct in 1880.
56	Eclectic Medical College of the City of New York	1866–1913	New York City	Eclectic. Incorporated by special act of the New York Legislature. Its president was William F. Havemeyer, former mayor; succeeded by Alexander Wilder in 1868. The *New York Eclectic Medical Review,* begun in 1866, was the official organ of the college.
57	New York Medical College and Hospital for Women	1866–1918	New York City	Homeopathic. Formerly New York Medical College for Women.
58	Georgia Eclectic Medical College	1866–18??	Atlanta	Eclectic. School did not begin in earnest until 1877 because of effects of Civil War. Recognized by the National Eclectic Medical Association in 1881.
59	American University of Pennsylvania	1867–1880	Philadelphia	Eclectic. Incorporated in 1867 and extinct by 1880. Begun as branch of Eclectic Medical College of Pennsylvania (John Buchanan) under pretense of educating African-Americans. Diploma mill.
60	Hahnemann Medical College of Philadelphia	1867–1885	Philadelphia	Homeopathic. Incorporated in 1867 and lectures commenced the same year. Classes graduated in 1868 and 1869. Merged with the Homeopathic Medical College of Pennsylvania in 1869 and kept name. Became Hahnemann Medical College and Hospital of Philadelphia in 1885.
61	Homeopathic Medical College for Women	1868–1870	Cleveland	Homeopathic. Incorporated in 1868 and opened the same year. Only one session held. Merged with the Homeopathic Hospital-College in 1870.

	Name of School	Years	Location	Comments
62	Bennett College of Eclectic Medicine and Surgery	1868–1908	Chicago	Eclectic. Name was chosen in honor of Dr. John Hughes Bennett (1812–1875) of Edinburgh whose reform tendencies were celebrated by eclectics. Its principal founders were Doctors John Forman, Anson L. Clark, H. K. Whitford, Robert A. Gunn, and Herod D. Garrison. Title of Bennett Medical College assumed in 1909, dropping "eclectic" form its title. Absorbed the Illinois Medical College and the Reliance Medical College in 1910. In same year, it affiliated with Loyola University becoming its medical department. In 1915, Bennett Medical College passed under the complete control of Loyola University. Official organ was the *Chicago Medical Times*.
63	St. Louis College of Homeopathic Physicians and Surgeons	1869–1882	St. Louis	Homeopathic. Formed in 1869 from faculty of the Alumni Association of Homeopathic Colleges of Missouri. Held two sessions. Suspended in 1871 and revived in 1880. Consolidated with Hering Medical College and the Homeopathic Medical College of Missouri in 1882.
64	New York Homeopathic Medical College	1869–1887	New York City	Homeopathic. First class graduated in 1870. Formerly Homeopathic Medical College of the State of New York. Became New York Homeopathic Medical College and Hospital in 1887.
65	Boston University School of Medicine	1869–1918	Boston	Homeopathic. Incorporated in 1869 and lectures commenced in 1873. First class graduated in 1874. Merged with the New England Female Medical College in 1874. Became non-sectarian in 1918.
66	Homeopathic Hospital-College	1870–1894	Cleveland	Homeopathic. Merged with Homeopathic Medical College for Women in 1870. First class graduated in 1871.
67	Central Michigan Homeopathic Medical College	1871–1873	Lansing	Homeopathic. Incorporated in 1871 and opened the same year. Also called Michigan Homeopathic College. Held only one session. Became extinct in 1873.
68	Eclectic Medical College of New Jersey	1871–188?	New Jersey	Eclectic. Faculty finally appointed in 1888 but misunderstandings between trustees and professors brought repeal of incorporation.
69	Homeopathic Medical College of Detroit	1872–1899	Detroit	Homeopathic. Suspended in 1876. Reorganized in 1899 as Detroit Homeopathic College. Extinct by 1912.
70	Pulte Medical College	1872–1910	Cincinnati	Homeopathic. Incorporated in 1872 and lectures commenced same year. First class graduated in 1873. Merged in 1910 with the Cleveland Homeopathic Medical College to form the Cleveland-Pulte Medical College.
71	Homeopathic College	18??–1874	Buffalo	Homeopathic. No information available. Extinct prior to 1874.

	Name of School	Years	Location	Comments
72	St. Louis Hahnemann Medical College	1873–1874	St. Louis	Homeopathic. Graduated one class of four students. Extinct by 1874.
73	Homeopathic Medical College of St. Louis	1873–1883	St. Louis	Homeopathic. Suspended after 1875. Extinct since 1883. Fraudulent.
74	American Medical College of St. Louis	1873–1910	St. Louis	Eclectic. Included Doctors George C. Pitzer, Edwin Younkin, Albert Merrell, John W. Thrailkill, W. V. Rutledge, and George H. Field. Dissension ensued and Dr. Field procured a separate charter in 1874 for the American Medical University that became rival institution. Official organ was the *American Medical Journal.* Dropped eclectic affiliation in 1910. In 1911, it absorbed Barnes Medical College to Become the Medical Department of the National University of Arts and Sciences. Suspended operations in 1919.
75	National University of Arts and Sciences Medical Department	1873–1918	St. Louis	Eclectic. Organized in 1873 as an eclectic college with the title American Medical College. First class graduated in 1874. Dropped eclecticism in 1910. In 1911 the Barnes Medical College was merged into it. Became the National University of Arts and Sciences Medical Department in 1912. Suspended operations in 1918.
76	Physio-Medical College of Indiana	1873–1909	Indianapolis	Physio-medical. Founded by George Hasty, a graduate of the Physio-Medical Institute at Cincinnati. Graduated 10 to 12 students annually, with at least one woman in each class. First class graduated in 1874. Known among supporters as the "mecca of physio-medicalism." Became extinct in 1909.
77	University of Michigan Homeopathic Medical College	1873–1922	Ann Arbor	Homeopathic. Created by special appropriation of Michigan Legislature in 1873–74. Lectures commenced in 1875 and first class graduated in 1877. Abolished by Board of Regents in 1922.
78	American Medical University	1874–1883	St. Louis	Eclectic. Organized by George H. Field who left the American Medical College of St. Louis. Title change a year later to St. Louis Medical College. Rejected by the Board of Health of the State of Missouri in 1883.
79	St. Louis Eclectic Medical College	1874–1883	St. Louis	Eclectic. Extinct 1883.
80	Physio-Eclectic Medical College	1876–1879	Cincinnati	Physio-medical. Held three terms of instruction and then united in 1879 with the American Eclectic Medical College of Cincinnati.
81	Alumni Association of Homeopathic Colleges of Missouri	1876–1880	St. Louis	Homeopathic. In 1880 a portion of faculty seceded and revived the St. Louis College of Homeopathic Physicians and Surgeons that held only two sessions.

	Name of School	Years	Location	Comments
82	American Eclectic Medical College	1876–1896	Cincinnati	Eclectic. Organized in 1876. Successor to Physio-Eclectic Medical College. Declared not in good standing by the Ohio State Medical Board in 1896. Last class graduated in 1896. Extinct.
83	Chicago Homeopathic Medical College	1876–1904	Chicago	Homeopathic. First class graduated in 1877. Consolidated with Hahnemann Medical College and Hospital in 1904.
84	Georgia Eclectic Medical College	1877–1886	Atlanta	Eclectic. Acquired charter of College of American Medicine and Surgery in 1884. Assumed title of Georgia College of Eclectic Medicine and Surgery in 1886. Extinct in 1916.
85	State University of Iowa, College of Homeopathic Medicine	1877–1919	Iowa City	Homeopathic. Incorporated in 1877 and lectures commenced in same year. First class graduated in 1878. Supported by state tax dollars. Offered a three-year graded course of study. Abolished in 1919.
86	United States Medical College	1878–1882	New York City	Eclectic. Faculty included Benjamin Stow, Robert A. Gunn, Paul W. Allen, Alexander Wilder, A. B. Woodward and others. First eclectic college to introduce a graded course of instruction. Extinct.
87	California Eclectic Medical College	1878–1915	Los Angeles	Eclectic. Organized at Oakland as California Medical College. First class graduated in 1880. Removed to San Francisco in 1887. Suspended operations in 1906. Reorganized at Los Angeles in 1907 and extinct in 1915.
88	Buffalo College of Rational Medicine	1879	Buffalo	Extinct. Fraudulent.
89	Homeopathic College of Physicians and Surgeons	1879–1880	Buffalo	Homeopathic. First and only class graduated in 1880.
90	College of Physicians and Surgeons	1879–1884	Buffalo	Homeopathic. Illegally organized. First class graduated 1881. Charter revoked in 1884.
91	Hering Medical College	1880–1882	St. Louis	Homeopathic. Organized in 1880 and held two sessions. In 1882 united with the Homeopathic Medical College of Missouri.
92	Indiana Eclectic Medical College	1880–1890	Indianapolis	Eclectic. Due to dissension in the state, a rival institution, the Beach Medical College, was organized in 1883 as the Beach Medical University. Merged with Beach Medical University in 1884. Suspended operations in 1890 after being disowned by National Eclectic Medical Association but revived in 1895 under title of American Medical College of Indianapolis. It represented the American Association of Physicians and Surgeons, a non-partisan medical organization. Dissension continued and classes suspended in 1895.

	Name of School	Years	Location	Comments
93	Michigan Eclectic Medical College	1880–1880	Detroit	Eclectic. Never recognized by the NEMA or by the Eclectic Medical and Surgical Society of the State. Did not go into operation.
94	Eclectic Medical College of Maine	1881–1887	Lewiston	Eclectic. Numerous changes in the faculty and chronic financial problems. Maine Legislature repealed charter following allegations of it being in close relations with the Druidic University at Lewiston whose charter was revoked in 1887.
95	Hahnemann Medical College	1881–1888	San Francisco	Homeopathic. Incorporated in 1881 and lectures commenced in 1884. First class graduated in 1884. Name changed to Hahnemann Hospital College of San Francisco. In 1902 name changed again to Hahnemann Medical College of the Pacific. Merged with University of California Medical School in 1915.
96	Curtis Physio-Medical Institute	1881–1900	Marion; Indianapolis	Physio-medical. Founded by Henly James and David B. Snodgrass. School moved to Indianapolis where it graduated classes in 1893 and 1894. Returned to Marion in 1894. Not recognized by the Indiana State Board of Medical Registration and Examination. Extinct in 1900.
97	Iowa Eclectic Medical College	1881–1894	Des Moines	Eclectic. Organized as a department within Drake University College of Medicine. First class graduated in 1882. Drake University severed relations with college in 1887 but institution continued to grant degrees until 1892.
98	King Medical College	1883–1889	De Moines	Eclectic. Rival to Iowa Eclectic Medical College. Incorporated by Dr. Oliver H. P. Shoemaker. Denied membership in National Eclectic Medical Association.
99	Women's Medical College of St. Louis	1883–1884	St. Louis	Homeopathic. Organized in 1883 and held only one course of lectures. Extinct by 1884.
100	College of Medicine, University of Nebraska	1883–1887	Lincoln	Mixed. The Nebraska Legislature authorized the establishment of three medical departments: regular, eclectic, and homeopathic. Departments merged in 1887.
101	University of Florida	1883–1886	Tallahassee	Eclectic. With the assistance of Dr. John Kost (former professor in the Reform Medical College at Cleveland, Ohio), a medical department was connected to the institution. Moved to Jacksonville in 1885 and closed in 1886.
102	Beach Medical College	1883–1886	Indianapolis	Eclectic. Merged with Indiana Eclectic Medical College in 1884. Six weeks later seceded and organized Beach Medical Institute which again merged into the Indiana Eclectic Medical College in 1885.

	Name of School	Years	Location	Comments
103	Homeopathic Department of the University of Nebraska College of Medicine	1883–1887	Lincoln	Homeopathic. Lectures commenced in 1883. First class graduated in 1884. Extinct by 1887.
104	American Eclectic Medical College of Ohio	1883–1896	Cincinnati	Eclectic. Organized as the successor of the institution of the same name. Extinct in 1896.
105	Beach Medical Institute	1884–1885	Indianapolis	Merged into Indiana Eclectic Medical College, Indianapolis.
106	Chicago Physio-Medical Institute	1885–1911	Chicago	Physio-medical. Founded by William H. Cook who had closed his Physio-Medical Institute in Cincinnati in 1885. In 1891 name changed to the Chicago Physio-Medical College. It 1899 it absorbed the Chicago College of Medicine and Surgery (Physio-Medical) and took its title. Combined with the Physio-Medical College of Dallas, Texas, in 1908. In 1911 it was absorbed by the College of Medicine and Surgery (Physio-medical).
107	Hahnemann Medical College and Hospital of Philadelphia	1885–present	Philadelphia	Homeopathic. Formerly Hahnemann Medical College of Philadelphia. Commenced lectures in 1886. Coeducational since 1941. Dropped required courses in homeopathy in 1945 and discontinued last elective class in 1959.
108	Minnesota Homeopathic Medical College	1886–1888	Minneapolis	Homeopathic. Incorporated in 1886 and commenced lectures the same year. Ceased to exist in 1888 and became the College of Homeopathic Medicine and Surgery of the University of Minnesota. Supported by the state.
109	Georgia College of Eclectic Medicine and Surgery	1886–1916	Atlanta	Eclectic. Organized by uniting College of American Medicine and Surgery (1874) and the Georgia Eclectic Medical College (1877). Member of National Confederation of Eclectic Medical Colleges.
110	New York Homeopathic Medical College and Hospital	1887–1909	New York City	Homeopathic. Formerly New York Homeopathic Medical College. Later named New York Homeopathic Medical College and Flower Hospital in 1909.
111	Hahnemann Hospital College of San Francisco	1888–1902	San Francisco	Homeopathic. Formerly Hahnemann Medical College. Name changed in 1902 to Hahnemann Medical College of the Pacific.
112	Kansas City Homeopathic Medical College	1888–1902	Kansas City	Homeopathic. Incorporated in 1888 and commenced lectures same year. First class graduated in 1889. United in 1902 with Hahnemann Medical College of the Kansas City University to form Kansas City Hahnemann Medical College.

	Name of School	Years	Location	Comments
113	College of Homeopathic Medicine and Surgery of the University of Minnesota	1888–1909	Minneapolis	Homeopathic. Absorbed Minnesota Homeopathic Medical College in 1888. First class graduated in 1889. Abolished by Board of Regents in 1909.
114	Lincoln Medical College of Cotner University	1889–1918	Lincoln	Eclectic. With the closing of the departments in the University of Nebraska, the eclectics negotiated with the Nebraska Christian University (Cotner University) for the organization of a medical department.
115	Eclectic College of Physicians and Surgeons	1890–1894	Indianapolis	Eclectic.
116	Eclectic College of Physicians and Surgeons	1890–1894	Indianapolis	Eclectic. The college was recognized by the National Eclectic Medical Association in 1891. Dissension broke out and sessions suspended in 1894.
117	Cleveland Medical College	1890–1898	Cleveland	Homeopathic. Incorporated in 1890 and commenced lectures that same year. First class graduated in 1892. Joined Cleveland University of Medicine and Surgery to form Cleveland Homeopathic Medical College in 1898.
118	Post-Graduate School of Homeopathics	1890–1900	Philadelphia	Homeopathic. Incorporated in 1890 and commenced lectures same year. Founded by James Tylor Kent and funded by John Pitcairn, founder of Pittsburgh Plate Glass and a leader in the Swedenborgian Church. The school trained thirty physicians over the course of its history and its free clinic treated more than forty thousand patients. In 1900, Kent moved the school to Chicago where he became dean of the Dunham Homeopathic College. In 1903 Dunham merged with Hering Medical College.
119	Southern Homeopathic Medical College and Hospital	1890–1907	Baltimore	Homeopathic. Incorporated in 1890. First class graduated in 1892. Coeducation established in 1902. Name changed in 1907 to Southern Homeopathic Medical College. Extinct in 1910.
120	National Homeopathic Medical College	1891–1895	Chicago	Homeopathic. Opened at 541 North Halstead Street in 1891. Coeducational. Offered a three-year course of study, each session being six months. First class graduated in 1892.

	Name of School	Years	Location	Comments
121	Chicago Physio-Medical College	1891–1899	Chicago	Physio-medical. Formerly Physio-Medical Institute. Reorganized in 1891 and merged into the College of Medicine and Surgery (Physiomedical) in 1899. Located at 605 West Van Buren Street, in the vicinity of Cook County Hospital, Presbyterian Hospital, Hospital for Women and Children, and the West Side Free Dispensary. Moved in 1895 to Milwaukee Avenue.
122	German Homeopathic Medical College	1891–1900	Chicago	Homeopathic. Located at 512–14 Noble Street near Milwaukee Avenue. Lectures commenced in 1891 and given in both English and German. Chartered by Johann Malok. Not recognized. Extinct.
123	German-American Homeopathic Medical College	1892	Chicago	Homeopathic. Chartered by Johann Malok. Fraudulent. Extinct.
124	Hering Medical College and Hospital and Postgraduate School of Homeopathy	1892–1913	Chicago	Homeopathic. Established ostensibly to teach what the founders believed to be the cardinal principles of homeopathy. Relations among faculty were strained. Noted for frequent faculty resignations and factionalism. First class graduated in 1893. Absorbed Dunham Medical College in 1903. Closed in 1913.
125	National Homeopathic Medical College	1893–1896	Washington, D.C.	Homeopathic. First class graduated in 1894. Merged into the Washington Homeopathic Medical College in 1896.
126	Southwestern Homeopathic Medical College and Hospital	1893–1910	Louisville	Homeopathic. First class graduated in 1894. Extinct in 1910.
127	Cleveland University of Medicine and Surgery	1894–1898	Cleveland	Homeopathic. Formerly Cleveland Homeopathic Hospital College.
128	Wisconsin Eclectic Medical College	1894–1898	Milwaukee	Eclectic. Not recognized by the Wisconsin Eclectic Medical Society; thought to be affiliated with the Health College of Chicago. Never graduated a class.
129	Denver Homeopathic Medical College	1894–1907	Denver	Homeopathic. First class graduated in 1896. In 1907 it became non-sectarian as the Westminster University College of Medicine. Changed name in 1908 to Denver College of Physicians and Surgeons. Extinct in 1909.

	Name of School	Years	Location	Comments
130	Dunham Medical College and Hospital	1895–1903	Chicago	Homeopathic. First class graduated in 1896. Merged with Hering Medical College in 1903.
131	Washington Homeopathic Medical College	1896	Washington, D.C.	Homeopathic. Closed for failure to meet legal requirements.
132	College of Homeopathic Medicine and Surgery of the Kansas City University	1896–1900	Kansas City	Homeopathic. First class graduated in 1897. Name changed to Hahnemann Medical College of the Kansas City University in 1901. United in 1902 with Kansas City Homeopathic Medical College to form Kansas City Hahnemann Medical College.
133	Chicago College of Medicine and Surgery, Physio-Medical	1897–1899	Chicago	Physio-medical. Formed by William H. Cook, and others who withdrew from the Chicago Physio-Medical College in 1897. No classes graduated. In 1899 it merged with the Chicago Physio-Medical College to form the College of Medicine and Surgery, Physio-Medical.
134	Cleveland Homeopathic Medical College	1898–1910	Cleveland	Homeopathic. Formed by union of Cleveland University of Medicine and Surgery and Cleveland Medical College. Merged in 1910 with Pulte Medical College to form Cleveland -Pulte Medical College.
135	Eclectic Medical University	1898–1918	Kansas City, Mo.	Eclectic. First class graduated in 1900. Removed to Kansas City, Kan. in 1907. In 1908 it assumed the name Western Eclectic College of Medicine and Surgery. Returned to Kansas City, Mo. In 1909 and resumed its first title. Not recognized by the Missouri State Board of Health. Last class graduated in 1918 when it became extinct.
136	Western Eclectic College of Medicine and Surgery	1898–1918	Kansas City, Mo.	Eclectic. Organized originally as the Eclectic Medical University. First class graduated in 1900. Removed to Kansas City, Kan in 1907. In 1908 it assumed the name Western Eclectic College of Medicine and Surgery. Returned to Kansas City, Mo. In 1909 and resumed its first title.
137	Missouri Eclectic Medical College	1898–1898	Kansas City, Mo.	Eclectic. Extinct about 1898.
138	Detroit Homeopathic College	1899–1912	Detroit	Homeopathic. Formerly Homeopathic Medical College of Detroit. First class graduated in 1900. Extinct in 1912.

	Name of School	Years	Location	Comments
139	College of Medicine and Surgery, Physio-Medical	1899–1911	Chicago	Physio-medical. Formed by merger of Chicago Physio-Medical College and Chicago College of Medicine and Surgery, Physio-Medical. By 1904 it claimed a faculty of 44 and a total registration of 70 students.
140	Twentieth Century Physio-Medical College	1900–1904	Guthrie, Oka.	Physio-medical. The school's dean, H. Warner Newby, advertised "correspondence departments" at Union City, Michigan, and Hatfield, Pennsylvania, where for ten dollars one could purchase shares in the Twentieth Century Health Association. These shares empowered their bearers to obtain diplomas permitting them to practice medicine. Declared fraudulent and charter revoked in 1904. No evidence that classes were ever held.
141	Eclectic Medical College of Indiana	1900–1908	Indianapolis	Eclectic. First class graduated in 1903. Suspended operations in 1908 when recognition withdrawn by the Indiana State Board of Medical Registration and Examination.
142	Hahnemann Medical College of the Kansas City University	1901–1902	Kansas City	Homeopathic. Formerly College of Homeopathic Medicine and Surgery of the Kansas City University. United in 1902 with Kansas City Homeopathic Medical College to form Kansas City Hahnemann Medical College.
143	Chicago College of Medicine and Surgery	1901–1917	Chicago	Eclectic. Organized in 1901 as American College of Medicine and Surgery (Eclectic). In 1902 it dropped its eclectic name and affiliated with the Medical Department of Valparaiso University. Dropped eclecticism in 1905. Assumed title of Chicago College of Medicine and Surgery in 1907. Absorbed the College of Medicine and Surgery, Physio-Medical in 1911. Purchased by Loyola University School of Medicine in 1917.
144	American College of Medicine and Surgery	1901–1907	Chicago	Eclectic. Eclecticism was dropped in 1905. In 1907 changed name to the Chicago College of Medicine and Surgery and became by affiliation the medical department of Valparaiso University in Indiana.
145	Physio-Medical College of Texas	1902–1908	Dallas	Physio-medical. Faculty drawn almost entirely from the Physio-Medical College of Indiana. By 1905 college had 39 students, six of whom were women. Combined in 1908 with the College of Medicine and Surgery, Physio-Medical, of Chicago. Had a 71.4 percent failure rate on state boards. Absorbed by the Chicago College of Medicine and Surgery (eclectic) in 1911 and thus ended the 72 year history of physio-medicalism in the United States. In 1917, the Chicago College of Medicine and Surgery was purchased by Loyola University School of Medicine.

	Name of School	Years	Location	Comments
146	Hahnemann Medical College of the Pacific	1902–1915	San Francisco	Homeopathic. Formerly Hahnbemann Hospital College. Merged with University of California Medical School in 1915.
147	Kansas City Hahnemann Medical College	1902–1915	Kansas City	Homeopathic. First class graduated in 1903. Formed by the union of the Kansas City Homeopathic Medical College and the Hahnemann Medical College of the Kansas City University. In 1915 name changed to Southwest School of Medicine and Hospital. Held one session under new name. Extinct in 1916.
148	Thomsonian Medical College	1904–19??	Allentown, Pa.	Independent Thomsonian. No evidence that classes were ever held.
149	Eclectic Medical and Surgical University	1905–19??	Dallas	Eclectic.
150	Southern Homeopathic Medical College	1907–1910	Baltimore	Homeopathic. Formerly Southern Homeopathic Medical College and Hospital. Extinct by 1910.
151	Reliance Medical College	1907–1910	Chicago	Eclectic. Last class graduated in 1910 when it was absorbed by the Bennett Medical College.
152	California Eclectic Medical College	1907–1915	Los Angeles	Eclectic. Originally California Medical College, Oakland. Removed to San Francisco in 1887. Suspended in 1906 and reorganized in 1907. Extinct by 1915.
153	Eclectic Medical University	1907–1908	Kansas City, Kan.	Eclectic.
154	Hospital Medical College	1908–1911	Atlanta	Eclectic. Organized in 1908. Merged with Georgia College of Eclectic Medicine and Surgery in 1912.
155	New York Homeopathic Medical College and Flower Hospital	1909–1936	New York City	Homeopathic. Formerly New York Homeopathic Medical College and Hospital. Renamed New York Medical College and Flower Hospital in 1936.

	Name of School	Years	Location	Comments
156	Cleveland-Pulte Medical College	1910–1914	Cleveland	Homeopathic. Formerly Cleveland Homeopathic Medical College. In 1910 absorbed Pulte Medical College. Property transferred to Ohio State University in 1914 to form Ohio State University College of Homeopathic Medicine.
157	Eclectic Medical College	1910–1938	Cincinnati	Eclectic. Formerly the Eclectic Medical Institute. Coeducational since 1871. School dissolved in 1939 and charter surrendered in 1942. Last class graduated in 1939. Official organ was the *Eclectic Medical Journal.* The first and the last eclectic medical school in the United States.
158	Maryland College of Eclectic Medicine	1912–1915	Baltimore	Eclectic. Organized in 1912 as the Eclectic School of Medicine of Milton University but in 1913 took the title of Eastern University School of Medicine. Changed to Maryland College of Eclectic Medicine in 1914. Its dean was reported as not licensed in Maryland. College not recognized by the Maryland State Board of Medical Examiners and corporation dissolved in 1915. Several diplomas reported sold in subsequent years.
159	Ohio State University College of Homeopathic Medicine	1914–1922	Columbus	Homeopathic. Organized with the property of the Cleveland-Pulte Medical College of Cleveland was transferred to the Ohio State University. Classes graduated from 1915 to 1922. College abolished in 1922 by Board of Trustees.
160	Kansas City College of Medicine and Surgery	1915	Kansas City	Eclectic. An offshoot of the Eclectic Medical University. First class graduated in 1916. Charter revoked 1926 under the name of American Medical University. Closed about 1940.
161	Southwest School of Medicine and Hospital	1915–1916	Kansas City	Homeopathic. Formerly Kansas City Hahnemann Medical College. Held one session. Extinct in 1916.

[Data obtained from *Polk's Medical Register and Directory of North America* (10th ed.; Detroit: R. L. Polk and Co., 1908); "Medical Schools of the United States," *Journal of the American Medical Association,* LI (1908), 594–603; and Virginia Dwyer (ed.), *American Medical Directory* (20th ed.; Chicago: AMA, 1958); Thomas Lindsley Bradford, *Homeopathic Bibliography of the United States* (Philadelphia: Boericke and Tafel, 1892), 466–82).]

APPENDIX C

Reform Medical Societies to 1900
(Botanic, Thomsonian, Physio-Medical, Homeopathic, and Eclectic)[1]

	Name	Year	Place	Comments
1	Friendly Botanic Societies	1811–1838	New England, South, and Middle West	These societies were established in towns across the nation by Samuel Thomson and continued until the schism in 1838. The earliest were organized at Eastport, Kittery, Portland, and York in Maine; Bridgewater, Georgia, Jericho, and Woodstock in Vermont; Alstead, Deerfield, Eastham, Exeter, Pelham, Portsmouth, Richmond, Salisbury, Surry, and Walpole in New Hampshire; and Beverly, Boston, Charlestown, Eastham, Newburyport, Petersham, Royalston, Salem, Salisbury, South Reading, and Warwick in Massachusetts. The societies were autonomous with rules and regulations that appeared in several versions. In 1832 Thomson reorganized and made them branch organizations of a single United States Thomsonian Friendly Botanic Society. By 1838 Thomson had appointed one to four agents in 91 towns in Massachusetts (43); Rhode Island (2); Vermont (6); New Hampshire (17); Maine (18); and Connecticut (5). Each of these towns had at least one branch of the United States Thomsonian Friendly Botanic Society. Outside of New England there were additional branch societies: New York (6); Pennsylvania (3); Indiana (8); Kentucky (1); Virginia (2); Tennessee (2); Ohio (2); North Carolina (1); South Carolina (1); Arkansas (1); Alabama (2); Georgia (2); Maryland (1); and Illinois (3).
2	Reformed Medical Society of the State of New York	1828	New York	Organized on January 23, 1828, in Rochester and continued until 1863 when it merged with the Eclectic Medical Society of the State of New York.

[1] Please note that while the numbers of Thomsonian, Eclectic, and Homeopathic societies identified in the appendix are reasonably accurate, it has been difficult to identify Botanic, Reform, and Physio-Medical organizations due to incomplete or missing data sources.

	Name	Year	Place	Comments
3	New York Association of Botanic Physicians	1828	New York	Organized in 1828 by Dr. Elisha Smith of New York City, the association looked regionally for its membership. It disbanded after Smith's death in 1831. Smith authored *The Botanic Physician: Being a Compendium of the Practice of Physic, Upon Botanical Principles* (1830), which represented an early synthesis of botanic practice.
4	Reform Medical Society of the United States	1829	New York	Formed by Wooster Beach (1794–1868) and his friends at the Reformed Medical College of the City of New York, it looked nationally for its membership. Represented the first national organization of physicians in the United States. The organization supported Beach's unchartered Reformed Medical College of the City of New York. Never really developed as anticipated, particularly with the dissolution of the college in 1838. The society's early membership included Beach and Washington Starrett of New York; John J. Steele and Thompson Richardson of Pennsylvania; Thomas Vaughan Morrow of Kentucky; Amzi Sanborn of Maine; and S. A. Stanley of Connecticut. Beach served as president of the association, Steele as vice president, and Starrett as secretary. Other members of the society included J. F. Daniel Lobstein, George W. Cheevers, John C. Kelly, A. Upham, James J. Vere, and Calvin Preston.
5	United States Thomsonian Friendly Botanic Society	1832	Massachusetts	Samuel Thomson replaced the earlier Friendly Botanic Societies with this centralized organization. Individual societies were now branch organizations of the parent society. Met annually as the United States Thomsonian Botanic Convention first in Columbus, Ohio, and later in Pittsburgh, Baltimore, Richmond, Nashville, Louisville, and Philadelphia. Represented the second national organization of a medical group in the United States. Lasted until 1838 when society was split by schism. Replaced by the Independent Thomsonian Botanic Medical Society of the United States (Independent Thomsonians) and the United States Thomsonian Society (Strict Thomsonians).
6	Genesee Union Botanical Society	1832	New York	Organized in Genesee, New York.
7	Reform Medical Society	1832	New York	Organized in Conesus, New York.
8	Reformed Medical Association of Western New York	1832	New York	Formed at Dansville in Livingston County.

	Name	Year	Place	Comments
9	Hahnemann Society	1833	Pennsylvania	Formed in Philadelphia, it was the earliest organization of homeopathy in Pennsylvania and the United States, and dates its history to April 10, 1833, when Drs. Ihm, Bute, Matlack, Hering and Wesselhoeft, with a few laymen, associated themselves for the purpose of disseminating knowledge of the history and doctrines of homeopathy and its advantages over other methods of medical treatment.
10	New York Homeopathic Medical Society	1834	New York	The society was organized September 23, 1834. Officers for 1834–85: President, John F. Gray; vice presidents, Edward A. Strong, George Baxter; corresponding secretary, Federal Vanderburgh; recording secretary, Daniel Seymour; treasurer, F. A. Lohse; registrar, A. Gerald Hull; librarian, F. L. Wilsey; finance committee, J. H. Patterson, Oliver S. Strong, L. M. H. Butler, William Bock. This society was composed of physicians and laymen. William Cullen Bryant (1794–1878), the famous journalist, served as an officer in the society.
11	Homeopathic Society of Northampton and Counties Adjacent	1834	Pennsylvania	Organized August 23, 1834, the society was formed by Drs. Wesselhoeft, Freytag, Romig, King, and Rev. Christian J. Becker, D. D. The object of the association was the advancement of homeopathy among its members and spread of the Law of Similia.
12	New York State Thomsonian Medical Society	1835	New York	Members included A. N. Burton, Thomas Lapham, Oliver Cook, and Abial Gardner. Opposed the Test Resolution (loyalty test) pushed by the friends and supporters of Samuel Thomson in 1838.
13	Medical Society of Botanic Physicians and Surgeons of the City of New York	1835	New York	Members including Isaac S. Smith, Abel Hanks, and Ives S. Barber. This society opened a college that continued until 1846.
14	Chester County Branch of the United States Thomsonian Friendly Botanic Society	1838	Massachusetts	Organized August 1838.
15	United States Thomsonian Society	1838	Massachusetts	Following the 1838 schism of the United States Thomsonian Friendly Society which met in Philadelphia, Samuel Thomson and his followers created their own separate society. Members were known as strict or "Old Light" Thomsonians. Adopted constitution on October 20, 1838. Met subsequently in New York City and in Wilmington, Delaware, before becoming extinct.

	Name	Year	Place	Comments
16	Independent Thomsonian Botanic Medical Society of the United States	1838	Ohio	In 1838 Alva Curtis split from Samuel Thomson and created his own Independent Thomsonian Botanic Medical Society whose constitution was adopted October 17, 1838, in Philadelphia. Like Thomson, Curtis rejected the heroic bleeding and purging therapeutics of the allopaths. Unlike Thomson, however, Curtis's followers began establishing colleges to train and credential sectarian practitioners, called physio-medical or physio-pathic practitioners. In 1841 the society separated into two districts: a northern district to include Maine, New Hampshire, Vermont, Massachusetts, Rhode Island, Connecticut, New York, New Jersey, Pennsylvania, Delaware, Maryland, Michigan, Upper and Lower Canada, Novia Scotia, and New Brunswick; and a southern district consisting of Virginia, Ohio, Indiana, Illinois, Kentucky, Tennessee, North and South Carolina, Georgia, Alabama, Louisiana, Mississippi, Missouri, all the Northwest Territory, Texas, and the Spanish provinces.
17	Homeopathic Medical Society of Philadelphia	1838	Pennsylvania	Succeeded the Hahnemann Society. Unlike its predecessor, laymen were excluded from membership. This was the first regularly constituted homeopathic society in the city of Philadelphia.
18	Homœopathic Fraternity of Massachusetts	1839	Massachusetts	During the ten years of its existence the members included Samuel Gregg, Josiah F. Flagg, John P. Spooner, Charles Wild, William W. Cutler, Luther Clark, Christopher Minot Weld, and Francis Clark, 1841; William Wesselhoeft, William Ingalls, Milton Fuller, Daniel Swan, George Russell, Robert Capen and William Gallup, 1842; John A. Tarbell, 1843; James M. Cummings, Schlegel, Eben Hale, 1844; Jehiel Abbott, George Baker, Daniel Holt, 1845; David Osgood, Isaac Colby, Hiram Luce Chase and Horace Dwight Train, 1846; Rufus Shackford, David Thayer and Christian F. Geist, 1847; J. L. Martin, Samuel W. Graves and George Barrows, 1848; James C. Neilson, 1850.
19	Dutchess Botanic Society	1839	New York	Worked with the New York State Thomsonian Medical Society and Friendly Botanic Society of the City of New York to establish college. Unsuccessful until 1852 when Metropolitan Medical College was established in New York City.
20	Friends of the Thomsonian System of Medical Practice	1840	Massachusetts	Organized to examine the claims of Thomson to the exclusive right to preparing, compounding, and vending his medicines.
21	Eclectic Medical Association of Pennsylvania	1840	Pennsylvania	No information available.
22	Botanic Medical Society of Connecticut	1841	Connecticut	No information available.

	Name	Year	Place	Comments
23	Milford Botanic Association	1841	Massachusetts	Organized in February, 1841.
24	New York Homeopathic Physicians' Society	1841	New York	Organized in the city and admitted only medical practitioners. Its life was short and it passed out of existence in the course of six or seven years. Responsible for calling a national convention of homeopathic physicians in 1844 to set standards for homeopathic physicians and provide information on the materia medica.
25	New England Thomsonian Society	1842	Massachusetts	Formed by delegates from Maine, New Hampshire, Vermont, Massachusetts, Connecticut and Rhode Island who drafted a constitution.
26	Tippecanoe County Botanic Medical Society	1844	Indiana	No information available.
27	Friendly Botanic Medical Society of Indiana	1844	Indiana	Organized January 15, 1844.
28	Western Reserve Botanico-Medical Reform Society	1844	Ohio	Organized on September 21, 1844, in Lake County, Ohio. Accepted as member any person having competent knowledge of the principles and practice of medicine as taught in the Botanico-Medical Colleges of Cincinnati and Georgia.
29	Thomsonian Botanico-Medical Society	1844	Ohio	Organized in February, 1844, in Summit County, Ohio. Elected I. P. Carpenter, president; William Lyon, vice president. Persuant to convention held in Akron, Ohio.
30	American Institute of Homeopathy	1844	Pennsylvania	Established April 10, 1844, the year after the death of homeopathy's German-born founder, Dr. C. F. Samuel Hahnemann. Became the third oldest national medical organization in the United States. The AIH held its first meeting at the Lyceum of Natural History in April 1844 and drew its charter members from Illinois, Indiana, Kentucky, Massachusetts, Michigan, New York, Ohio, Pennsylvania, and Rhode Island.

	Name	Year	Place	Comments
31	Homeopathic Medical Society of Western New York	1845	New York	The society was organized at Waterloo, in Seneca County, in 1845. The first officers were C. D. Williams of Geneva, president; H. H. Cator of Syracuse, vice president; A. Childs of Waterloo, secretary. The society published its proceedings in 1852 when it occupied a position of prominence in homeopathic medical circles in Western New York and enjoyed the honor of having taken the first steps toward the establishment of a homeopathic medical college in New York State. The undertaking failed and the society became inactive after a few years, but was revived at a meeting held in Buffalo, February 28, 1852, when it took the name of Homeopathic Association of Western New York and Branch of the American Institute of Homeopathy.
32	Pittsburgh Eclectic Medical Society	1845	Pennsylvania	Introduced by Doctors Oldshue and Henry Yeagley
33	Susquehanna Eclectic Medical Society	1845	Pennsylvania	Introduced by Dr. A. B. Woodward.
34	Uxbridge Thomsonian Botanic Society	1846	Massachusetts	Dedicated to the cause of Thomsonism and urged the establishment of Wooster Medical School which graduated its first class in 1846. School renamed Wooster Medical Institution in 1849. School eventually became eclectic.
35	New Jersey Branch of the American Institute of Homeopathy	1846	New Jersey	Dr. J. Richardson Andrews was chairman; M. J. Rhees, secretary; Drs. John A. Paine and J. C. Boardman, censors. The constitution and bylaws were published and promulgated in 1846, and the society was in existence in 1850, but became inactive and not recognized as a legally organized body.
36	Society of Homeopathic Physicians (Cleveland)	1846	Ohio	Reports of the organization are found in the *American Journal of Homeopathy*, Vol. I, p. 46, and also in the *Michigan Journal of Homeopathy* for June, 1849. The society was continued only a short time, and then dissolved.
37	Philadelphia Branch of the American Institute of Homeopathy	1846	Pennsylvania	Organized June 6, 1846
38	Michigan Institute of Homeopathy	1847	Michigan	An offshoot and branch of the American Institute of Homeopathy. Formed October 20, 1847, by eight physicians. Its first officers were Dr. C. A. Lamb of Pontiac, president; Dr. Thomas Blanchard of Ann Arbor, vice president; Dr. P. M. Wheaton of Detroit, secretary; Dr. John Ellis of Detroit, treasurer. Passed out of existence in 1855 and was succeeded in 1866 by another society of the same name, the history of which dates from October 3, 1866, to May 16, 1871, when it was merged with the newly organized Homeopathic Medical Society of the State of Michigan.

	Name	Year	Place	Comments
39	Rhode Island Homeopathic Society	1847	Rhode Island	Organized and incorporated in 1847, and for a short time held quarterly meetings. On May 1, 1850, Drs. A. H. Okie and H. C. Preston issued a circular to all homeopathic physicians in the state inviting them to meet in Providence for the purpose of forming a new state homeopathic society. In response to this request a meeting was held in that city May 11, 1850, with eleven physicians present.
40	New Hampshire Botanic Medical Society	1848	New Hampshire	Charter obtained by Oran P. Warren, M.D..
41	County Botanic Medical Society	1848	New Jersey	Founded by Alexander Wilder (1823–1908) in opposition to regular medicine. Although friendly to Thomsonism, Wilder ultimately turned to eclecticism.
42	American Eclectic Medical Association	1848	Ohio	Hearing of the formation of the new American Medical Association, practitioners representing the different elements of Reformed medical practice met at the Eclectic Medical Institute in Cincinnati on May 25, 1848, to take up the issue of organizing a national association. Forty-three individuals attended the convention, representing Illinois, Indiana, Iowa, Kentucky, Missouri, New York, Ohio, and Pennsylvania. Original members included T. V. Morrow, Wooster Beach, Joseph R. Buchanan, Lorenzo E. Jones, Ichabod Gibson Jones, John King, Orin Davis, Thomas Cooke, Benjamin L. Hill, and John H. Jordan. The association elected Morrow as president, and doctors John King and L. E. Jones as secretaries. The association, which also included Alva Curtis's Independent Thomsonians, urged the formation of state and local societies and the compilation of statistics to document the successes of Reformed medical practice. Changed name the following year to National Eclectic Medical Association.
43	Wisconsin Institute of Homeopathy	1848	Wisconsin	Branch of the American Institute of Homeopathy. Organized in Milwaukee and continued a few years. On June 16, 1858, the homeopathic profession in the state held a meeting in Milwaukee and organized the Homeopathic Medical Association of the State of Wisconsin, a larger and stronger body than its predecessor though the period of its existence was comparatively brief.
44	Kentucky State Homeopathic Society	1849	Kentucky	Little is now known of this society except that it was among the earliest institutions of its kind in the upper South. The Kentucky State Homeopathic Medical Society was its successor and organized in Louisville, May 7, 1873.
45	New York Eclectic Medical Society	1849	New York	Formed at the office of Dr. Hermes M. Sweet in New York City.

	Name	Year	Place	Comments
46	American Medical Association	1849	New York	Organized on the western side of New York City. Included Dr. Elijah Whitney, Dr. Van Doren, Dr. Atkinson, and Dr. Wooster Beach.
47	Central New York Homeopathic Medical Society	1849	New York	A branch of the American Institute of Homeopathy. Organized at Utica in June, 1849, and was a means of union of the homeopathic physicians in the vicinity and also the cause of rapid growth of the system. Called the "Syracuse and Utica Convention of Homeopathic Physicians." The first informal meeting was held in Utica, September 13, 1849.
48	Eclectic Medical Society of Brooklyn	1849	New York	Formed by Doctors Dennis E. Smith, P. S. Lapham, Grover Coe, and others. In 1861 it took the name of the Brooklyn Academy of Medicine.
49	National Eclectic Medical Association	1849	Ohio	Founded with the aim of researching and promoting the use of herbal medicines. Officially sanctioned coeducation as early as 1852. However, its annual meetings were discontinued after the eighth convention held in June 1857 at Cincinnati. So few attended the meeting that there was not even a notification canceling the 1858 meeting. Revived again in 1870. By 1900, it had thirty-two societies and associations in several states, with local and district organizations in twelve states, and seven medical colleges that were represented in the organization.
50	Homeopathic Society of Cincinnati	1849	Ohio	The society was composed largely of laymen and its purpose was to vindicate homeopathy and to uphold the truth regarding the cholera epidemic; to petition the assembly of 1849 for an act establishing a homeopathic college; to promulgate the lectures by Storm Rosa in 1849; to organize a college at Cleveland in 1850; and to promote the advancement of the system throughout the towns of the state.
51	Eclectic Medical Society of Cincinnati	1849	Ohio	No information available.
52	Hahnemann Medical Institute	1849	Pennsylvania	Student organization in Philadelphia.
53	Homeopathic Medical Society of Alabama	1850	Alabama	In 1850 Drs. Lingen of Mobile, Angell of Huntsville, and Ulrich, Henry, and Albright of Montgomery formed the society. It was predecessor to the Homeopathic Medical Association of Alabama (1889), although a number of years passed after the dissolution of the old society before the new one came into existence.
54	Massachusetts Physo-Medical Society	1850	Massachusetts	No information available.

	Name	Year	Place	Comments
55	Schuyler County Homeopathic Medical Society	1850	New York	No information available.
56	Academy of Medicine of the State of New York	1850	New York	See Homeopathic Medical Society of the State of New York
57	Homeopathic Medical Society of the State of New York	1850	New York	The first gathering of physicians for the purpose of forming a homeopathic medical society in New York state was held at the common council room in city hall in Albany, May 15, 1850. The organization was called Academy of Medicine of the State of New York. At the first annual meeting held in Albany, February 19, 1851, the name was changed to Homeopathic Medical Society of the State of New York. It was composed of individual members and was not a representative body. The meeting was called to order by Dr. John F. Gray of New York City. Dr. D. Chase of Palmyra was chosen president, and Dr. H. D. Paine of Albany, secretary. The society held annual meetings at different places.
58	Connecticut Institute of Homeopathy	1851	Connecticut	The first society of homeopathic physicians in Connecticut was formed in Hartford, November 17, 1851. At this meeting seven were in attendance: Drs. Jeremiah T. Dennison, of Fairfield; W. W. Rodman, of Waterbury; W. C. Bell, of Middletown; C. H. Skiff and E. T. Foote, of New Haven; and C. A. Taft and George S. Greene, of Hartford. At a meeting held June 10, 1864, a reorganization was effected, and the society was incorporated under the name of Connecticut Homeopathic Medical Society.
59	Western Institute of Homeopathy	1851	Illinois	Organized in the office of Drs. Skinner and Hoyne, Chicago, June 3, 1851. At a meeting held June 4, at Warner's Hall, the following officers were elected: Dr. L. M. Tracy of Milwaukee, president; Drs. T. G. Comstock of St. Louis, D. S. Smith of Chicago, Lewis Dodge of Cleveland and A. Giles of Southport, Wisconsin, vice presidents (one for each western state represented); Dr. George E. Shipman of Chicago, secretary. The institute was not incorporated, and met annually in May. It admitted students of homeopathy as junior members. Continued but a short time.
60	Indiana Physio-Medical Association	1851	Indiana	No information available.
61	New Hampshire Homeopathic Medical Society	1851	New Hampshire	Organized at a meeting of homeopathic physicians held in Concord, June 3, 1851. On January 8, 1853, it was incorporated under the laws of the state.

	Name	Year	Place	Comments
62	Ohio College of Homeopathic Physicians	1851	Ohio	Organized in Columbus on September 23, 1851. The first officers were Drs. O. A. Blair, president ; J. H. Coulter of Columbus and John Tifft of Norwalk, vice presidents; C. A. Leuthstrom of Columbus, secretary; G. St. C. Hussey of Portsmouth, corresponding secretary; C. D. Williams of Cleveland, H. P. Gatchell of Cincinnati, J. W. Dennis of Portsmouth, Jacob Bosler of Dayton and L. K. Rosa, censors. In 1852 and 1853 meetings were held in Cleveland, the next year in Columbus, but none were afterward held until 1864 when the homeopathic physicians of the state met in convention in Columbus, revived the dormant organization, and brought into existence the Homeopathic Medical Society of the State of Ohio.
63	Eclectic Medical Society of Philadelphia	1851	Pennsylvania	No information available.
64	Southern Reform Medical Association	1851	Tennessee	Member states included Alabama, Arkansas, Kentucky, Mississippi, Tennessee, and Virginia. Continued to meet until the outbreak of the Civil War. After the war, the surviving elements of Reform medicine and their respective colleges coalesced around the "eclectics" and became known as the American Reform School of Medical Practice in the South.
65	Caledonia County Homeopathic Medical Society	1851	Vermont	Organized chiefly through the efforts of Dr. Beniah Sanborn.
66	Connecticut Physo-Medical Society	1852	Connecticut	No information available.
67	Baltimore Convention	1852	Maryland	Meeting organized by Alva Curtis and the reform wing of the Thomsonians. Included delegates from Connecticut, Delaware, Georgia, Maryland, Massachusetts, New York, Ohio, Pennsylvania, South Carolina, and Virginia. Organized the Reformed Medical Association of the United States with Curtis as President.
68	Washington and Warren County Homeopathic Medical Society	1852	New York	Organized October 16, 1852
69	Orange County Homeopathic Medical Society	1852	New York	Organized February 28, 1852
70	Eclectic Medical Society of the State of New York	1852	New York	No information available.

	Name	Year	Place	Comments
71	Homeopathic Medical Society of Northern New York	1852	New York	Organized at Fort Ann on October 16, 1852. Seven homeopathic physicians residing in Washington and Saratoga counties had formed an association called the Homeopathic Medical Society of the Counties of Washington and Saratoga, of which the society here considered is the outgrowth. To this society belongs the honor of originating the movement to secure legal rights for the homeopathic societies in New York.
72	Homeopathic Medical Society of the Counties of Washington and Saratoga	1852	New York	Originally organized October 16, 1852. Later became Homeopathic medical Society of Northern New York.
73	Homeopathic Association of Western New York	1852	New York	Formerly known as the Homeopathic Medical Society of Western New York. Organized in Buffalo February 28, 1852. Became branch of the American Institute of Homeopathy.
74	Hahnemann Academy of Medicine	1852	New York	No information available.
75	Reformed Medical Association of the United States	1852	Ohio	Organized by Alva Curtis and the reform wing of the Thomsonians as a result of the Baltimore Convention of 1852. Initiated the Baltimore Platform hoping to resolve philosophical and sectional differences left after the 1838 schism. Convention elected Alva Curtis as President.
76	Philadelphia County Homeopathic Medical Society	1852	Pennsylvania	Organized April 13, 1859.
77	Missouri Institute of Homeopathy	1853	Missouri	In June, 1853, this state medical society was formed with Dr. Thomas Houghton president and Dr. T. G. Comstock secretary. The society dissolved in the course of a few years. Reorganized under same name in 1876.
78	Homeopathic Medical Academy of the State of New York	1853	New York	The Homeopathic Medical Academy of the State of New York, included physicians from Yates, Ontario, Steuben, and neighboring counties. It was organized at Penn Yan, January 1, 1853, under the law of 1848. First officers: President, Geo. W. Malin, Jerusalem; vice president, Richard Huson, Dundee, secretary, Samuel K. Huson, Dundee; treasurer, O. W. Noble, Penn Yan. The academy met quarterly in April, July, and October at different places. The annual meeting was held in January.
79	Eclectic Medical Society of the State of Ohio	1853	Ohio	No information available.
80	American Provers' Union	1853	Pennsylvania	Organized in Philadelphia on August 15, 1853.

	Name	Year	Place	Comments
81	Middle States Reformed Medical Society	1853	Pennsylvania	Met in Philadelphia on May 18, 1854. Membership came from New Jersey, Pennsylvania, Delaware, Virginia, and Maryland. Established platform of principles. Officers included Palemon John, John Prettyman, William Williams, William Fields, and William Armstrong.
82	Convention of Physio-Medical Reformers for Kentucky and Tennessee	1854	Kentucky	Met third Monday in May, 1854, in Cadiz, Kentucky.
83	Convention of Physio-Medical Reformers of Mississippi, Alabama, Louisiana, and Arkansas	1854	Mississippi	Met May 1, 1854, in Yazoo City, Mississippi.
84	Hahnemann Medical Society of Rhode Island	1854	Rhode Island	Succeeded the Rhode Island Homeopathic Society. Organized in Providence, October 21, 1854, with these officers: Dr. A. Howard Okie, president; Dr. G. C. McKnight, vice president; Dr. N. Francis Cooke, secretary and treasurer; Drs. J. J. DeWolf and Washington Hoppin, censors. The society began its history with seventeen members, but was discontinued about 1862.
85	Green Mountain Homeopathic Medical Association	1854	Vermont	In 1858 changed its name to the Vermont State Homeopathic Medical Society.
86	Eclectic Medical Society of Connecticut	1855	Connecticut	Incorporated by act of the legislature in 1855. Holds semiannual meetings in New Haven.
87	Illinois State Homeopathic Medical Society	1855	Illinois	One of the oldest and strongest organizations of homeopathic practitioners in the West. Organized in Peoria on December 6, 1855, and was incorporated October 24, 1881. Meetings were held annually in May and generally in Chicago, and semiannually in November, in the same city.
88	Northern Illinois Homeopathic Medical Association	1855	Illinois	Organized at a convention of physicians held at Haskill Hall in Peoria on December 6, 1855. First annual meeting held in Elgin, January 1, 1856.

	Name	Year	Place	Comments
89	New Jersey State Homeopathic Medical Society	1855	New Jersey	Organized at a meeting held in Trenton, February 13, 1855. Its officers included: Dr. Thomas Lafon of Newark, president; Drs. William A. Durrie of Jersey City, J. R. Andrews of Camden and J. C. Boardman of Trenton, vice presidents; Dr. J. B. Petherbridge of Trenton, recording secretary; Dr. J. J. Youlin of Jersey City, provisional secretary; Dr. J. B. Scott of New Brunswick, corresponding secretary; Dr. P. E. Vastine of Trenton, treasurer; Drs. J. D. Annin, J. D. Moore, R. M. Wilkinson, J. S. Bassett and R. Titsworth, censors. The society continued to hold meetings until 1858, after which there is no record. On February 4, 1868, a reorganization meeting was held in Jersey City, and on April 15, the old society was revived, with Dr. Youlin president and Dr. Thompkins secretary. The society was incorporated on February 9, 1870.
90	Hahnemann Society of Cincinnati	1855	Ohio	Organized April 10, 1855.
91	Massachusetts Homeopathic Medical Society	1856	Massachusetts	The society held several informal meetings to settle upon a plan of permanent organization, and on September 24, 1856, elected its first officers: Dr. Samuel Gregg of Boston, president; Dr. Charles Weld of Brookline and Dr. William Wesselhoeft of Boston, vice presidents; Dr. G. W. Swazey of Springfield, corresponding secretary; Dr. David Thayer of Boston, recording secretary; Dr. William F. Jackson of Roxbury, treasurer; Dr. George Russell of Boston, librarian, Drs. C. M. Weld, of Jamaica Plain, and B. H. West, Luther Clark, Milton Fuller and L. M. Barker, of Boston, censors.
92	Union Eclectic Medical Society	1856	Ohio	Organized October 18, 1856. Meets at Amelia in Clermont County in April and October of each year.
93	Chicago Homeopathic Medical Society	1857	Illinois	Organized April 2, 1857, but was not incorporated. Continued in existence only a few years.
94	New York County Homeopathic Medical Society	1857	New York	Organized August 13, 1857.
95	Oneida County Homeopathic Medical Society	1857	New York	Organized October 20, 1857.
96	Livingston County Homeopathic Medical Society	1857	New York	Organized December 1, 1857.
97	Kings County Homeopathic Medical Society	1857	New York	Organized November 12, 1857.

	Name	Year	Place	Comments
98	Homeopathic Medical Society of Northern New York	1857	New York	In 1855 an act passed the senate to authorize the incorporation of homeopathic societies, but the bill remained in the lower house and failed to pass. In the next year, however, the act was revived, passed both branches of the legislature, and was approved by the governor, April 13, 1857. This resulted in the creation of several societies in the state, including this society.
99	Homeopathic Medical Society of Chester and Delaware Counties	1858	Delaware	The society was organized in October, 1858, by the meeting of Drs. Duffield, of New London; Hawley, of Phoenixville; Hindman, of Cochranville; Johnson, of Kennett Square; Wood and Jones, of West Chester. It held four meetings annually, which are held in January, April, July, and October. Dr. Duffield was its first president. Its membership numbered thirty-four.
100	Société Hahnemannienne De La Nouvelle Orleans	1858	Louisiana	Organized sometime between 1858 and 1860. It published a monthly paper called *L'Homoion*, which, like the society itself, was soon discontinued.
101	Boston Academy of Homeopathic Medicine	1858	Massachusetts	Organized November 30, 1858. Consolidated in May, 1873, with Boston Homeopathic Society and taking the latter's name.
102	New York County Homeopathic Medical Society	1858	New York	No information available.
103	New York State Association of Reformed Physicians	1858	New York	Formally known as the Botanic Medical Society of the State of New York.
104	Hahnemann Academy of Science	1858	New York	No information available.
105	Chester County Homeopathic Medical Society	1858	Pennsylvania	Organized September 5, 1858.
106	Vermont State Homeopathic Medical Society	1858	Vermont	Formerly known as the Green Mountain Homeopathic Medical Association. The first officers of the society were Dr. Thomas Bigelow of Burlington, president; Dr. C. B. Currier of South Troy, corresponding secretary; Dr. G. E. Sparhawk of Rochester, recording secretary; Dr. T. C. Taplin of Montpelier, treasurer; Dr. C. W. Scott of Irasburg, auditor.
107	Homeopathic Medical Association of State of Wisconsin	1858	Wisconsin	Organized June 16, 1858, when the homeopathic profession in the state held a meeting in Milwaukee. It was a larger and stronger body than its predecessor (Wisconsin Institute of Homeopathy) though the period of its existence was comparatively brief.
108	Rensselaer County Homeopathic Medical Society	1859	New York	Organized June 9, 1859.

	Name	Year	Place	Comments
109	Erie County Homeopathic Medical Society	1859	New York	Organized December 14, 1859.
110	Boston Eclectic Gynecological and Obstetrical Society	186?	Massachusetts	No information available.
111	Otsego County Homeopathic Medical Society	1860	New York	Organized June 20, 1860.
112	Cayuga County Homeopathic Medical Society	1860	New York	Organized February 16, 1860.
113	Albany County Homeopathic Medical Society	1860	New York	Organized January, 1860.
114	Lucas County Homeopathic Medical Society	1860	Ohio	No information available.
115	Miami Valley Homeopathic Medical Society	1860	Ohio	Organized June 14, 1860.
116	Eclectic Medical Society of the State of Massachusetts	1861	Massachusetts	Incorporated by act of the legislature on March 1, 1861. Annual meetings were held in Boston. Had three auxiliary societies: the Boston District Eclectic Medical Society; the Boston Eclectic Gynacological and Obstetrical Society; and the Worcester North Eclectic Medical Society.
117	Brooklyn Academy of Medicine	1861	New York	Organized March 26, 1861 under the name of the Brooklyn Academy of Medicine. Incorporated by act of the legislature on April 24, 1865. Reorganized September 4, 1867 under the name of the Brooklyn Academy of Eclectic Medicine.
118	Homeopathic Medical Society of Oneida County	1861	New York	Meeting was held at Albany, February 28, 1861. An act of incorporation was procured April 17, 1862, and at a meeting held in Albany, May 6, 1862, it was decided to proceed as if the society had not before existed. At this meeting the following officers were elected: President, Jacob Beakley. New York; vice presidents, A. R. Wright, Buffalo, E. A. Munger, Waterville, W. S. Searle, Troy; secretary, H. M. Paine, Clinton; treasurer, L. B. Wells, Utica. Met annually in February at Albany, and semiannually in various cities in September.
119	Chemung (including Steuben and Schuyler) County Homeopathic Medical Society	1861	New York	Organized February 5, 1861.

	Name	Year	Place	Comments
120	Columbia and Green County Homeopathic Medical Society	1861	New York	Organized October 1, 1861.
121	Dutchess County Homeopathic Medical Society	1861	New York	Organized November 27, 1861.
122	Oswego County Homeopathic Medical Society	1861	New York	Organized January 23, 1861.
123	Indiana State Physio-Medical Society	1862	Indiana	No information available.
124	Iowa Homeopathic Medical Association	1862	Iowa	Organized at a meeting of physicians held in Davenport, May 21, 1862, and while from the first the interest shown in its welfare was commendable, the disturbed conditions which then prevailed throughout the country on account of the civil war made the continuance of the society impracticable.
125	Boston District Eclectic Medical Society	1862	Massachusetts	Organized January 20, 1862. Met annually in January in Boston.
126	Onondaga County Homeopathic Medical Society	1862	New York	No information available.
127	Ontario and Yates County Homeopathic Medical Society	1862	New York	No information available.
128	Cincinnati Homeopathic Medical Society	1862	Ohio	No information available.
129	Ladies' Association of the Homeopathic Hospital of Philadelphia for Sick and Wounded Soldiers	1862	Pennsylvania	Organized October 15, 1883.
130	Broome County Homeopathic Medical Society	1863	New York	No information available.
131	Chautauqua and Cattaraugas County Homeopathic Medical Society	1863	New York	No information available.
132	Eclectic Medical Society of the State of New York	1863	New York	Organized October 13, 1863, and incorporated by act of the legislature on April 24, 1865. Meetings held annually in Albany. Had numerous auxiliary societies.
133	Saratoga County Homeopathic Medical Society	1863	New York	No information available.

	Name	Year	Place	Comments
134	Connecticut Homeopathic Medical Society	1864	Connecticut	Formerly the Connecticut Institute of Homeopathy. A reorganization was effected, and the society was incorporated under the name of Connecticut Homeopathic Medical Society. A new constitution was adopted in 1880.
135	Indiana Eclectic Medical Association	1864	Indiana	Organized at Indianapolis in 1864. Held annual meetings at Indianapolis. Reported 587 eclectic physicians in the state in 1884. A committee of the association met in 1890 to procure a charter for the Indiana College of Eclectic Physicians and Surgeons.
136	Wayne County Homeopathic Medical Society	1864	New York	Organized February 9, 1864.
137	Homœopathic Medical Society of the State of Ohio	1864	Ohio	The officers were as follows: Dr. A. O. Blair of Cleveland, president; Drs. E. C. Witherill of Cincinnati and W. W. Webster of Dayton, vice presidents; Dr. Charles Cropper of Cincinnati, secretary; Dr. C. C. White of Columbus, treasurer; Drs. A. Shepherd of Springdale, G. H. Blair of Columbus, Charles Osterlin of Findlay, T. P. Wolson of Cleveland, Lewis Barnes of Delaware, T. M. Miller of Stubenville and E. C. Beckwith of Zanesville, censors. At first the society met annually at Columbus, but later adopted the rule of meeting in different cities. The society was incorporated in 1878.
138	Northeastern Ohio Homeopathic Medical Society	1864	Ohio	No information available.
139	State Eclectic Medical Association of Ohio	1864	Ohio	Organized in 1864 with annual meetings. Had about 100 active members out of approximately 600 eclectic physicians in the state. Included four auxiliary societies: the Northwestern Ohio Eclectic Medical Association; the Central Ohio Eclectic Medical Association; the Miami Valley Eclectic Medical Association; the Clermont Eclectic Medical Association.
140	Maine Eclectic Medical Society	1865	Maine	Organized at Portland, June 28, 1865. Incorporated by act of the legislature on June 24, 1868.
141	Eclectic Medical Society of the Thirty-Second Senatorial District	1865	New York	Auxiliary to the Eclectic Medical Society of the State of New York. Established by act of the legislature on April 24, 1865.

	Name	Year	Place	Comments
142	Madison County Homeopathic Medical Society	1865	New York	Organized January 4, 1865.
143	Ulster County Homeopathic Medical Society	1865	New York	Organized May 10, 1865.
144	Westchester County Homeopathic Medical Society	1865	New York	Organized February 1, 1865.
145	Eclectic Medical Society of the State of New York	1865	New York	Incorporated by act of the legislature on April 22, 1865, after existing as a voluntary association for two years. Had fifteen auxiliary societies.
146	Eclectic Medical Society of the City of New York	1865	New York	Organized November 14, 1865 and incorporated by act of the legislature on April 24, 1865. Auxiliary of the New York State Eclectic Medical Society. Its meetings were held at the Eclectic Medical College, 223 E. 26th Street, on the third Wednesday of each month.
147	Eclectic Medical Society of the Twenty-Third Senatorial District	1865	New York	Auxiliary to the Eclectic Medical Society of the State of New York. Established by act of the legislature on April 24, 1865.
148	Eclectic Medical Society of the Thirteenth Senatorial District	1865	New York	Auxiliary to the Eclectic Medical Society of the State of New York. Established by act of the legislature on April 24, 1865.
149	Eclectic Medical Society of the Eighteenth Senatorial District	1865	New York	Auxiliary to the Eclectic Medical Society of the State of New York. Established by act of the legislature on April 24, 1865, and organized on January 11, 1866.
150	Eclectic Medical Society of the Twelfth Senatorial District	1865	New York	Auxiliary to the Eclectic Medical Society of the State of New York. Established by act of the legislature on April 24, 1865 and organized September 19, 1865.
151	Eclectic Medical Society of the Twenty-Ninth Senatorial District	1865	New York	Auxiliary to the Eclectic Medical Society of the State of New York. Established by act of the legislature on April 24, 1865.
152	Eclectic Medical Society of the Twenty-Sixth Senatorial District	1865	New York	Auxiliary to the Eclectic Medical Society of the State of New York. Established by act of the legislature on April 24, 1865, and organized September 12, 1865.

	Name	Year	Place	Comments
153	Eclectic Medical Association of the State of Ohio	1865	Ohio	Organized May 31, 1865.
154	Cleveland Medical Association	1865	Ohio	No information available.
155	Cuyahoga County Homeopathic Medical Society	1865	Ohio	Organized November, 1865.
156	Wisconsin State Homeopathic Medical Society	1865	Wisconsin	Dates its history from October 18, 1865. The first officers were Dr. T. J. Patchin of Fond du Lac, president; Dr. E. L. Ober of La Crosse, vice president; Dr. H. B. Dale of Oshkosh, secretary; Dr. P. Moore of Nenah, treasurer; Drs. Pierce of Green Bay, Page of Appleton and Swetting of Berlin, censors. The society was incorporated in 1868.
157	Washington Medical and Surgical Club	1866	District of Columbia	Never incorporated.
158	Cook County Homeopathic Medical Society	1866	Illinois	Organized in the Hahnemann Medical College building, May 11, 1866. It was not incorporated but maintained a healthful existence until 1873 when it merged into the Chicago Academy of Homeopathic Physicians and Surgeons.
159	Central Homeopathic Medical Association of Maine	1866	Maine	Meetings of which were held quarterly in different towns.
160	Bristol County Homeopathic Medical Society	1866	Massachusetts	Organized October 3, 1866.
161	Worcester County Homeopathic Medical Society	1866	Massachusetts	Organized June 27, 1866.
162	Michigan Homeopathic Institute	1866	Michigan	Its history dates from October 3, 1866, to May 16, 1871, when it was merged in the then newly organized Homeopathic Medical Society of the State of Michigan.
163	Central District Homeopathic Medical Society	1866	Michigan	Organized in Lansing.

	Name	Year	Place	Comments
164	Central New York Homeopathic Medical Society	1866	New York	Outgrowth of a convention of homeopathic physicians of the counties of Broome, Cayuga, Cortland, Jefferson, Madison, Ontario, Oneida, Onondaga, Oswego, Seneca and Wayne, held at Syracuse on May 1, 1866. Officers elected: President, Lyman Clary, Syracuse; vice president, E. A. Potter, Oswego; secretary, E. R. Heath, Palmyra. Had 40 members in 1903.
165	Monroe County Homeopathic Medical Society	1866	New York	Organized January 2, 1866.
166	Homeopathic Medical Society of the Seventeenth Congressional District	1866	Ohio	Organized August 1, 1866.
167	Homeopathic Medical Society of the State of Pennsylvania	1866	Pennsylvania	The society was organized at a convention of physicians held June 5, 1866, in the Homeopathic Hospital of Pittsburgh and in response to a call from the Allegheny County Homeopathic Medical Society. In 1903 the society numbered three hundred and fifty-eight members, which represented about one-half the strength of the profession in the state.
168	Cumberland Valley Homeopathic Medical Society	1866	Pennsylvania	Organized May 8, 1866.
169	Dauphin County Homeopathic Medical Society	1866	Pennsylvania	No information available.
170	Northwestern Pennsylvania Homeopathic Medical Society	1866	Pennsylvania	Organized July 5, 1866.
171	Eclectic Medical Society of the State of Vermont	1866	Vermont	Incorporated by act of the legislature on June 6, 1866. President was A. G. Brush of Fairfax.
172	Connecticut and Passumpsic Valley Homeopathic Medical Society	1866	Vermont	No information available.
173	Indiana Homeopathic Institute	1867	Indiana	On May 23, 1867, a number of homeopathic physicians met in the senate chamber in the state house in Indianapolis and organized the Indiana Homeopathic Institute, with officers as follows: Dr. O. P. Baer, president; G. T. Parker and P. M. Leonard, vice presidents; J. T. Boyd, recording secretary; N. G. Burnham, corresponding secretary; W. Eggert, J. T. Boyd, G. H. Stockham, A. J. Compton, M. H. Waters, censors. On May 11, 1870, the society was reorganized under the name of Indiana Institute of Homeopathy, which it still bears, and under which it was incorporated in 1882.

	Name	Year	Place	Comments
174	Iowa State Eclectic Medical Society	1867	Iowa	Incorporated in 1867 and held annual meetings at Des Moines. Helped to organize the Iowa Eclectic Medical College in 1881.
175	Eclectic Medical Society of the State of Maine	1867	Maine	Operating in 1867 with N. K. Martin of Westbrook as president.
176	Maine Homeopathic Medical Society	1867	Maine	Formed from the Central Homeopathic Medical Association of Maine which met at Augusta, January 15, 1867, and was incorporated May 23 following. Its first officers were Dr. William E. Payne of Bath, president; Drs. C. H. Burr of Portland and Hosea B. Eaton of Rockport, vice presidents; Dr. N. G. H. Pulsifer of Waterville, recording secretary; Dr. J. B. Bell of Augusta, corresponding secretary; Drs. Eliphalet Clark of Portland, George P. Jeffords of Bangor, Richmond Bradford of Auburn, Moses R. Pulsifer of Ellsworth and M. S. Briry of Bath, censors.
177	Worcester North Eclectic Medical Society	1867	Massachusetts	Operating in 1867 with A. W. Sidney as president.
178	Eclectic Medical Society of Michigan	1867	Michigan	Dissolved due to admission of "illiterate, worthless and objectionable members." Reconstituted in 1876 as the State Eclectic Medical and Surgical Society of Michigan.
179	Minnesota State Homeopathic Institute	1867	Minnesota	Organized February 13, 1867.
180	Missouri Homeopathic Institute	1867	Missouri	Was short lived. Reorganized in 1876 with same name. Became one of the strongest homeopathic organizations in the Southwest, having about 250 members.
181	Brooklyn Academy Eclectic Medicine	1867	New York	Formerly the Brooklyn Academy of Medicine, organized March 26, 1861. Reorganized under new name September 4, 1867.
182	Steuben County Homeopathic Medical Society	1867	New York	Organized May 25, 1867.
183	Muskingum Valley Homeopathic Medical Society	1867	Ohio	No information available.
184	Boenninghausen Club of Philadelphia	1867	Pennsylvania	Organized November, 1867.

	Name	Year	Place	Comments
185	Boston Homeopathic Society	1868	Massachusetts	Consolidated with the Boston Academy of Homeopathic Medicine in May, 1873.
186	Ingham, Shiawassee, Clinton and Eaton Counties Homeopathic Society	1868	Michigan	Organized June 18, 1868.
187	Wayne County Homeopathic Institute	1868	Michigan	No information available.
188	Eastern District Homeopathic Medical Society	1868	New Jersey	Organized February 6, 1868.
189	Loraine and Medina County Homeopathic Medical Society	1868	Ohio	Organized July 18, 1868.
190	Montgomery County Homeopathic Medical Society	1868	Ohio	Organized November 6, 1868.
191	Union Homeopathic Medical Society of Northern Ohio	1868	Ohio	Organized June 6, 1868.
192	Luzerne County Homeopathic Medical Society	1868	Pennsylvania	No information available.
193	Central Illinois Homeopathic Medical Association	1869	Illinois	Organized in Jacksonville, October 12, 1869, and comprised physicians representing the central counties of the state. On July 1, 1873, the society was reorganized under the name of Central Illinois Medical Society, and afterward held quarterly meetings in different places until 1882 when it merged in the state society.
194	Chicago Academy of Medicine	1869	Illinois	Originally formed April 10, 1869 and was a well managed institution. It continued until 1873 when it was merged with another society to form the Chicago Academy of Homeopathic Physicians and Surgeons.
195	Chicago Pedological Society	1869	Illinois	Organized at the Foundlings' Home in Chicago, October 14, 1869, and afterward held monthly meetings, generally at the residence of one of its members.

	Name	Year	Place	Comments
196	Illinois State Eclectic Medical Society	1869	Illinois	Organized at Springfield, May 26, 1869. Its annual meetings were held in Springfield, East St. Louis, Chicago, Lincoln, Bloomingdale, and Decatur.
197	Montgomery County, Illinois, Eclectic Medical Society	1869	Illinois	Organized in 1869 and held semiannual meetings.
198	Homeopathic Medical Society of Kansas	1869	Kansas	Organized in Leavenworth, April 14, 1869, and incorporated in 1871.
199	Central Michigan Homeopathic Medical Society	1869	Michigan	Organized in East Saginaw, July 13, 1869.
200	Western District New Jersey Homeopathic Medical Society	1869	New Jersey	Organized in Camden, May 19, 1869. Officers elected: Dr. D. R. Gardiner of Woodbury, president; Dr. R. M. Wilkinson of Trenton, vice president; Dr. Wallace McGeorge of Hightstown, secretary; Dr. J. G. Streets of Bridgton, treasurer; Drs. W. H. Maline, H. F. Hunt and Isaac Cooper, censors. Incorporated in May, 1872.
201	New Jersey Medical Club	1869	New Jersey	Organized March 29, 1969.
202	Montgomery (including Fulton) County Homeopathic Medical Society	1869	New York	Organized February 4, 1869.
203	Ohio Physio-Medical Association	1869	Ohio	No information available.
204	Berks and Schuylkill Counties Homeopathic Medical Society	1869	Pennsylvania	Organized November 9, 1869.
205	Kent County and Grand Valley Homeopathic Medical Society	187?	Michigan	Dissolved in 1879.
206	Newark, Union and Hudson Counties Homeopathic Medical Society	187?	New Jersey	No information available.
207	Washington Homeopathic Medical Society	1870	District of Columbia	Organized in the District of Columbia, May 20, 1870. Its first officers were Dr. Tullio S. Verdi, president; Dr. C. W. Sonnenschmidt, secretary; Dr. G. W. Pope, treasurer; and Drs. J. Brainerd, J. T. O'Connor and S. J. Grout, censors.

	Name	Year	Place	Comments
208	Military Tract Homeopathic Society	1870	Illinois	Organized by the homeopathic physicians of Knox and adjoining counties in Galesburg, on November 1, 1870. Its first officers were T. Bacmeister of Toulon, president; W. C. Anthony of Princeton, vice president; J. H. Miller of Abingdon, secretary; G. W. Brewington of Wataga, provisional secretary; T. J. Merryman of Aledo, treasurer. The society held semiannual meetings in different places until 1872, when it became stationary in Galesburg. It continued until 1885 when it passed out of existence.
209	National Convention of Eclectic Physicians	1870	Illinois	Assembled in Chicago in September, 1870, for the purpose of organizing an association "which shall comprise all physicians of the New School on the Western Continent." Organized by officers of several state eclectic medical societies and colleges acting by the direction and approval of their societies and institutions.
210	Indiana Institute of Homeopathy	1870	Indiana	Formerly the Indiana Homeopathic Institute. Reorganized on May 11, 1870 and incorporated in 1882.
211	Society of Homeopathic Physicians of Iowa	1870	Iowa	Organized in Des Moines, May 31, 1870.
212	Eclectic Medical Association of the State of Missouri	1870	Missouri	Organized at Chillicothe on May 11, 1870. Replaced by the Eclectic Medical Society of Missouri in 1877 which was incorporated under the influence of the American Medical College.
213	Tioga County Homeopathic Medical Society	1870	New York	Organized July 29, 1870.
214	Perry County Homeopathic Medical Society	1870	Ohio	Organized October 26, 1870.
215	Alumni Society of the Physio-Medical Institute	1870	Ohio	Organized in Cincinnati, Ohio, in 1870.

	Name	Year	Place	Comments
216	California State Medical Society of Homeopathic Practitioners	1871	California	Organized in San Francisco, March 24, 1871, and was incorporated April 10, 1872. Because of disagreements a reorganization was effected as the result of a conference, and on August 8, 1874, the Pacific Homeopathic Medical Society of the State of California was brought into existence.
217	Chicago Eclectic Medical and Surgical Society	1871	Illinois	Organized in 1871 and held monthly meetings.
218	Marion County Homeopathy Medical Society	1871	Indiana	Organized at Indianapolis on December 10, 1871, but was not incorporated. Its meetings were held semiannually until 1881, when the society passed out of existence.
219	Kansas Eclectic Medical Association	1871	Kansas	Organized on February 14, 1871, and incorporated by an act of the legislature on February 15, 1871. Its auxiliary society was the Eclectic Medical Society of Central Kansas.
220	Eclectic Medical Society of Central Kansas	1871	Kansas	Auxiliary society to the Kansas Eclectic Medical Association.
221	Homeopathic Medical Society of the State of Michigan	1871	Michigan	Founded at a meeting held in Jackson, November 10, 1869, and soon afterward was incorporated. It was re-incorporated February 18, 1900.
222	Southern Minnesota Homeopathic Medical Society	1871	Minnesota	Organized in October, 1871, but later was merged into the state society.
223	Hudson County Homeopathic Medical Society	1871	New Jersey	Organized March 8, 1871.
224	Newark Homeopathic Medical Union	1871	New Jersey	Lasted until 1885.
225	Chenango County Homeopathic Medical Society	1871	New York	Organized September 27, 1871.
226	Niagara and Orleans County Homeopathic Medical Society	1871	New York	Organized October 3, 1871.
227	St. Lawrence County Homeopathic Medical Society	1871	New York	Organized October 4, 1871.

	Name	Year	Place	Comments
228	National Eclectic Medical Association	1871	New York	Incorporated in New York, March 27, 1871. By 1900 there were thirty-two affiliate societies and associations in fourteen states, with local and district organizations in twelve, and seven medical colleges that were admitted to representation at the meetings.
229	Homeopathic Medical Association of Summit and Portage Counties	1871	Ohio	Organized June, 1871.
230	Physio-Medical Association of Warren County	1871	Ohio	
231	Illinois Valley Homeopathic Medical Society	1872	Illinois	Organized in La Salle in March or April, 1872, but never incorporated. It held at first bimonthly meetings, which afterward became semiannual upon reorganization in 1888.
232	Essex County Homeopathic Medical Society	1872	Massachusetts	Organized May 1, 1872.
233	West Jersey Homeopathic Medical Society	1872	New Jersey	Formerly the Western District New Jersey Homeopathic Medical Society. Incorporated under new name in May, 1872.
234	Seneca County Homeopathic Medical Society	1872	New York	Organized September 26, 1872.
235	Cleveland Academy of Medicine and Surgery	1872	Ohio	No information available.
236	Chicago Academy of Homeopathic Physicians and Surgeons	1873	Illinois	Organized in Chicago in 1873, a consolidation of the Cook County Homeopathic Medical Society and the Chicago Academy of Medicine.
237	Fourteenth District Homeopathic Medical Society of Illinois	1873	Illinois	Organized in Naperville, May 13, 1873, and included in its membership the physicians of the school living in Du Page and Kane counties.

	Name	Year	Place	Comments
238	Kentucky State Homeopathic Medical Society	1873	Kentucky	Formerly the Kentucky State Homeopathic Society. the present organization and probably the successor to the society just mentioned, was organized in Louisville, May 7, 1873, with these officers: Dr. Henry W. Kohler of Louisville, president; Dr. W. H. Blakeley of Bellevue, vice president; Dr. J. W. Kline of Louisville, secretary. The organization, like its predecessor, declined and was finally revived and reorganized in Lexington, July 14, 1886, with about thirty constituent members. Incorporated in 1888.
239	Boston Homeopathic Society	1873	Massachusetts	Consolidated in May, 1873, with the Boston Academy of Homeopathic Medicine.
240	Nebraska State Homeopathic Medical Society	1873	Nebraska	Organized in September, 1873, and known as the Nebraska State Homeopathic Medical Association.
241	Eclectic Medical Society of New Jersey	1873	New Jersey	Organized in 1873 and maintained semiannual meetings. The society had about thirty members.
242	Queens County Homeopathic Medical Society	1873	New York	Organized June, 1873.
243	Homeopathic Medical Society of Eastern Ohio	1873	Ohio	Organized April 2, 1873, by union of the Homeopathic Medical Society of the Seventeenth Congressional District and the Homeopathic Medical Association of Summit and Portage Counties.
244	Susquehanna Eclectic Medical Society	1873	Pennsylvania	One of four auxiliary societies of the Eclectic Medical Association of the State of Pennsylvania.
245	Eclectic Medical Society of Northwestern Pennsylvania	1873	Pennsylvania	One of four auxiliary societies of the Eclectic Medical Association of the State of Pennsylvania.
246	Central Eclectic Medical Society of Pennsylvania	1873	Pennsylvania	One of four auxiliary societies of the Eclectic Medical Association of the State of Pennsylvania.

	Name	Year	Place	Comments
247	Philadelphia Eclectic Medical Society	1873	Pennsylvania	One of four auxiliary societies of the Eclectic Medical Association of the State of Pennsylvania.
248	Eclectic Medical Association of the State of Pennsylvania	1873	Pennsylvania	Organized at Titusville, April 15, 1873. Incorporated the following autumn. Had four auxiliary societies: the Susquehanna Eclectic Medical Society; the Eclectic Medical Society of Northwestern Pennsylvania; the Central Eclectic Medical Society of Pennsylvania; and the Philadelphia Eclectic Medical Society.
249	Pacific Homeopathic Medical Society of the State of California	1874	California	Brought into existence through reorganization of the California State Medical Society of Homeopathic Practitioners on August 8, 1874.
250	Eclectic Medical Society of the State of California	1874	California	Organized at San Francisco, December 8, 1874, with an initial membership of twelve.
251	Delaware State Homeopathic Medical Society	1874	Delaware	Organized in Wilmington in November, 1874. It was not incorporated and held its annual meetings in different parts of the state. The first officers were Dr. L. Lukens of Newport, president; Dr. L. Kittinger of Wilmington, vice president; Dr. J. M. Curtis of Wilmington, secretary and treasure; Dr. C. H. Lawton of Wilmington, corresponding secretary; Drs. J. R. Tantum, J. R. Shaw and C. H. Lawton, censors. The society held for several years, but later there came a decline followed by a reorganization in 1884 under the name of Homeopathic Medical Society of Delaware and the Peninsula.
252	Georgia Eclectic Medical Association	1874	Georgia	Organized in March, 1874 and incorporated by a special act of the legislature that same year; held its annual meetings in Atlanta.
253	Baltimore Homeopathic Medical Society	1874	Maryland	Organized at Baltimore September 24, 1874, and continued until 1883, when it was dissolved.
254	Northern New Hampshire Homeopathic Medical Society	1874	New Hampshire	No information available.

	Name	Year	Place	Comments
255	Southern Tier Homeopathic Medical Society	1874	New York	Organized at Elmira, January 20, 1874. First officers: President, Henry Sayles, Elmira; vice president, W. S. Purdy, Corning; secretary and treasurer, W. J. Bryan, Corning. Iincorporated April 16, 1878, and published for a short time a journal *The Regular Physician,* Dr. A. P. Hollett, editor. The annual meeting were held at Corning in January; quarterly meetings in April, July and October in different places. Had twenty-one members in 1903.
256	Hudson River Homeopathic Medical Society	1874	New York	Organized at Poughkeepsie in 1874.
257	Tompkins, Cortland and Tioga County Homeopathic Medical Society	1874	New York	Organized September 25, 1874.
258	Hahnemann Club of Philadelphia	1874	Pennsylvania	Organized January, 1874.
259	Northwestern Pennsylvania Homeopathic Medical Society	1874	Pennsylvania	Organized January 13, 1874.
260	Rhode Island Homeopathic Medical Society	1874	Rhode Island	Formerly the Hahnemannian Medical Society of Rhode Island. Held its first session January 2, 1874. At that time the officers elected were: Dr. Ira Barrows, of Providence, president; Dr. J. E. Wheaton, of Pawtucket, vice president; Dr. G. A. Wilcox, of Providence, treasurer; Dr. Edward B. Knight, of Providence, secretary.
261	Texas Homeopathic Medical Association	1874	Texas	Reorganized in Galveston, March 18, 1874, at which time officers were chosen: Dr. H. C. Parker of Houston, president; Dr. William M. Mercer of Galveston, secretary; Dr. James H. Blake of Houston, treasurer; Dr. Edward P. Angell of Double Bayou, essayist. The association was incorporated in May, 1874, and continued in existence about ten years. It was reorganized, however, at a meeting held in Austin, May 1, 1884.
262	Champlain Valley Homeopathic Medical Society	1874	Vermont	No additional information.

	Name	Year	Place	Comments
263	Pacific Medical Society	1875	California	Lost its charter but united with another society of the same name to form the California State Homeopathic Medical Society. Its first officers were: Dr. G. M. Dixon, president; Drs. J. N. Eckel and A. A. Thiese, vice presidents; Dr. George H. Jenks, secretary; Dr. A. Liliencrantz, treasurer; Drs. T. C. Coxhead, J. A. Albertson, J. M. Selfridge, C. W. Breyfogle, H. H. Lyon, censors. The society was incorporated December 22, 1877.
264	Kankakee and Des Plaines Valley Homeopathic Medical Association	1875	Illinois	Included Will and Grundy counties and organized in Joliet in February, 1875. Dissolved in 1882.
265	Cedar Valley Homeopathic Medical Society	1875	Iowa	Organized at Waterloo, September 30, 1875.
266	Hardin County Society of Homeopathic Physicians	1875	Iowa	No information available.
267	Linn County Homeopathic Medical Society	1875	Iowa	Organized at Marion, June 23, 1875.
268	Northeastern Iowa Homeopathic Medical Society	1875	Iowa	Organized at Waterloo, October 28, 1875.
269	Maryland Homeopathic Society of Baltimore City	1875	Maryland	A state society notwithstanding the local character implied by its name. The society last mentioned was organized in Baltimore on December, 16, 1875.
270	Grand Rapids Society	1875	Michigan	No information available.
271	Nebraska Eclectic Medical Association	1875	Nebraska	Closely associated with the medical department of the Nebraska State University.

	Name	Year	Place	Comments
272	Homeopathic Medical Society of Tennessee	1875	Tennessee	Organized at a convention assembled in Nashville, December 1, 1875, when officers were elected: Dr. J. P. Dake of Nashville, presiden ; Dr. L. D. Morse of Memphis and Dr. E. H. Price of Chattanooga, vice presidents; Dr. Eugene R. Smith of Edgefield, secretary; Dr. T. E. Enloe of Edgefield, treasurer; Drs. R. M. Lytle, Charles R. Doran and H. Falk, all of Nashville, censors. The society held meetings until 1877, after which none were held until September 10, 1890, when a reorganization was effected at Lookout Mountain, Chattanooga. Incorporated that same year.
273	Northern Indiana Homeopathic Institute	1876	Indiana	Known as the Northwestern Indiana Society and organized at Elkhart, February 1, 1876. Enjoyed a brief career until about 1882, when it was dissolved, not having published its transactions and leaving only a meager record.
274	North Missouri Valley Homeopathic Medical Society	1876	Iowa	Organized at Hamburg, Iowa, June 1, 1876.
275	Massachusetts Surgical and Gynecological Society	1876	Massachusetts	Organized in Boston December 6, 1876.
276	Organon Society of Boston	1876	Massachusetts	Organized December 8, 1887.
277	Detroit Institute of Homeopathy	1876	Michigan	Organized April 12, 1876, and was subsequently a part of the College of Physicians and Surgeons, and still later of the Homeopathic Medical Association of Detroit.
278	Jackson County Homeopathic Medical Society	1876	Michigan	Organized March, 1876.
279	Homeopathic Medical Society of Southern Michigan and Northern Indiana	1876	Michigan	No information available.
280	Homeopathic Medical Society of Tuscola and Adjacent Counties	1876	Michigan	No information available.
281	Thayer Homeopathic Medical Society of Southern Michigan	1876	Michigan	No information available.

	Name	Year	Place	Comments
282	State Eclectic Medical and Surgical Society of Michigan	1876	Michigan	Organized at Kalamazoo on May 31, 1876. Eligibility for membership limited to graduates of reputable medical colleges only. Incorporated by act of the legislature in 1877. Recognized that same year by the National Eclectic Medical Association.
283	Oregon State Homeopathic Medical Society	1876	Oregon	Organized and incorporated in 1876. Its first officers were Dr. H. McKennell, president; Drs. William Geiger and A. Pohl, vice presidents; Dr. G. A. Wilcox, recording secretary; Dr. T. J. Sloan, corresponding secretary; Dr. Francis C. Paine, treasurer.
284	Society of Homeopathic Practitioners	1877	California	Incorporated and served as board of state medical examiners; scrutinized all diplomas and issued certificates of qualification for practice.
285	Eclectic Medical Society of Missouri	1877	Missouri	Incorporated in 1877 and replaced the Eclectic Medical Association of the State of Missouri that had been organized in 1870.
286	Philadelphia Homeopathic Clinical Society	1877	Pennsylvania	No information available.
287	Tennessee Eclectic Medical Society	1877	Tennessee	Formed in 1877 but sustained only a precarious existence. Incorporated the same year.
288	Wisconsin State Eclectic Medical Society	1877	Wisconsin	No information available.
289	Rock River Institute of Homeopathy	1878	Illinois	Organized in Dixon, Illinois, in 1878, held quarterly meetings in different places.
290	Homeopathic Medical Association of Wabash Valley	1878	Illinois	Organized in Paris, Illinois, May 1, 1878, and held semiannual meetings until 1884, when it was dissolved.
291	Fox River Eclectic Medical Association	1878	Illinois	Organized in 1878 and had a membership of twenty active physicians who held quarterly meetings.

	Name	Year	Place	Comments
292	Hughes Medical Club of Boston	1878	Massachusetts	Organized October 23, 1878.
293	The Homeopathic Medical Society of Western Massachusetts	1878	Massachusetts	Organized at Greenfield on May 23, 1878.
294	College of Physicians and Surgeons	1878	Michigan	Organized in Detroit, October 21, 1878.
295	Homeopathic Medical Society of Camden	1878	New Jersey	No information available.
296	Women's Homeopathic Medical Society of Chicago	1879	Illinois	Organized April 17, 1879, and was the first society of its kind in the country which was formed and governed exclusively by women.
297	Homeopathic Clinical Society of Rock Island, Henry and Whiteside Counties, Illinois, and Scott County, Iowa	1879	Illinois	Organized in Rock Island, October 22, 1879, and held its meetings quarterly in different places.
298	Central Homeopathic Medical Association	1879	Iowa	Organized at Cedar Rapids, January 29, 1879.
299	Hahnemann Medical Society of Eaton and Barry Counties	1879	Michigan	No information available.
300	Dayton City Homeopathic Medical Society	1879	Ohio	No information available.
301	Central Ohio Eclectic Medical Association	1879	Ohio	Formed in December 1879 and met bimonthly at the St. James Hotel at Springfield.
302	Germantown Homeopathic Medical Society	1879	Pennsylvania	Organized October, 1879.
303	Michigan State Physio-Medical Association	188?	Michigan	Organized at Grand Rapids, Michigan. Dr. A. Nyland was the organization's president in 1891.
304	St. Louis Eclectic Medical Society	188?	Missouri	One of four auxiliary societies to the Eclectic Medical Society of the State of Missouri.
305	Southwestern Medical Society of Missouri	188?	Missouri	One of four auxiliary societies to the Eclectic Medical Society of the State of Missouri.

	Name	Year	Place	Comments
306	Kansas City Eclectic Medical Society	188?	Missouri	One of four auxiliary societies to the Eclectic Medical Society of the State of Missouri.
307	Clermont Eclectic Medical Society	188?	Ohio	Held semiannual meetings at Amelia and had a list of 21 active members.
308	Miami Valley Eclectic Medical Association	188?	Ohio	Met at Hamilton and had a membership of 88 with about 25 active members.
309	Physio-Medical Association of Washington	188?	Washington	Operating in 1890.
310	Hahnemann Medical Association of Louisiana	1880	Louisiana	This society was succeeded in 1885 by the Southern Homeopathic Medical Association.
311	Hering Club of Philadelphia	1880	Pennsylvania	Organized December 20, 1880.
312	Homeopathic Medical Council of Pennsylvania	1880	Pennsylvania	Organized November 24, 1880.
313	Lippe Society of Philadelphia	1880	Pennsylvania	Organized January 5, 1880.
314	State Eclectic Medical Association of Tennessee	1880	Tennessee	Organized on May 15, 1880.
315	Hahnemann Medical Society of the Old Dominion	1880	Virginia	Organized at Richmond in 1880. The first officers were Dr. Joseph V. Hobson, president; Dr. James H. Patton, secretary. The society met annually for several years, after which there were occasional lapses and interest in its affairs declined. A reorganization, however, was effected in 1893, and on December 13, a number of physicians met in Danville and re-established the society.
316	Eclectic Medical Association of Arkansas	1881	Arkansas	After a failed attempt to organize in 1878, the endeavor was renewed in 1879 and eventually succeeded in January, 1881.
317	Colorado State Homeopathic Medical Society	1881	Colorado	Organized June, 1881, and reorganized in May, 1891.
318	Topeka Homeopathic Medical Society	1881	Kansas	Organized in 1881 and incorporated in 1882.
319	Kentucky State Eclectic Medical Association	1881	Kentucky	Organized at Newport in 1881.

	Name	Year	Place	Comments
320	Medical Investigation Club of Baltimore	1881	Maryland	Organized November 5, 1881, with five members, for the special purpose of promoting the investigation of medical and scientific subjects.
321	Lowell Hahnemann Club	1881	Massachusetts	Organized November 22, 1881.
322	Boston Gynecological Club	1881	Massachusetts	Organized March 23, 1881.
323	Lehigh Valley Homeopathic Medical Society	1881	Pennsylvania	Organized March 24, 1881.
324	Pennsylvania Homeopathic Pharmaceutical Association	1881	Pennsylvania	Organized April 9, 1881.
325	Pittsburgh Microscopical Society	1881	Pennsylvania	No information available.
326	Homeopathic Medical society of the Twenty-Third Ward, Philadelphia	1881	Pennsylvania	Organized October 21, 1881.
327	Homeopathic Medical Society of Western Pennsylvania	1881	Pennsylvania	Organized August 3, 1881.
328	Terre Haute Homeopathic Medical Society	1882	Indiana	No information available.
329	Polk County Homeopathic Medical Society	1882	Iowa	Organized at Des Moines in May, 1882.
330	Eclectic Medical Association of Kentucky	1882	Kentucky	Organized in 1882 and showed much initial energy. Reorganized in 1890 to become the West Kentucky Eclectic Medical Society.
331	Medical Institute of Homeopathy	1882	Maryland	Became the Maryland State Homeopathic Medical Society around 1887.
332	Medical Club of Northern New Jersey	1882	New Jersey	No information available.
333	American Association of Physio-Medical Physicians and Surgeons	1882	Ohio	Organized in 1882 in Toledo, Ohio. Known as "The American." Cfficers in 1890 were J. E. Roop, president; and Loomis and Marks, vice presidents. Included representatives from twenty-three states but primarily from Indiana, Ohio, New York, Illinois, Iowa, and Minnesota.

	Name	Year	Place	Comments
334	Northwestern Ohio Eclectic Medical Association	1882	Ohio	Formed December 21, 1882. Held quarterly meetings.
335	Crawford County Homeopathic Medical Society	1882	Pennsylvania	Organized July 28, 1882.
336	Hahnemann Medical Society of Reading	1882	Pennsylvania	Organized November 23, 1882.
337	Northern Pennsylvania Homeopathic Medical Society	1882	Pennsylvania	Organized June 20, 1882.
338	Philadelphia Medical Club	1882	Pennsylvania	No information available.
339	West Philadelphia Homeopathic Medical Association	1882	Pennsylvania	No information available.
340	Wilmington Medical Club	1883	Delaware	Otherwise known as the Hughes Club, was organized in Wilmington in 1883 and was incorporated under the laws of the state in 1889. Its meetings, held weekly, were social in character.
341	Medical Science Club of Chicago	1883	Illinois	Organized in that city in 1883, did not incorporate, and made provision for semimonthly meetings.
342	Rockford Homeopathic Medical Society	1883	Illinois	Organized in Rockford, November 12, 1883, but was continued only a few years. It was not incorporated and did not publish its transactions.
343	Scott County Homeopathic Medical Society	1883	Iowa	Organized at Davenport.
344	Allegheny County Homeopathic Medical Society	1883	New York	Organized July 10, 1883
345	Beaver County Homeopathic Medical Society	1883	Pennsylvania	Organized January 8, 1883.
346	Northeastern Philadelphia Society of Homeopathic Physicians	1883	Pennsylvania	Organized February 9, 1883.
347	Women's Homeopathic Association of Pennsylvania	1883	Pennsylvania	No information available.
348	Schuylkill County Homeopathic Medical Society	1883	Pennsylvania	Organized July 28, 1883.

	Name	Year	Place	Comments
349	Eclectic Medical Association of Alabama	1884	Alabama	Organized in Montgomery, May 6, 1884, by Dr. J. W. Raleigh Williams of Opelika; and Drs. R. J. Thornton and William H. Lamar.
350	Dakota Homeopathic Medical Association	1884	Dakota Territory	Organized June 25, 1884. On the admission of South Dakota as a state, the society ceased to exist, and the South Dakota State Homeopathic Medical Society was organized and incorporated on May 16, 1893.
351	Homeopathic Medical Society of Delaware and the Peninsula	1884	Delaware	Formerly the Delaware State homeopathic Medical Society which reorganized in 1884. Incorporated in 1889.
352	Wayne County Homeopathy Medical Society	1884	Indiana	Organized at Richmond on September 16, 1884, and discontinued in 1888.
353	Southern Homeopathic Medical Association	1885	Louisiana	The society has enjoyed a continuous existence to the present time, although a re-organization was affected in 1890. Annual meetings were held in New Orleans in January, with bimonthly meetings in the same city. The membership in 1903 was twenty-two physicians.
354	Essex County Homeopathic Medical Society	1885	New Jersey	No information available.
355	Hahnemann Medical Club of Plainfield	1885	New Jersey	Dissolved in 1889.
356	Western New York Homeopathic Medical Society	1885	New York	Organized at the Tifft house, Buffalo, April 10, 1885. First officers: President, L. M. Kenyon, Buffalo; vice presidents, J. F. Baker, Batavia, W. B. Gifford, Attica; recording secretary, Jos. T. Cook, Buffalo; treasurer, E. P. Hussey, Buffalo; censors, A. R. Wright, F. D. Ormes, S. W. Hurd, J. D. Zwetsch, A. M. Curtis. Quarterly meetings were held in different places in July, October and January. The annual meeting was held in April in Buffalo and Rochester, alternately.
357	Homeopathic Club of Cincinnati	1885	Ohio	Organized December, 1885.

	Name	Year	Place	Comments
358	Summit County Homeopathic Clinical Society	1885	Ohio	Organized January 15, 1885.
359	Mutual Aid Society of the National Eclectic Medical Association	1885	Ohio	Organized June, 1885. Intended for the mutual aid and benefit of families and patrons of Eclectic physicians.
360	Eclectic Medical Association of Texas	1885	Texas	Organized in 1885 out of meeting held in Dallas. Barely maintained its existence.
361	Southern Kansas Homeopathic Medical Association	1886	Kansas	Organized December 15, 1886.
362	Huron District Medical Society	1886	Michigan	No information available.
363	Northern Michigan Homeopathic Medical Association	1886	Michigan	No information available.
364	Saginaw Valley Homeopathic Association	1886	Michigan	No information available.
365	Homeopathic Medical Society of Southwestern Michigan	1886	Michigan	Organized in December, 1886.
366	Western Michigan Institute of Homeopathy	1886	Michigan	No information available.
367	Communipaw Medical Society	1886	New Jersey	No information available
368	Hudson Homeopathic Medico-Chirurgical Society	1886	New Jersey	Organized December 8, 1886.
369	Pulaski County Homeopathic Medical Society	1887	Arkansas	Organized in Little Rock, May 24, 1887, was the first and for a long time the only society of homeopathic physicians in the state. Eventually reorganized as the Arkansas State homeopathic Medical Association in Little Rock, April 12, 1903.
370	New Haven Homeopathic Medical Society	1887	Connecticut	Organized February 24, 1887, at the residence of Dr. C. B. Adams in the city of New Haven. The society was not incorporated.

	Name	Year	Place	Comments
371	Maryland State Homeopathic Medical Society	1887	Maryland	Formerly the Medical Institute of Homeopathy.
372	Plymouth County Homeopathic Medical Society	1887	Massachusetts	Organized March 3, 1887.
373	Chester Organon Club	1887	Pennsylvania	No information available.
374	Hahnemannian Association of Pennsylvania	1887	Pennsylvania	Organized in Philadelphia on October 11, 1887.
375	Adams County Homeopathic Medical Association	1888	Illinois	Organized in Quincy in December, 1888, elected officers, but did not incorporate, and in the course of a few years passed out of existence, leaving little record of its history or works.
376	Homeopathic Medical Society of Woodbury County	1888	Iowa	Organized at Sioux City, December 27, 1888.
377	West Kentucky Eclectic Medical Society	1888	Kentucky	Organized in 1888 with Dr. G. T. Fuller, of Lowes, as president. After discouraging period, it reorganized in May, 1892.
378	Trenton Club of Homeopathic Physicians	1888	New Jersey	No information available.
379	Farrington Materia Medica Club of Allegheny County	1888	Pennsylvania	No information available.
380	Organon and Materia Medica Society	1888	Pennsylvania	Organized November 6, 1888.
381	Homeopathic Medical Association of Alabama	1889	Alabama	Formerly the Homeopathic Medical Association of Alabama. Dates its history from May 15, 1889, and at the organization meeting these officers were elected: Dr. F. F. DeDerkey of Mobile, president; Dr. A. N. Duffield of Huntsville, vice president; Dr. George G. Lyon of Mobile, secretary; Dr. A. P. Myers of Mobile, treasurer. The society was incorporated on November 13, 1889, when a reorganization was effected.
382	Grace Homeopathic Medical Society of New Haven	1889	Connecticut	Incorporated June 21, 1889, and at once became an active organization in promoting the interests of the homeopathic profession in Connecticut.

	Name	Year	Place	Comments
383	State Homeopathic Medical Society of Florida	1889	Florida	Organized in Jacksonville, January 19, 1889, with these first officers: Dr. H. R. Stout of Jacksonville, president; Dr. Ada F. Bruce of Tampa, vice president; Dr. C. W. Johnson of Jacksonville, secretary; Drs. T. J. Williamson, Blanding and E. Johnson, censors.
384	Illinois State Physio-Medical Society	1889	Illinois	Reorganized June 20, 1889. President was W. F. Tait.
385	Hahnemann Club of Terre Haute	1889	Indiana	Organized in 1889, and was a social organization devoted chiefly to the study of Hahnemann's .
386	Indianapolis Homeopathy Institute	1889	Indiana	Organized November 25, 1889, and flourished for several years, then declined.
387	First District Physio-Medical Association	1889	Indiana	Organized in Newcastle, Indiana, in 1889.
388	Sioux City Homeopathic Medical Association	1889	Iowa	Formerly the Homeopathic Medical Society of Woodbury County. Name changed on May 7, 1889.
389	State Homeopathic Medical Society of Mississippi	1889	Mississippi	Its constituent members were Drs. Eugene A. Guilbert, H. J. Coleman, J. C. French, A. O. Hardenstein, B. D. Chase, H. P. Cook, H. Bewlay and Jesse R. Jones.
390	Northwestern Ohio Homeopathic Medical Society	1889	Ohio	Organized June, 1889.
391	Cincinnati Homeopathic Lyceum	1889	Ohio	Organized October 28, 1889.
392	Round Table Club	1889	Ohio	Organized August 28, 1889.
393	Germantown Homeopathic Medical Club	1889	Pennsylvania	No information available.
394	Washington State Homeopathic Medical Society	1889	Washington	Organized in Seattle in November, 1889.
395	Homeopathic Medical Society of King County	1889	Washington	Organized September, 1889.

	Name	Year	Place	Comments
396	Liberal Medical Society of the State of Oregon	189?	Oregon	Physicians professing to be eclectics but "employ questionable modes of advertising and are so quackish in their methods as to be ineligible" for membership in the Oregon State Eclectic Medical Association. Their only requirement for membership is the payment of a fee.
397	Eclectic Medical Association of Colorado	1890	Colorado	Organized in 1890 but succumbed to the financial depression of 1893.
398	Des Moines Homeopathic Clinical Society	1890	Iowa	No information available.
399	Shawnee County Homeopathic Medical Society	1890	Kansas	Organized October 29, 1890.
400	Homeopathic Clinical Society of Maryland and the District of Columbia	1890	Maryland	Organized October 1, 1890, a union of the Homeopathic Society of Maryland and the Homeopathic Medical Society of the District of Columbia.
401	College of Homeopathic Physicians and Surgeons, Grand Rapids	1890	Michigan	Organized April 26, 1890.
402	Columbus Clinical Club	1890	Ohio	Organized June 2, 1890.
403	Oregon State Eclectic Medical Association	1890	Oregon	Organized and became incorporated on September 14, 1890.
404	Tacoma Homeopathic Academy of Medicine	1890	Washington	No information available.
405	Eclectic Medical Association of the State of Washington	1890	Washington	Formed in 1890 but fell on hard times.
406	Central Illinois Homeopathic Medical Society	1891	Illinois	Organized in Champaign, January 21, 1891.
407	La Salle County Homeopathic Society	1891	Illinois	Organized by physicians of La Salle county at a meeting held in Streator, August 7, 1891.
408	Provers' Union and Materia Medica Club	1891	Illinois	Organized at the Grand Hotel in Chicago, August 8, 1891, and provided for the admission to membership of medical students as well as graduate physicians.

	Name	Year	Place	Comments
409	Homeopathic Medical Society of Northern Indiana and Southern Michigan	1891	Indiana	Organized at Elkhart, September 22, 1891. It met semiannually.
410	Northwest Missouri Eclectic Medical Society	1891	Missouri	Organized at Cameron, Missouri, on September 10, 1891. One of four auxiliary societies to the Eclectic Medical Society of the State of Missouri. Held first annual meeting at Cameron on June 7, 1892.
411	Cleveland Academy of Medicine	1891	Ohio	Organized February 4, 1891.
412	Cleveland Homeopathic Maternity Society	1891	Ohio	Organized October 12, 1891.
413	Erie County Homeopathic Medical Society	1891	Pennsylvania	Organized July 1, 1891.
414	Doctors' Round Table Club of Allegheny County	1891	Pennsylvania	No information available.
415	State Eclectic Medical Society of South Dakota	1891	South Dakota	Organized and incorporated in June, 1891.
416	Western Kentucky Homeopathic Medical Society	1892	Kentucky	Organized in Princeton, January 10, 1892. Its membership in 1903 was 35.
417	Scranton Homeopathic Clinical Club	1892	Pennsylvania	Organized March 1892.
418	Utah Homeopathic Medical Association	1892	Utah	Organized in Salt Lake City on January 21, 1892, and was incorporated the same year. For several years the society maintained a healthful existence, but declined after 1895.
419	Eclectic Medical Society of Utah	1892	Utah	Formed in 1892 and incorporated on March 14.
420	South Dakota State Homeopathic Medical Society	1893	South Dakota	Organized May 16, 1893.
421	Eclectic Medical Society of West Virginia	1893	West Virginia	An earlier organized formed at Brownstone in October, 1870, and held several annual meetings, with Dr. Daniel Mayer of Charlestown as president. Formerly organized in 1893.

	Name	Year	Place	Comments
422	National Association of Eclectic Medical Colleges	1894	New York	Created by the National Eclectic Medical Association at its meeting at Niagara Falls. Association was to determine the prospects and opportunities of future institutions of instruction in the eclectic school of medicine.
423	Toledo Clinical Society	1894	Ohio	No information available.
424	New England Eclectic Medical Association	1895	Vermont	Formed in June, 1895, and incorporated by the Vermont legislature in November, 1896. Comprised the six northeastern states.
425	Southern California Eclectic Medical Association	1896	California	Held well attended meetings.
426	Medico-Chirurgical Society of Central New York	1896	New York	Organized in 1896, but is not incorporated. It met annually in Syracuse in June, and semiannually in different places in December. Membership was 72 in 1903.
427	West Virginia Homeopathic Medical Society	1898	West Virginia	Organized on May 49, 1898, at Wheeling, and its first officers were Dr. M. L. Casselbury, president; Drs. C. M. Boger and J. M. Fawcett, vice presidents; Dr. C. A. Roberts, secretary; Dr. C. H. Wilsey, treasurer; Dr. John W. Morris, necrologist. The society held its annual meetings in different cities.
428	Northwestern Ohio Eclectic Medical Association	18??	Ohio	No information available.
429	Pennsylvania Association Medical Society of Botanic Physicians	18??	Pennsylvania	No information available.

[Sources include National Library of Medicine, *Index-Catalogue of the Library of the Surgeon-General's Office, United States Army, Series III* (10 volumes; Washington D.C.: Government Printing Office, 1918–1952); Thomas Lindsley Bradford, *Homeopathic Bibliography of the United States, From the Year 1825 to the Year 1891, Inclusive* (Philadelphia: Boericke and Tafel, 1892); William Harvey King, *History of Homeopathy and Its Institutions in America: Their Founders, Benefactors, Faculties, Officers, Hospitals, Alumni, etc., With a Record of Achievement of Its Representatives in the World of Medicine* (4 volumes; New York: Lewis Publishing Company, 1905); Alexander Wilder, *History of Medicine; A Brief Outline of Medical History and Sects of Physicians, from the Earliest Historic Period* (New Sharon, Maine: New England Eclectic Publishing Co., 1901); *Transactions of the National Eclectic Medical Association*; *American Eclectic Medical Review*; *American Eclectic Medical Register*; *First Search Database; Google Search Engine.*]

Index

Abbott, Jacob, 62
Ackerknecht, Erwin H., 17, 26
Ackerley, George, 62
Albany Medical College, 98
Alcott, Amos Bronson, 23
Alcott, William A., 62
Alison, William Pulteney, 22
Allopathy. *See* Regular medicine
American Association of Anatomists, 122
American Association of Pathologists and Bacteriologists, 122
American Association of Physio-Medical Physicians and Surgeons, 120
American Institute of Homeopathy, 55, 107–8, 130
American Journal of Homeopathy, 83
American Magazine of Homeopathy, 83
American Medical Association, xvi, 68, 102, 108–10; admits sectarians, 132; Code of Ethics of, 89, 109–10, 125, 132; on consultation, 109–10, 132; controls examining boards, 124; Council of Medical Education of, 122, 128; on sectarian medicine, 47, 90, 109–10, 111, 117, 125, 128
American Medical College, 125, 126, 128
American Medical Institute and Botanico-Medical College of Ohio, 175
American Physiological Society, 122
American Provers Union, 84
American Reformed School, 103
American Reformed School of Medical Practice in the South, 115
American Surgical Association, 122
Anatomy, 41
Andral, Gabriel, 18, 25, 54, 160
Angell, James, 122
Animal magnetism, 19, 55–56
Arsenic, 5, 6
Arthur, Timothy Shay, 62

Association of American Medical Colleges, 122–23
Association of American Physicians, 122
Athenaeus of Attaleia, 15
Athenian, 80
Atlantic Medical College, 133
Atlee, J. L., 109–10

Bacon, Francis, 2, 87
Bankston, Lanier, 92, 103
Barber, Ives S., 103
Barnes Medical College, 128
Barrow, Logie, 37
Bartlett, Elisha, 26, 38, 58, 166
Barton, Benjamin S., 8
Barton, William P. C., 8
Bayle, Gaspard Laurent, xii
Beach, Wooster, 8, 33, 64, 110, 112, 172, 173; as eclectic, 31–32, 88; as medical reformer, 30–32; plant medicines of, 51; society founded by, 102–3, 104
Beecher, Henry Ward, 62
Bennett, John Hughes, 21–23
Bichat, Xavier, xii
Bigelow, Jacob, 8, 21
Biomedicine, 117
Bloodletting, 3, 4, 5, 48, 77, 157, 158; eclectics on, 18, 21, 22, 112; homeopaths avoid, 50; regulars use, 11, 80
Boerhaave, Hermann, xii, 1, 3, 54, 93
Boericke and Tafel, 64–65
Boisliniere, L. C., 6
Boston University, 132
Botanic College of Medicine, 91
The Botanic Medical Reformer and Home Physician, 47
Botanic Medical Society of the State of New York, 115
Botanic medicine, 46–47; eclectics use, xiv, 36, 47, 90; education in, 46, 91–93, 118–21; informs medical reform, 36; societies of, 47, 68, 115. *See also* Physio-medicals; Thomsonians
Botanico-Medical College and Infirmary, 91
Botanico-Medical College of Memphis, 92, 93
Bouillaud, Jean Baptiste, 18, 19, 25, 54
Bowditch, Henry I., 26
Bretonneau, Pierre Fidele, 19, 54
Brooks, Silas S., 94
Broussais, François J. V., 4, 40, 54
Brown, John, xii, 93; on disease origin, 3; followers of, 3–4, 110; irritability theory of, 3–4, 11
Buchan, William, 8, 46
Buchanan, Joseph Rodes, 56, 96, 98, 110, 111, 177
Butler, Nicholas Murray, 122

California Medical College, 125, 128
Calomel, 77, 80–81
Capsicum, 119
Cassedy, James, 38
Castleton Medical College, 34
Caventou, Joseph, 7
Central Free Medical College of America, 96
Central Homeopathic Pharmacy, 108
Central Medical College of New York, 91, 94
Chase, Hiram L., 94
Chase, Philander, 88
Chase, Thomas J., 47
Chatterton, W. A., 64
Chevers, George W., 30, 103
Chicago Medical Times, 23
Chicago Physio-Medical Institute, 92

Childs, Henry H., 32
Cholera, 66, 52
Chomel, Auguste François, 18
Chrono-thermal system, 47, 90
Cinchona, 49
Clark, A. A., 70–72
Clark, Alonzo, 26
Cleveland, Charles S., 51
Clifford, John D., 29
Close, Stuart, 36
College of Homeopathic Medicine, State University of Iowa, 133
College of Medicine, 91
College of Medicine and Surgery of Chicago, 93
College of Medicine and Surgery, Physio-Medical, of Chicago, 121
Consultation, 109–10, 132
Cook, William H., 33–34, 92, 121
Cooke, Thomas, 47, 110, 111
Cooper, James Fenimore, 61
Corresponding Journal for Homeopathic Physicians, 52
Corvisart, Jean-Nicolas, xii
Cotner University Medical College, 126, 128
Cousin, Victor, 18, 38; as eclectic, 16–17, 28; influence of, 23–24, 25, 39
Crowe, Charles, 23–24
Cruveilhier, Jean, xii
Cullen, William, xii, 54, 93; medical system of, 2–3
Culpeper, Nicholas, 7–8
Curtis, Alva, 30, 32, 114, 174, 175; as journal publisher, 64, 65; medical college of, 91, 92, 121; medical society of, 105, 111
Curtis, G. W., 62
Curtis Physio-Medical Institute of Indiana, 92, 121
Cutler, Manasseh, 8, 29

Dake, Jabez P., 55, 108
Darwin, Charles, 119
Darwin, Erasmus, 40
Davis, Orin, 110
Detroit Homeopathic College, 133
Dewey, Orville, 62
Dickson, Samuel, 47, 90
Diet, 50, 65
Digitalis, 4
Dilution, high v. low, 49, 50, 65–66
Diploma mills, 121, 123
Disease, 48, 53; origin, xii, 3–4, 13, 48–49, 119; specificity, 18; as unitary, 11–12, 43, 57
Dispensaries, 52
Drake, Daniel, 6
Dudley, Benjamin W., 26
Dudley, Pemberton, 94
Duke, Richard J., 77
Dynamization, 49–50

Eberle, John, 34
Eclectic Conciliators, 16
Eclectic Medical College of Cincinnati, 91
Eclectic Medical College of the City of New York, 91, 125, 126–27
Eclectic Medical College of Pennsylvania, 47
Eclectic Medical College of Philadelphia, 94, 180
Eclectic Medical Institute (EMI), 31, 56, 81, 94, 97, 125; A.M.A. on, 128; Flexner on, 127; homeopathy taught at, 98–99, 111; influence of, 89–90, 96; transfer students at, 123

Eclectic Medical Institute of Memphis, 93
Eclectic Medical Institute of New York, 91
Eclectic Medical Journal, 111
Eclectic Medical School of Chicago, 23
Eclectic Medical Society of the State of New York, 102
Eclectico-homeopathists, 55
Eclectics, 15–36; A.M.A. on, 90, 125, 128; on bloodletting, 18, 21, 22, 112; British, 20–23, 28; education of, 23, 31, 32, 47, 56, 81, 88–91, 93, 94, 96, 97, 98–99, 111, 124, 125–27, 180; failure of, xiii–xiv; feuds among, 112, 113; French, 16–20, 28, 45–46; generational shift among, 127; German, 28; on heroic medicine, 21, 112; homeopaths merge with, 99–100; on homeopaths, 99–100, 111; influence of, 16, 23, 24–25, 92–93; journals of, 111 (*see also* Appendix A); licensed, 128; origins of theories of, xiv, 15–16, 28–30; pharmacy of, 90, 97, 120; physio-medicals merge with, 97, 99, 105, 112, 115, 121; plant-based medicines of, xiv, 28, 29–30, 36, 47, 51, 90, 97; positive medicine of, 20; reconcile competing theories, 18; regulars become, 99; social standing of, 58; societies of, 31, 102, 103–4, 110–15, 123, 124, 128; Swedenborg influenced, 56–57; Thomson and, 33–34, 44–45, 88; transcendentalism and, 23, 24–25; on vitalism, 127
Education, medical, 87–100, 117–34; botanic, 46, 91–93, 118–21; British, 26, 27; dissension in, 92–93, 96, 98; eclectic, 23, 31, 32, 47, 56, 81, 88–91, 93, 94, 96, 97, 98–99, 111, 124, 125–27, 180; Flexner on, 117, 121, 125–27, 129, 132–33; funding problems in, 96, 98, 122, 123, 124; German, 20, 27, 122, 134; homeopathic, 55, 93–95, 96, 97–98, 111, 128–34; lab/science based, xiii, 118, 122, 134; mixed, 98; Paris Clinical School influenced, xii, 13, 19, 25–28, 35, 38, 42–43, 45, 54, 77, 84–85, 118, 129, 134; physician-patient focus in, 118; physio-medical, 33, 91–93, 97, 105, 118–21; as post-graduate, 94, 133; proprietary, 97–98, 118, 122, 130; regular, 93–94, 107, 108, 123, 124–25, 130; regulars on, 88, 90, 128; as single national infirmary, 95–96; standards raised in, 39–43, 117, 122–23, 132; student demographics of, 123–24; texts in, 1, 40; university-based, 121–22, 124, 132. *See also* Appendix B
Eliot, Charles, 122
Emerson, Ralph Waldo, 23, 24–25, 62–63
Empiricism, 27–28
Esrey, William P., 94
Everest, Thomas R., 51

Felter, Harvey Wickes, 111
Fever, 6–7, 49; yellow, 11, 12
Firth, H. E., 31
Fishbein, Morris, 16, 28, 29
Five Hutchinsons, 80

Flagg, Josiah F., 94
Flexner, Abraham, xv, xvi, 58; on sectarian medical education (*Medical Education in the United States and Canada*), 117, 121, 125–27, 129, 132–33
Forbes, John, 20–21, 130, 163
Foucault, Michel, 26
Fowler, Stephen F., 80
Fowler and Wells, 65
France: electicism in, 16–20, 28, 45–46; medical education in (Paris Clinical School), xii, 13, 19, 25–28, 35, 38, 42–43, 45, 54, 77, 84–85, 118, 129, 134
Friendly Botanic Societies, 44, 45, 46, 51, 92, 102, 104–6, 107

Gaillard, Peter C., 26
Gardiner, William A., 58, 83, 84, 85, 107
Gatchell, H. P., 83
Gavarret, Jules, xii, 18, 38
Geary, John F., 84–85
Genesee Union Botanical Society, 103
Georgia College of Eclectic Medicine and Surgery, 125, 126, 127
Gerhard, William W., 26
Germany: eclecticism in, 28; homeopathy in, 84, 85; medical education in, 20, 27, 122, 134; laboratory medicine in, xiii, 122, 134
Gersdorff and Birnstill, 83
Gillman, J. B., 94
Godman, John, 26
Grahamites, 65
Gram, Hans Birch, 52
Graves, Robert J., xii
Great Britain: eclecticism in, 20–23, 28; medical education in, 26, 27
Greeley, Horace, 62
Gregg, Samuel, 55
Guernsey, H. N., 94

Haeckel, Ernst, 119
Hahnemann, Samuel, 16, 19, 21, 40, 47, 54, 55, 57, 181; on animal magnetism, 56; on cause of disease, 48–49; on dynamization, 49–50; influence of, 83; *Organon* of, 130–31, 132; plant materia medica of, 51; on regular medicine, 48, 101; spiritualism of, 129; on symptoms, 40, 49; treated fever, 49
Hahnemannianism, 129
Hahnemann Medical College and Hospital of Philadelphia, 133
Hahnemann Medical College of the Pacific, 133
Hall, Marshall, xii, 21, 162
Halsey and King, 64
Hammond, William, 80
Hanks, Abel, 103
Harrison, William Henry, 77
Harvey, William, 1, 16
Hasty, George, 92
Headley, Joel, 62
Hegel, G. W. F., 17
Helmuth, William Tod, 94, 130
Hempel, Charles J., 50–51, 84, 182
Henry, Caleb Sprague, 23
Henry, Samuel, 46
Hering, Constantine, 52, 83, 84, 85
Hering Medical College, 133
Hill, Benjamin J., 110
Hippocrates, 16, 44
Hoffmann, Friedrich, xii, 3, 40, 93
Holbrook, Josiah, 62
Hollembaek, Henry, 47

Holmes, Oliver Wendell, 7, 18, 21, 26, 62, 130
Homeopathic Medical College of Missouri, 95, 133, 184
Homeopathic Medical College of Pennsylvania, 94
Homeopathic Recorder, 36
Homeopaths, 13, 22, 23, 47–55; A.M.A. on, 47; aspire to specialty within regular medicine, 47–48, 95, 128, 132, 133; began as regulars, 107, 108, 128; on bloodletting, 50; cholera treated by, 52; consult with regulars, 110; on diet, 50; on disease, 53; dispensaries of, 52; drug provings by, 54; eclectics merge with, 99–100; eclectics on, 98–100, 111; education of, 55, 93–95, 96, 97–98, 111, 128–34; feuds/schisms among, 49, 50, 65–66, 83–85, 129, 130, 132; Flexner on, 129, 132–33; German, 84, 85; hospitals of, 52; journals of, 36, 58, 64–66, 82–85, 127 (*see also* Appendix A); lay, 52, 82–83, 107, 108, 133–34; Mesmer influenced, 56; pharmacies of, 52, 108; poem on, 66–67; Paris Clinical School influenced, 54, 129; popularity of, 21, 39; principles of, 53–54; and regulars, 47, 108, 128–29; similars, law of, 47, 49, 50, 53, 55, 83, 187; social standing of, 57–58; societies of, 52, 55, 107–8, 127, 130–31; spiritualism of, 95, 129, 130, 134; Swedenborg influenced, 56–57, 129; on symptoms, 54–55; texts of, 132; women, 95
Hooker, Worthington, 130
Hope, John, 20
Horner, William E., 41
Hosack, David, 30
Hospital Medical College, 125, 126
Houard, J. E., 94
Howard, Horton, 45, 51, 64
Howell, John B., 47
Hufeland, Christoph Wilhelm, 16, 64
Humoral theory, 1
Huxley, Thomas, 119
Hydropathy, 55, 67–68

Illinois Medical College, 23
Independent Thomsonian Botanic Society, 105
Independent Thomsonians. *See* Physio-medicals
Infirmaries, 105
Ingalls, William, 94
International Hahnemannian Association, 130–31

Jackson, James, 38, 110
Jackson, James, Jr., 26
Jackson, Samuel, 39–43, 51, 108, 167
Jahr, Gottlieb H., 51
Jefferson, Thomas, xi–xii, 10, 17, 64, 76
Jefferson Medical College, 44, 58, 94
Jenner, Edward, 16
Johnson, Paul, xi
Jones, Ichabod Gibson, 30, 88, 89, 110
Jones, Lorenzo E., 51, 110
Jordan, John H., 110
Josselyn, John, 8
Jourdan, A. J. L., 16
Journals, 83–86; eclectic, 111; education via, 63–66;

homeopathic, 36, 58, 64–66, 82–85, 127; owners of, 64–65; on regular medicine, 63; Swedenborgian, 64–65; Thomsonian, 105. *See also* Appendix A

Kansas City College of Medicine and Surgery, 128
Kansas City Hahemann Medical College, 133
Karsner, C., 94
Kelly, John C., 30, 103, 106
King, John, 51, 110
King, Lester S., 1
Kirby, S. R., 83
Koch, Edward, 119

Laennec, René T. H., xii, 38
Lapham, Thomas, 105
Latham, Peter M., 20
Lay practitioners, 64; homeopathic, 52, 82–83, 107, 108, 133–34; Thomsonian, 105
Leeuwenhoek, Antoni van, 1, 16
Lerminier, T. N., 18
Lewis, Winslow, 55
Licensing, xii, 97, 117; scandals, 128; by societies, 101, 106–7; by state legislation, 106–7
Lincoln Medical College, 125, 126, 128
Lippe, Adolph, 84, 183
Literary and Botanico-Medical Institute of Ohio, 91
Little and Brown, 21
Lloyd, Curtis Gates, 97
Lloyd, John Uri, 36, 97
Lloyd, Nelson A., 97
Lloyd Brothers, Pharmacists, Inc., 97
Lobelia, 43–44, 45, 119
Lobstein, J. F. Daniel, 30, 103
Longshore, Joseph S., 90
Loomis, Joseph Griswold, 94
Louis, Pierre C.A., xii, 25, 38, 54; on bloodletting, 18; numerical system of, 111
Low, Seth, 122
Lowell, James Russell, 25
Loyola University School of Medicine, 23
Lyceum movement, 62–63

Malpighi, Marcello, 1
Marcy, E. E., 53, 83, 84
Materia medica, 4–7; botanic, xiv, 7, 8, 28, 29–30, 36, 43–44, 46–47, 51, 90, 97; eclectic, xiv, 28, 29–30, 36, 47, 51, 90, 97; heroic/mineral-based, 5–6, 21, 77, 80–81, 112; homeopathic, 52, 54, 108
Matlack, Charles F., 94
McClellan, George, 34, 44, 168
McClintock, James, 34–36, 179
Medical Department of the National University of Arts and Sciences, 128
Medical Repository, 10
Medical School of Fredonia, 91
Medical Society of Botanic Physicians and Surgeons of the City of New York, 103
Medicine: organic, 40, 41; physiological, 40; preventive, 13; rational v. empirical, 12–13; regional differences in, 11; as science, xiii, 38–39; symptomatic, 40–41; system-building in, 2–4
Mercury, 5–6, 21, 112
Merrell, William S., 90, 97
Mesmer, Franz Anton, 21, 55–56
Metcalf, J. W., 83

Metropolitan Medical College of the City of New York, 90, 98, 178
Middle States Reformed Medical Society, 120
Millspaugh, Charles F., 51
Mintzer, St. John H., 47
Mitchell, Samuel Latham, 29
Mitchell, Thomas D., 35
Morrow, Thomas Vaughan, 30, 103, 110, 111, 176; at EMI, 88, 89; plant medicines of, 51, 88
Mott, Valentine, 26, 30

National Eclectic Medical Association, 31, 110–14, 123, 128
New England Botanico-Medical College, 93
"New Light." *See* Physio-medicals
Newton, Calvin, 32, 33, 111
Newton, R. S., 64
New York Association of Reformed Physicians, 122
New York Homeopathic College, 95, 132
New York Homeopathic Dispensary, 52
New York Homeopathic Medical College and Flower Hospital, 133
New York Medical College and Hospital for Women, 98
New York State Association of Reformed Physicians, 115
Nicely, William, 121
North American Academy of Homeopathy, 52, 84, 85, 94
North American Homeopathic Journal, 107
North American Journal of Homeopathy, 83, 84, 96
North-Western Journal of Homeopathy, 83

Opium, 5, 11, 21, 77
Osler, William, 129

Packard, Francis R., 30
Paine, W., 64, 99
Paracelsus, 15, 16, 57
Pediatric Society, 122
Pelletier, Pierre, 7
Penn Medical College, 90, 98
Pennock, C. W., 26
Pepper, William, 122
Pharmacies: eclectic, 90, 97, 120; homeopathic, 52, 108
Philadelphia College of Medicine, 35
Philadelphia Journal of Homeopathy, 58, 83, 84–85
Physio-Eclectic Medical College, 121
Physio-Medical College of Indiana, 92, 119
Physio-Medical Institute of Cincinnati, 33, 92, 121
Physio-medicals, 32, 90; botanic medicines of, 119–20; on disease, 119; education of, 33, 91–93, 97, 105, 118–21; feuds among, 46, 120 (*see also* Thomsonians); merge with eclectics, 97, 99, 105, 112, 115, 121; on regulars, 119; social standing of, 58; societies of, 103–4, 105, 120; on vitalism, 119
Physiopaths. *See* Physio-medicals
Physopathic Medical College of Ohio, 92
Pidoux, Hermann, 19
Pinel, Philippe, xii, 18
Piorry, Pierre A., 18, 19
Platt, A. H., 105

Porcher, Francis P., 26
Post, Wright, 30
Potter, Stephen H., 47, 64
Poughkeepsie Thomsonian, 105
Preston, Calvin, 30, 103
Preston, Henry C., 99–100
Pretsch, Curt, 84
Priessnitz, Vincent, 55
Pulte, Joseph H., 83
Pulte Medical College, 133

Quarterly Homeopathic Journal of Boston, 83
Quarterly Homeopathic Magazine, 83
Quinine, 7

Radde, William, 16, 64
Redemacher, Johann, 83
Rafinesque, Constantine S., 29–30, 33, 46, 64
Rasori, Giovanni, 4, 6, 38, 40
Rayer, Pierre F. O., xii, 18–19
Reading, J. R., 94
Reformed Medical Academy, 30–31
Reformed Medical Association of the United States, 114–15, 120
Reformed Medical Association of Western New York, 103
Reformed Medical College of the City of New York, 102–3, 173
Reformed Medical Department at Worthington College, 88
Reformed Medical Journal, 64
Reformed Medical School of Cincinnati, 89
Reformed Medical Society of the State of New York, 102
Reformed Medical Society of the United States, 31, 64, 88, 102–3, 104
Reform Medical College of Georgia, 93, 115
Reform Medical College of New York, 88
Reform Medical Physicians, 112
Reform Medical Society, 103
Regular medicine: and homeopaths, 47, 108, 128–29; homeopaths merge with, 132, 133; homeopathy as specialty within, 47–48, 95, 128, 132, 133; on sectarian medicine, 47, 89, 90, 109–10, 111, 117, 121, 125–27, 128, 129, 132–3; sectarian opposition to, 48, 63, 67, 77–79, 101, 119
Reid, Thomas, 17
Reliance Medical College, 23, 30–31, 103
Resurrection riot, 89
Reynaud, A. C., 18
Richardson, Thompson, 103
Riley, Woodbridge, 23
Ripley, George, 23–24
Robertson, John Dill, 33
Robinson, Samuel, 45–46
Robinson, William, 44
Rokitansky, Karl, 20
Roorbach, Orville, 62
Rosa, Storm, 98, 111
Rosenstein, I. G., 50, 65
Rostan, Léon, 18, 19, 159
Rothstein, William G., xv
Royer-Collard, P. P., 18
Rush, Benjamin, 8, 43, 45, 164; unitary disease theory of, 11–12

Sanborn, Amzi, 103
Sarcognomy, 56
Savannah Medical College, 93–94
Schelling, F. W. J. von, 17

Schoepf, Johann D., 8
Schönlein, Johann L., xii, 20
Scudder, John Milton, 64, 90
Senscopathy, 68
Shattuck, George C., 26
Sheek, Jacob F., 83
Sheppard, David, 111
Sheppard, H. D., 64
Sherwood, William, 51
Shipman, George E., 83
Short, Thomas, 8
Shryock, Richard, 26
Similars, law of (*similia similibus curantur*), 47, 49, 50, 53, 55, 83, 187
Simpson, James Y., 130
Sites, Joseph, 47
Skoda, Josef, xii
Smith, Adam, 2, 12
Smith, Elisha, 46–47, 91, 102
Smith, Isaac S., 46, 91, 103, 106
Smith, Sydney, 9
Societies, medical, 101–15; Beach's, 102–3, 104; become national, 102; botanic, 47, 68, 115; eclectic, 31, 102, 103–4, 110–15, 123, 124, 128; homeopathic, 52, 55, 107–8, 130–31; licensing via, 101, 106–7; membership criteria for, 107–8; physio-medical, 103–4, 105, 120; schisms in, 46; Thomsonian, 44, 45, 46, 52, 92, 102, 103–6, 107. *See also* Appendix C
The Southern Botanic Journal, 70
Southern Botanico-Medical College, 92, 93, 103, 115, 121
Southern Reform Medical Association, 115, 120
Southwestern Homeopathic Medical College, 133
Sperry, Isaac J., 31
Spurzheim, Johann G., 38
Stahl, George Ernst, xi, 40
Stanley, S. A., 103
Starrett, Washington, 103
Stearns, Samuel, 8
Steele, John J., 30, 88, 103
Stennert, Daniel, 16
Stillé, Alfred, 26
Stokes, William, xii, 20
Swedenborg, Emanuel, 56–57, 64–65, 129
Sweet, P. F., 47
Sydenham, Thomas, 93
Symptoms, 40, 49, 54–55

Tarbell, John A., 94
Tartar emetic, 4, 5, 6, 21, 38, 112
Taylor, Bayard, 62
Tessier, Jean Paul, 85
Thacher, James, 46
Thomas, Rolla, 125
Thomson, Cyrus, 171
Thomson, Samuel, 11, 43–46, 64, 65, 169; compared to Rush, 45; on disease, 43; and eclecticism, 33–34, 44–45, 88; patents of, 104, 105, 170; poems/acrostics on, 68–72, 80; on professional classes, 73–76; remedies of, 43–44, 51, 69–72, 91, 119; on single national infirmary, 95–96
Thomsonians, 43–46; Paris Clinical School influenced, 45; poems on, 68–72; on regulars, 78–79; social standing of, 58; societies of, 44, 45, 46, 52, 92, 102, 103–6, 107; split among, 92–93, 105–6, 118 (*see also* Physio-medicals)

Thoreau, Henry David, 62
Thurston, Joseph M., 119
Tidd, Jacob, 8, 30
Tocqueville, Alexis de, xv, 102
Tommasini, Giacomo, 4
Townsend, Peter S., 26
Transcendentalism, 23, 24–25
Trites, D. T., 94
Trousseau, Armand, xii, 18, 19, 161
Tully, William, 44
Twain, Mark, 63
Twentieth Century Physio-Medical College of Guthrie, Oklahoma, 121

Union Medical Journal, 89
United States Journal of Homeopathy, 83–84
United States Thomsonian Society, 105
University of the Literary and Botanico-Medical College of the State of Ohio, 91
University of Nebraska, 90–91
University of Pennsylvania, 94
Upham, A., 103

Vanderburg, Federal, 52
van Helmont, Jan Baptista, 40, 93
Vere, James J., 103
Vesalius, Andreas, 16
Vitalism, 57, 112, 119, 127
von Haller, Albrecht, 3

Ware, John, 38–39, 58
Warner, John Harley, 12–13, 19, 26–27
Warren, John C., 26
Washington, George, 64, 77
Waterhouse, Benjamin, 44–45, 165
Waters, G. H., 94
Watson, Thomas, 20
Wesley, John, 8, 64
Wesselhoeft, J. G., 64
Western College of Homeopathic Medicine, 111
Western Eclectic College of Medicine and Surgery, 125, 126, 128
Western Homeopathic College, 94–95
Western Medical Reformer, 88
Whipple, E. P., 62
Whorton, James, 28–29
Wilder, Alexander, 33, 36, 56, 103–4, 114, 188
Wisconsin Eclectic Medical College, 123
Wistar, Caspar, Jr., 10
Wood, James R., 30
Worcester Botanico-Medical College, 32
Worcester Medical College, 93
Worthington College, 88–89
Wright, J. I., 94
Wyman, Jeffries, 55